DYING, DEATH, AND GRIEF

A Critically Annotated Bibliography and Source Book of Thanatology and Terminal Care

Michael A. Simpson

Academic Department of Psychiatry
Royal Free Hospital
London, England

PLENUM PRESS • NEW YORK AND LONDON

Library of Congress Cataloging in Publication Data

Simpson, Michael A
  Dying, death, and grief.

  Includes index.

  1. Death — Bibliography. 2. Terminal care — Bibliography. 3. Grief — Bibliography.
I. Title.
Z5725.S55 [BD444]   016.128'5   78-27273
ISBN-13: 978-1-4684-3470-5   e-ISBN-13: 978-1-4684-3468-2
DOI: 10.1007/978-1-4684-3468-2

© 1979 Plenum Press, New York
A Division of Plenum Publishing Corporation
227 West 17th Street, New York, N.Y. 10011

Softcover reprint of the hardcover 1st edition 1979

This book is dedicated
in cheerful affection to

Jeff

and those like him
who had to learn too much
about all this too soon

Introduction

Death is a very badly kept secret; such an unmentionable
and taboo topic that there are over 750 books now in print
asserting that we are ignoring the subject.At no time in
history has there been so much attention paid to death as
a subject for scholarly and literary study,clinical and
research attention,or for cynical commercial exploitation.

We have exceeded even the literary genre of the Ars
Moriendi,which advanced the study of the art of dying
some 500 years ago.Such an interest has a long and
distinguished history,as we have demonstrated in the
recent Arno Press series of reprints of classic works.
Those who naively believe that the onlie begetter of
Thanatology lived in Manhattan,or who snobbishly frown
on the very term Thanatology as ugly modern jargon,should
attend to their study of history.The earliest use I have
encountered of this term in its modern sense is in the
book,in the Bibliotheque Imperial,Paris: THANATOLOGIA—
Sive in Mortis Naturam Causas,Genera ac Species,et
diagnosi Disquisitiones;published in Goettingen,in 1795.

The student,teacher,clinician and researcher in this
area now has need for a guide to the massive literature,
which contains some gems and so much dross;for one can
easily waste scarce time and money on the wrong books and
resources.As funds are limited,it becomes increasingly
important to buy books wisely.This Bibliography grew from
the listings I have prepared for my students at various
times and in various countries,and from a common concern
among members of the International Work Group on Death
Dying and Bereavement,and of the Forum for Death Education
and Counselling,for the need for better bibliographic
resources for all of us working in this field.

This is the Fourth Edition of my Annotated,Critical
Review Bibliography of books in print (or otherwise still
obtainable) dealing with dying,death,grief,and related

subjects.Encouraged by the very positive responses and
support from the wide range of distinguished experts who
have received,read,and used earlier editions,I have made
this edition far more comprehensive and detailed,and more
widely available than any other.In the Second Edition,I
listed 147 books;in the Third,276.In this edition,I list
over 750 books-as well as over 200 films,audio-and video-
tapes and cassettes,teaching materials,journals and other
relevant publications and resources.

　　Any Bibliography that provides more than a skeletal
listing,especially one based on critical reviews,is
subjective.(Man is an animal that is inherently and
absolutely incapable of wholly objective perceptions,though
he likes to pretend that he has this facility). Any
critic is licensed to be overtly subjective,and should
never be ashamed of his personal tastes and opinions,
for he can try to stifle them only at the expense of
becoming both dishonest and unreadable (to display
either of these failings is regrettable;to display both
is unforgiveable).To complain that a critic is critical,
is like complaining that water is wet.If it isn't,you've
been cheated.Although the degree and extent of general
expert agreement with my ratings in previous editions
has been both surprising and agreeable,any intelligent
reader is bound to disagree with at least some of the
opinions expressed.That is inevitable.One advantage of
having one reviewer for a large body of books,is that
you can more readily calibrate his opinion to yours.Compare
my ratings with your own on those books with which you
are already familiar,and calibrate my ratings.If we
generally agree,then my ratings will be a reasonably
reliable guide for you.If we usually disagree,simply
invert my rating scale,and you will still have a reliable
guide when seeking,purchasing,or recommending books.

　　No one is helped by the "positive" and
"encouraging" attitude some critics feel obliged to adopt
towards rubbish.Some of the literature on death is frank
rubbish---some mawkish and ghoulish,some over-simplified
beyond any relation to the reality of the phenomena
described;some is well-meaning (one hopes) but very ill-
informed,and written by people with no personal experience
of the situation of the dying or the bereaved.Some authors
simply seek to take advantage of the sad,the naive,the needy,
and the bereft.Some may be simply jumping on the great

Terminal Band-wagon,but simply unequal intellectually or stylistically to the challenge.Some publishers seem to function almost as a vanity press.All readers should be encouraged to have the confidence to recognize bad books when they encounter them,and not to tolerate them.It is not "negative" to do so;this is what the undisciplined and over-exuberant growth of literature in this area has needed badly for years.

I have included a reference to every relevant book about which I have received any information;and such information as is absent,was not provided by the Publishers, nor available from other sources.I have included an indication of the most recent prices made available to me: although in inflationary times such prices may be outdated by publishers who seem better at re-pricing than at copy-editing;I believe it is useful to indicate approximate and relative prices. I apologise in advance for inaccuracies and errors;although every attempt has been made to avoid these, it is inevitable that some will slip through.Neither I nor the publishers can be responsible in any way for problems arising from over-literal reliance on this guide.

The main section of the book which follows,is a numbered listing of books,arranged by title in alphabetical order,with reviews and a general indication of quality by a 5-star rating system,as follows:

***** Strongly recommended. Buy and read.
**** Useful for general reference work,very good
       in parts.
*** Useful for special reference,or for those making
      a special study of this area.
** I find it hard to get excited about this book;
      but it's relatively harmless.
* Not recommended.Not suitable for use at all.

The abbreviation PB indicates the paperback edition. Then there is an Extra Listing of more recently identified and reviewed books,and other books without review,many of which are not recommended for use,and are not considered to merit even a one-line review.

There follows an Index of Authors,by which the works of individual authors may be located in the Main Listing and the Extra Listing; and a Subject Index,which locates

books on particular subjects,and identifies the best books
in each category. Further Listings identify Journals in
this field; and Films (including a list of film distributors
and sources); Audiotapes and Videotapes/cassettes; other
teaching materials,filmstrips,packages and kits; and a list
of publisher's addresses.

The next section provides a series of carefully
selected references from the journal literature and of
books not in print,on various thanatological topics of
particular interest where there is not as yet a definitive
book. A penultimate section lists European works of
Thanatology---Scandinavian,French,Dutch and German.While
these may not be fully accurate or comprehensive listings,
they are included because of the importance of such works,
and the regrettable Anglo-American tendency to ignore
non-English works.

Finally,there is a Stop-Press listing of books and
materials reviewed or notified as we are going to press.

Despite frequent discussions of schemes for
collaborating in the production of such Bibliographies,I
have produced this edition,like the previous editions,alone.
Colleagues whose advice has been especially helpful have
included Prof.Loma Feigenberg of Stockholm with regard to
the Scandinavian and general literature,Prof.Georges Heuse
of Paris with regard to the French literature,Prof.Jurgen
Harms of Bloemfontein with regard to the German and
Dutch literature,and Joan McNeil with regard to films.

I hope this book will help guide you to the books and
other resources you need (and help you to avoid those you
don't need)and will aid you in all the good work that remains
to be done in all these areas.

London   Michael A. Simpson

Contents

Contents

CATEGORIES USED IN CLASSIFICATION

1. BIBLIOGRAPHIES

2. DEATH
   2.1 General Books on Death
   2.2 Death and Philosophy
   2.3 Death and History
   2.4 Death and Art,Literature,Novels
   2.5 Death and Religion
   2.6 Death and Culture,Anthropology,Cross-Cultural Aspects
   2.7 Eschatology,Life after Death,Reincarnation
   2.8 Death and Disaster,Violence,Mass Death

3. DYING
   3.1 Psychology of Death,Attitudes to Death
   3.2 Sociology of Death
   3.3 Personal Accounts
   3.4 Death and Children
   3.5 Death and the Old
   3.6 Miscellaneous,Including Self-Help Books

4. DEATH EDUCATION
   4.1 General
   4.2 Children,Junior School
   4.3 High School,College
   4.4 University
   4.5 Clinical,Counselling Training

5. TERMINAL CARE AND COUNSELLING
   5.1 General
   5.2 Medical
   5.3 Nursing
   5.4 Psychological,Social
   5.5 Religious

6. LOSS,GRIEF,& BEREAVEMENT
   6.1 General
   6.2 Personal Accounts,Widowhood
   6.3 Professional & Clinical Aspects & Help
   6.4 Counselling,Consolation,Self-Help
   6.5 Wills,Probate,Law

7. BURIAL,FUNERALS
    7.1 General Accounts
    7.2 Burial & Funeral Customs -- Historical and Cross-
        Cultural Aspects
    7.3 Burial & Funeral Customs -- Criticisms,Alternatives
        to Present Practices
    7.4 Funeral Directors & Directing

8. EUTHANASIA

9. SUICIDE
    9.1 General
    9.2 Clinical Management,Counselling & Prevention
    9.3 Suicide & Art,Philosophy,Literary Accounts
    9.4 Personal Accounts

10. MEDICAL ETHICS
    Death and Medical Technology,Decision-Making,Priorities;
    Ethical Dimensions of Death & Dying

————oOo————

Annotated List of Books

1. <u>ABOUT DYING.</u> Sara Bonnett Stein. Open Family Series.
   Walker & Co.,New York. 1974. 48 pp. Illus. $ 5.95

   Slim,brief,story of the deaths of a bird and a grand-
   -father,with dual narratives for parent and child.
   **

2. <u>AN ABSOLUTE GIFT.</u> Ned Rorem. Simon & Schuster,New York.
   1978

   A rather superficial and unconvincing novel dealing
   with death.
   **

3. <u>ACQUAINTED WITH GRIEF.</u> A.C.Rose.Westminster Press,
   Philadelphia. 1967. 96 pp. $ 4.50

   A woman's description of her experiences after her son's
   sudden death, her views on grief & consolation.
   ***

4. <u>ACT OF LOVE.</u> Paige Mitchell. Alfred A.Knopf,New York.
   1976. $ 8.95

   The Zygmanik case.George,paralyzed from the neck down in
   a motorcycle accident,and expecting a shortened life of
   physical and mental torment,pleaded with his brother Lester
   to kill him.On June 20,1973,Lester went to the Intensive
   Care Unit and fatally shot his brother.Defense Lawyer
   entered the plea of temporary insanity;and Lester was
   acquitted. Clear account of a controversial case.
   ***

5. <u>ACUTE GRIEF AND THE FUNERAL.</u>ed.Vanderlyn Pine,Austin
   Kutscher,David Peretz,Robert Slater,Robert De Bellis,
   Robert Volk & Danial Cherico. C.C.Thomas,Springfield,Ill.
   1975. 301 pp. $ 16.50.
No book can have 7 editors,surely?Another Thanatology book,
with a cast of thousands,written by dozens of authors &
edited by too many cooks.Funerals & the work of those who
deal with the remains & the remaining.Some good chapters,such
as Pine,but very variable "standards".
*

6. ADJUSTMENT TO WIDOWHOOD,& SOME RELATED PROBLEMS. A
Selected,Annotated Bibliography. Cecile Strugnell.
Health Sciences Publishing Corp.,New York.1974.
210 pp. $ 6.50. PB.

Unmemorable-neither very thorough nor very helpful.
*

7. ADMISSION TO THE FEAST. Gunnel Beckman. Rinehart &
Winston,New York. 1971.

A 19 year-old,knowing she is dying of leukemia,writes to
a friend about her life and the meaning of life and death.
Too ambitious a project,and rather precious in effect.No,no.
*

8. ADULTHOOD AND AGING.D.C.Kimmel. Wiley & Sons,New York.
1974. 484 pp. $ 11.95

A competent,interdisciplinary and developmental study of
man--adulthood,maturity,aging,retirement,dying and
bereavement.Draws together many important themes quite ably.
Well illustrated,and includes case-histories.
***

9. AFTERLIFE:REPORTS FROM THE THRESHOLD OF DEATH.Archie
Matson. Harper & Row,New York.Fitzhenry & Whiteside,
Toronto. 1977. 151 pp. $ 2.95 PB.

Old-fashioned superstition in the guise of "science".Re-
-tells many dated & uncritically accepted stories,without
adequate verification of the facts.Purports to answer such
questions as "Will we meet our loved ones after death? What
is heaven like? Do we have a physical shape in the next
world? " Naive,simplistic,totally unscientific while
assuming scientific status,selective in its use of data.
Less scientific than Swedenborg.
*

10. AFTER SUICIDE. S.E.Wallace.Wiley,New York. 1973.

After the suicides of 12 men;an analysis of in-depth
interviews with the surviving widows,with an emphasis on
aspects of the genesis of suicide rather than on the
processes of bereavement.
**

11. ALONE & SURVIVING : A GUIDE FOR TODAY'S WIDOW.Rae
    Lindsay. Walker Publ.Co.,New York.(Fitzhenry &
    Whiteside,Canada) 1977. $ 9.95

A very routine Widowbook,with nothing special to commend it.
**

12. THE AMERICAN FUNERAL : A STUDY IN GUILT,EXTRAVAGENCE,
    AND SUBLIMITY. LeRoy Bowman. Public Affairs Press,
    Washington D.C. 1959;Greenwood,1973. $ 11.75.

A well researched and documented sociological study of
American funerals and the economics of the industry.
***

13. THE AMERICAN VIEW OF DEATH (Acceptance or Denial?)
    Richard G.Dumont & Dennis C.Foss. Schenkman Publishing
    Co.,Cambridge,Mass.(Distrib.General Learning Press)
    1972. 117 pp. $ 2.95 PB

A somewhat overambitious sociological review,superficial in
parts,when it over-reaches itself,but adequately critical
in general.Surveys American attitudes to death,patterns of
acceptance and denial,with some consideration of
methodological problems in death attitude research.Wide-
-ranging,with a competent list of references.
***

14. THE AMERICAN WAY OF DEATH. Jessica Mitford. 1963.280 pp.
    Simon & Schuster,New York,1963.Fawcett/Crest PB $ 1.95.

Justly famous,witty,well-documented and merciless exposure
of the multi-million dollar Death Industry and American
Funeral practices.
*****

15. AND A TIME TO DIE. Mark Pelgrin.Edited Sheila Moon &
    Elizabeth B.Howes. Re-Quest Books,Theosophical
    Publishing House, Wheaton,Ill. 1976. 160 pp.PB $ 2.95.

Re-issue of the experiences of Pelgrin,who lived with an
equivocal diagnosis of cancer and then died of it,and the
insights he gained at the end of his life through Jungian
psychotherapy.An encouraging exploration of a search for
meaning and faith.
***

16. ANGUISH. Anselm Strauss & Barney Glaser. Sociology Press, California. 1970. 193 pp. $ 4.95 PB

Exemplifying their earlier work,this book describes the dying trajectory of one patient in great detail.Repetitious. **

17. ANNOTATED BIBLIOGRAPHY OF BIOETHICS: Selected 1976 Titles. ed.M.M.Nevins. Information Planning Associates, Rockville,MD. 1977. 91 pp. PB $ 12.00

Over 1200 briefly annotated references from the Journal literature of bioethics for 1976,under the categories used by the Bioethics Digest:General works,mental health,death & dying,medical research,professional/patient relationship, genetics/fertilization & pregnancy,population control, medical technology,& health care.A valuable resource guide for those interested in the ethical dimensions of health care & research.The area of death is reasonably dealt with, though neither in great depth or breadth. ***

18. ANTICIPATORY GRIEF.ed.Schoenberg,Carr,Kutscher,Peretz and Goldberg.Columbia University Press,New York. 1974. 380 pp. $ 12.50, £ 11.55

Another of those tragically unselective Foundation of Thanatology books.Some good essays on anticipatory grief and its management,almost smothered by the weight of trivia. If well-edited to a fraction of its present hypertrophied bulk,this could have been a useful book. **

19. ANTITRUST ASPECTS OF THE FUNERAL INDUSTRY. 1.Hearings Before the Subcommittee on Antitrust & Monopoly of the Committee on the Judiciary,U.S.Senate,88th Congress, Second Session.U.S.Govt.Printing Office,Washington,D.C. 1964. and 2. Views of the Subcommittee on Antitrust & Monopoly to the Committee on the Judiciary,U.S.Senate. U.S.Govt.Printing Office,Washington D.C. 1967.

Volume 1.is a most useful source book on funeral industry economic practices,including sales techniques,pricing,and advertising bans,etc.Statements by religious,labor,consumer & industry officials. Vol.2. No consensus was reached by the Subcommittee;this document records the different views of its members. ***

20. THE ART OF DYING.Ian Crichton. Peter Owen,London ;
    Humanities Press,New York. 1976. 166 pp. £5.00,$ 9.00

Amateurish,very general and uninteresting account of this
and that about death.Absolutely unusable for educational
purposes,or by anyone who knows much about death.
*

21. THE ART OF DYING. Robert E.Neale. Harper & Row,New York.
    1973. 158 pp. $ 5.95. 1976,PB $ 3.95.

Slightly unorthodox specimen of the genre of Death Lit.A
competent review of existing literature,interspersed with
rather eager exercises & quizzes (What type of awareness
context would you hope to set up?...Which of the following
categories pertains most to your way of fearing death?
Check only one...) But generally integrative & positive.
***

22. AS I LAY DYING. William Faulkner. Penguin PB 30 pence;
    Random PB,New York, $ 1.95.

Episodes in the death & burial of Addie Bundren in the
South,during the Depression;glum writing,and I find it
awfully dull.
**

23. ASSASSINATION IN AMERICA. James McKinley. Harper & Row,
    New York; Fitzhenry & Whiteside,Toronto.1977.
    243 pp. $ 13.25.

An unusually interesting account of eleven major American
assassinations & assassination attempts: Lincoln,Garfield,
McKinley,Theodore Roosevelt,Franklin Roosevelt,Huey Long,
John Kennedy,Malcolm X,Martin Luther King,Robert Kennedy,
and George Wallace,with the briefest mention of the attempts
on Gerald Ford. He draws illuminating parallels between the
circumstances of each case,between the assassins:Booth,
Guiteau,Czolgosz,Schrank,Zangara,Weiss,Oswald,Ray,Sirhan &
Bremer;the strategies,background issues,& the shoddy
investigations & management of each case.For a Professor
of English,the author's style is at times confusing,and his
grammar and phraseology and use of obsolete words,is
curiously inept,but the stories make compulsive reading.
***

24. ATTACHMENT AND LOSS. Volume 1.ATTACHMENT.John Bowlby.
    Basic Books,New York. (orig.1969) 1977.428 pp. $ 4.95
    reprint PB. Penguin PB 1978 re-issue,£ 1.50.

The definitive work on the child's attachment to his mother,
seeing attachment in an ethological perspective as
functional in preserving the individual and,ultimately,the
species.Research & empirical work has advanced well beyond
the stage represented by this book,but its theoretical
importance remains substantial. The obverse of loss.
***

25. AT THE HOUR OF DEATH:The Results of Research on over
    1,000 Afterlife Experiences. Karlis Osis & Erlendur
    Haraldsson. Avon Books,New York.1977.244 pp. $ 3.95 PB

The only recent attempt at scientific study of the
possibility of afterlife experiences;the only recently
published book on the subject to present assessable data on
the matter.Continuing Osis' earlier work on death-bed
visions & related experiences,on an international scale,
co-ordinated by the American Society for Psychical Research.
A unique book whose reasonable methods & discussion will
convince some readers of the validity of the authors'
conclusions,and will lead many more to keep the question
open,rather than dismissing it too readily.
****

26. AUTOPSY. James R.Adams & Robert D.Mader.Lloyd-Luke,
    London. 1976. 196 pp. £ 15.60.

Deals with the technique of post-morten examination,with
detailed description and illustration.Absurdly expensive.
**

27. AWARENESS OF DYING.Barney G.Glaser & Anselm L.Strauss.
    Aldine,Chicago. 1965. 305 pp. $ 7.50

A classical sociological study,in which the authors advance
a reasonably useful model of contexts of awareness of death;
the problems that arise when there's "nothing more to do",
and how we handle them. Interesting,and with many practical
examples.Would have benefitted from some tighter editing.
****

B
28.   BEFORE THE GREAT SILENCE. Maurice Maeterlinck.(Transl.
      B.Miall) Arno Press,New York.1976. (1st Edn,NY,1937)
      200 pp. $ 14.00

Is death to be conquered--or embraced as "more beautiful
than life"? From a disillusioned old age,Maeterlinck
produced a stylistic,unfinished,aphoristic soliloquoy on
death and the violence of the 20th century.His meditations
are fresh and thought-provoking.Samples: "The majority of
human beings live only in order not to die ; If you were
not dead,what would you do during eternity? ; Eternity is
the ocean,time is the wave ; The living are the dead on
holiday ; and What misfortune could be comparable to that
of remaining oneself for a million years? "
***

29.   BEGINNINGS: A BOOK FOR WIDOWS.Betty Jane Wylie.
      McClelland & Stewart,Toronto.1977. 144 pp. $ 7.95

Probably the best widow-book.Wise,wry and realistic;succinct
and sensitive without being too sorry for herself.Briefly
deals with many topics including finances and jobs,relations
with friends & children,loneliness,companionship and sex,
insurance, repairs,and living as a widow.
****

30.   BEHAVIORAL METHODS FOR CHRONIC PAIN AND ILLNESS.
      Wilbert E.Fordyce.C.V.Mosby,St Louis.1976.
      (Henry Kimpton,London) 236 pp. £ 7.75

A book that will be valuable for all involved in chronic &
terminal care.Successive chapters provide authoritative
reviews of pain as a clinical problem,psychogenic pain,
operant conditioning as a factor in pain,techniques of
behavioral analysis & behavior change,treatment goals and
biofeedback,assessment of pain,selection of patients and
treatment methods including orientation of patient & family,
managing pain medications & pain cocktails,generalization &
maintenance of performance. The bibliography is valuable.
****

31.   THE BELL JAR. Sylvia Plath. Bantam ,NY.PB $ 1.75

A brilliant novel,autobiographical in many respects,about a
19 year old girl who attempts suicide,finding life difficult
to bear. One of the best evocations of suicidal thinking
in literature.
*****

32.   BENIFICANT EUTHANASIA. Ed.Marvin Kohl. Prometheus Books,
      Buffalo. 1975.   255 pp. $ 10.95.

This book argues the case for euthanasia,active & passive,
though giving some room to counter-arguments.The dangers &
problems are discussed and safeguards proposed,including the
Living Will.The case of "Hopelessly abnormal children" is
considered. 10 of the 19 papers have already been published
elsewhere,but the collection is readable and clear,without
becoming verbose.It examines religious,moral & ethical,&
philosophical aspects of the problem,with contributors that
include Maguire,Fletcher,Summerskill & Engelhardt.There are
some ugly jargon inventions,including Benemortasia,the
unhelpful 'beneficent',and deliveration('compassionate
complicity in suicide") & its spawn:deliverator,self-
-deliverationer,deliverist,etc.Deliver us from such
terminology! Very short bibliography,and regrettably
no index.
***

33.   THE BEREAVED PARENT: A Book of Counsel for Those Who
      Suffer This Heartbreaking Experience. Harriet Sarnoff
      Schiff. Crown Publishers,New York.1977.140pp.$7.95.

Neither very inspiring,stylish or helpful.
**

34.   BEREAVEMENT. Colin Murray Parkes. Tavistock,London,1972.
      International Universities Press,NY. $ 10.00   233 pp.
      Penguin PB $ 3.95

The major study of grief in adult life,its phenomena and
consequences,by the man who has condicted many of the best
studies in this area.Includes discussion of the "broken
heart"phenomenon,atypical grief reactions,and ways of
helping the bereaved.A very important work.
****

35.   BEREAVEMENT : ITS PSYCHOSOCIAL ASPECTS.Ed.Schoenberg,
      Gerber,Wiener,Kutscher,Peretz and Carr. Columbia
      University Press,New York. 1975. 380 pp. $ 18.75

Just when one had been beginning to wonder whether the
Columbia University Press were Academic Publishers,a book
that is really rather good.It shares the usual faults of
the Foundation of Thanatology books:too many editors,too
little editing;uneven quality and bittiness.But unlike others
in the series,this contains a good proportion of genuinely

35 - ctd)   original and useful fragments: Lerner on War
Widows,Danto on the widows of slain police officers,
Rosenblatt on Ethnography,Welu on the prevention of
pathological bereavement.'Fundamental concepts'are too
briefly reviewed,and the section on Health Professionals is
also disappointingly trite.Unpleasant & unnecessary jargon
appears,such as 'conjugal bereavement' & the 'maternal
orphan'. One of the best of the series,though,implying the
beginnings of a concern for quality as well as quantity.
***½

36. BETWEEN SURVIVAL AND SUICIDE. ed.B.J.Wolman. Gardner
     Press,New York. 1976. 195 pp. £ 11.55 $ 19.60
Scholarly and consistently interesting,this book collects 8
essays dealing with non-clinical views of suicide as a social
& philosophical challenge.Of particular interest are chapters
by Medard Boss on the existential meaning of suicide,the
flight into death,compared with the flight from death into
mere survival;Robert Jay Lifton on death & the continuity of
life,proposing a new paradigm (not really new,but very well
expressed);Barbara Suter on suicide & Women;Thomas Szasz on
the ethics of suicide (as passionate and as glib as ever);
and Mamoru Iga on the personal situation as a factor in
suicide,citing Yasunari Kawabata & Yukio Mishima.More routine
chapters are contributed by Krauss,Wolman & Bernstein.
***½

37. BEYOND AND BACK:Those Who Died...And Lived to Tell It.
     Ralph Wilkerson. Melodyland Productions,Anaheim. 1977
     and Bantam,NY (in press) 275 pp. illus. $ 8.95
Odd.A revivalist Christian,gossipy,anecdotal book about
life after death.Its stories provide equivocal date,in which
resuscitation,recovery from illness,or even sudden death,are
construed as proofs of the reality of life after death and
of resurrection;whatever the outcome,it is interpreted as
"proving" the original hypothesis.Interesting as an example
of Cognitive Dissonance phenomena.Addresses itself to some
of the awkward questions that can be asked about such
experiences,but chooses easy answers.
**

38. BIATHANATOS. John Donne.(Reproduced from the first
     Edition,1646) Arno Press,New York.1976.218pp. $ 17.00
Written in 1608,considers the paradox of'self-homicide'.A
great landmark in the study of suicide & death,of great and
lasting influence.
***

39. A BIBLIOGRAPHY OF BOOKS ON DEATH,BEREAVEMENT,LOSS AND
     GRIEF : 1935-1968. Ed.A.H.Kutscher. Health Sciences
     Publ.,New York.1969. 84 pp. $ 10.00, $ 4.95 PB.

A moderately comprehensive,very uncritical,not always
relevant,unannotated bibliography of books.Too unselective
to be very useful.
**
     Supplement I. Includes citations 1968-1972. Health
     Sciences,NY. 1974. 94 pp. $ 4.95 PB.
**

40. A BIBLIOGRAPHY ON DEATH EDUCATION. The Celo Press in
     collaboration with the Forum for Death Education and
     Counselling. Celo Press,Burnsville,NC.1977.20pp.$1.00

Intended as a basic reference guide for students,teachers &
"serious laypersons".Briefly annotated titles of books,some
for children,a few films & filmstrips.Desultory & regrettably
sloppy in execution (especially inadequate in referencing &
publishing details of books).Limited in range & extent.Also,
this is not a bibliography on or about death education at
all---most of the available literature on death education
is totally ignored.It is a bibliography for death
educators,listing some books that may be useful to them in
learning something about death.Some very surprising
omissions,such as no reference to the journal 'Death
Education".
*

41. A BIBLIOGRAPHY ON DEATH,GRIEF AND BEREAVEMENT 1845-1973.
     Compiled by Robert Fulton.3rd revised edition.1973.
     Center for Death Education & Research,Minnesota.173pp.PB

Quite simply the very best & most comprehensive bibliography
on the subject available. Lists 2,639 items,& efficiently
corss-references them in a useful index.Not fully
comprehensive,but has only relatively minor omissions &
errors. Generally excludes journalistic,literary and
principally theological works,& much of the material on
suicide. Very useful for any serious student of the subjects.
*****

42. A BIOETHICAL PERSPECTIVE ON DEATH & DYING :Summaries
    of the literature. Ed.Madeline M.Nevins. Information
    Planning Associates,Rockville,MD. June 1977.
    88 pp. PB $ 8.95

A special supplement of the Bioethics Digest,containing the
217 abstracts from its first 12 issues on: attitudes to
death,death education,definitions of death,euthanasia,care
of the dying,bereavement,and suicide.Efficient but
uncritical annotations,with an emphasis on ethical
dimensions.Reasonably wide-ranging,though not fully
comprehensive,guide to the Journal literature of 1973-1976.
***

43. THE BIOETHICS DIGEST.: Summaries of Literature on
    Biomedical Ethics. ed.M.M.Nevins.Information Planning
    Associates,Rockville,MD. Monthly,PB. 63 pp. $6.00 per
    copy, $ 48. per year,subscription.

Efficiently abstracted uncritical summaries of bioethical
literature in several disciplines.Especially competent in
the areas of ethics of health care,resource allocation and
research.Less thorough with regard to the death literature.
***

44. BIOMEDICAL ETHICS AND THE LAW. Ed.James M.Humber and
    Robert F.Almeder.Plenum Press,New York. 1976.

An odd volume of reprinted articles which fails to meet
its absurd claim to "cover every social problem caused by
the revolution in medical technology",and which is not
well-suited for use as a text in courses in biomedical
ethics.Separate sections deal with Abortion (reasonably
competently);Mental Illness (much less so,with an excess of
Szasz); Human Experimentation (very well indeed,including
the NIH Guidelines on Research with Human Subjects,which
should be carefully read by research thanatologists) and
Human Genetics (welldone,& with more new material). The
final section on Dying,is very poor indeed.It includes a
faulty piece by Robitscher and a boring reprint of Morison.
It shows no real understanding of the area at all,& only
the articles by Rescher on allocation of exotic medical
life-saving therapy,& by Capron & Kass on definitions of
death,are worthwhile.The bibliography for this section is
especially bodly done.Very uneven in readibility,
originality,and in value and quality of contributions;
very weakly edited.
**

45. BODY,MIND AND DEATH.ed.Antony Flew. Macmillan,New York.
     1971. 305 pp. $ 1.95 PB

A useful anthology of philosophical speculations regarding
death,the meaning of mind,relations between mind and body,
and speculations about an after-life. Ranges from Plato
and Aristotle to William James,Gilbert Ryle and A.J.Ayer,
via Hume,Huxley and Descartes.
***

46. THE BODY SNATCHERS. Daniel Cohen.J.B.Lippincott,
     Philadelphia. 1975. 155 pp. $ 5.95, $ 2.95 PB.

Lively though macabre account of the history of grave-
-robbing.Of considerable historical,sociological and
psychological interest.
***

47. THE BOOK OF THE CRAFT OF DYING and Other Early English
     Tracts Concerning Death:Taken from Manuscripts and
     Printed Books in the British Museum and Bodleian
     Libraries. Ed. Frances M.M.Comper. Arno Press,New
     York,1976 (1st edn,London,1917). 174 pp. $ 15.00

The last period of great public concern with death was
during the 14th & 15th centuries,amid bubonic plague,war,
persecution and famine.Brief guidebooks by popular
preachers dealt with the"art"of dying.The Craft of Dying
(about 1450),of uncertain authorship,is derived from
various European sources.This edition includes other
related pieces including selections from Richard Rolle and
Heinrich Suso.
***

48. A BOY THIRTEEN.(Reflections on Death).Jerry Irish.
     Westminster Press,Philadelphia. 1975. 62 pp. $ 3.95.

A slim,honest book by a theologian who faced the sudden death
of his oldest son soon after another son died of congenital
heart disease.The three main chapters face:'Anger:Death as
Utterly Unacceptable','Aloneness:Death as Complete
Abandonment',loss & the challenge of all one's assumptions;&
'Freedom:Death as Occasion to Love'.With contributions by
other family members,the author traces his path through
bereavement ,and how he was able to find something positive
in the experience.
****

49. <u>BREAK-THROUGH</u>. Konstantin Raudive. Zebra Books,New York.1977 391 pp. $ 2.25 PB (orig.Taplinger,1971)

"Electronic Communication with the Dead may be possible! " Based on the earlier work of the Swede Friedrich Jurgenson, Raudive uses a technique of recording on tape--via microphone, radio or diode--and later claims to hear voices of the dead speaking at a distinct rate and rhythm,polyglot messages. Despite its attempt to be convincing in scientific terms, this seems to be an audio version of the Rorschach Ink Blot, in which crackles & static are interpreted by wishful thinking.Even if life after death were a proven reality,and communication with the dead an established fact,I don't believe that the illustrious dead (his examples include Goethe,Kennedy,Churchill,Stalin,Pasternak & Jung) would choose to talk such utter drivel in distorted combinations of Latvian,German,Russian,Spanish and French. "Breakfast, Please--send ink.Otherwise swamp",as some transcripts read. How banal!
*

50. <u>BUT NOT TO LOSE : A Book of Comfort for Those Bereaved</u>. Austin H.Kutscher.Frederick Fell,New York. 1969 288 pp. $ 5.95 (Also via MSS Information Corp).

Offers advice from various health professionals and also from lawyers,clergy and funeral directors.Very unremarkable, vapid,unimpressive.
**

51. <u>BY THE HIGHWAY HOME</u>. Mary Stolz. Harper & Row,New York. 1971. $ 4.95.

Fiction for the younger reader.Catty's brother dies in Vietnam,but no-one will talk about him,no-one understands her feelings. The relationships within the family,and how they are affected by the death,are well described.
**$\frac{1}{2}$

C

52. CANADIAN GUIDE TO DEATH AND DYING.Jill Watt.
       International Self-Counsel Press,Vancouver & Toronto.
       1974. 156 pp. $ 3.50 PB

A good idea,variably achieved. Some woolly writing on
attitudes to death,for example.But some soundly practical
guidance on pre-arranging funerals,estate planning,and what
to do after a death occurs.Realistic comments on funeral
expenses and costs,with review of local provincial laws,and
a summary of Catholic,Anglican & United Church practices.
Specific advice on organ donation & death benefits in
Canada,with relevant addresses.
**$\frac{1}{2}$
(The same publishers produce a series of booklets:The
Layman's Guide to Drafting Wills (Probate Procedure),
relating the laws of British Columbia,Alberta & Ontario,
at $ 2.95 each).

53. CANCER CARE NURSING. Marilee Ivers Donovan & Sandra
       Girton Pierce. Appleton-Century-Crofts. 1976.
       272 pp. PB $ 13.35 £ 8.40

An outstanding contribution to practical cancer care.Its
chapters deal with the meaning of cancer,and aspects of
dying-and problems related to pain,infection,nutrition,
elimination (and ostomies),and identity and body image.
Useful references and selective bibliographies cover a wide
range of literature.The details of palliative care,including
sexual difficulties,are quite comprehensively,if briefly,
discussed.
****

54.   CANCER: THE BEHAVIORAL DIMENSIONS.Ed.J.W.Cullen,B.H.Fox,
        & R.N.Isom.(National Cancer Institute Monograph).
        Raven Press,New York. 1976. 408 pp. $ 23.70.

A unique monograph examining the interface between the
behavioral sciences and cancer prevention,detection,diagnosis,
treatment,rehabilitation and chronic care.Good chapters
review the psychosocial epidemiology of cancer,delay factors,
the effectiveness of cancer-detection & anti-smoking
programs,physician attitudes,& the effects of mass media on
health behavior. Holland writes on coping with cancer,Krant
on the problems of presenting the diagnosis & team approaches.
The Browns write cogently about decision making for the
terminally ill patient,& Weisman on coping behavior and

54 ctd) suicide in cancer,in two especially valuable
chapters.Some of the discussion from the original conference
is presented.While the quality is variable,the general
standards are high and much of the content is not readily
available elsewhere.
***½

55. CANCER WARD. A.Solzhenitsyn. Bantam,New York. 1969.
     560 pp. $ 1.25

A great novel,about life in the Cancer Ward of a Russian
hospital,that defies any brief review.
*****

56. CARE FOR THE DYING. Ed. Richard N.Soulen. John Knox
     Press,Atlanta. 1975. 141 pp. PB $ 4.95

An unusually effective discussion of the problems of
counselling the dying and suicidal,from a theological
point of view.Using verbatim transcripts of counselling
sessions,it discusses the issues raised in the light of
the concepts of Christian ethics,pastoral & systematic
theology,and even Black and Third-World theology.
Realistic and stimulating.
***½

57. CARE OF PATIENTS WITH FATAL ILLNESS. Ed. L.P.White.
     Annals of the New York Academy of Sciences. 1969
     Vol.164,Art.3,pp.635-896. Monograph.

A wide-ranging seminar,with some excellent and some
mediocre material.Especially good are:Gifford on some
psychoanalytic theories about death,Feifel on perception
on death,Strauss,Hackett & Weisman on Denial in Heart
Disease & Cancer patients,LeShan on Mobilizing the Life
Force,& Racy on Death in an Arab culture.
***

58. THE CARE OF THE AGED,THE DYING,AND THE DEAD.Alfred
     Worcester. 2nd Edition. (1st published 1950)
     Arno Press,New York. 1976. 77 pp. $ 10.00

A practical and compassionate work that was one of the
first books in the current wave of interest in
Thanatology.Brief and lucid,with a genuine concern for
the dying,the survivors,and the aged.
***

59.   CARE OF THE CHILD FACING DEATH. Ed.Lindy Burton.
      Routledge & Kegan Paul,London & Boston.   1974.
      225 pp. $ 15.85.

Very practical and sound,looking at the problems faced
by the child and the parents,the staff & the sibs,from a
broad interdisciplinary basis.Variable in quality but
contains some excellent & unusual material.Relatively
limited reference to the general literature,but records
some original observations.
***

60.   CARE OF THE DYING. Richard Lamerton. Priory Press,
      London. 1973. 140 pp. $ 9.25

A very disappointing book. Watery,simplistic,bitty.Relies
heavily on often extensive quotations from other sources.
Not very sound theoretically,and very much less practically
helpful than it claims to be.Amateurish. Nice series of
engravings of terminal care and cancer clinics;if you
like that sort of thing,it's the sort of thing you'd like.
Strongly not recommended for use.
*

61.   CARE OF THE DYING. Cicely Saunders. Nursing Times
      Publications Section.2nd Edn.1976. 24pp.PB.
      50 pence ; 90 cents U.S.

A collection of reprints of gentle,mild,not very detailed
articles written by Dr Saunders for the Nursing Times.They
include her essays on 'The problem of Euthanasia','Should
a Patient Know?',mental distress in the dying patient,the
nursing of patients dying of cancer,and a valuable article
on the control of pain. Also lists the addresses of Hospices
& similar institutions in the United Kingdom.A gentle,
concerned approach with some useful practical advice.
An appetizer,though not an entree.
***

62.   CARETAKER OF THE DEAD (The American Funeral Director)
      Vanderlyn R.Pine. Irvington Publishers,N.Y. (Halsted
      Press Divn of John Wiley & Sons,distrib.) 1975
      220 pp. $ 12.95

American funeral practices have long deserved proper
sociological study.So far,they have tended to be the
subject either of absurdly uncritical and monotonously
laudatory descriptions (often originating within or

62. ctd) sponsored by the funeral industry),or of shrill,
acid,uniformly critical journalism.Though decorated with
stray facts,these works have been principally elaborate
statements of opinion,either prepared to find no faults,or
prepared to find nothing but fault.
Van Pine,with a background in the funeral service and now
and academic position in sociology,is unusually well-placed
to produce the sort of competent & dispassionate study that
is needed.This book is a promising start,though one hopes
Dr.Pine will add to it,for he has whetted our appetite
without entirely satisfying it.Deeply influenced by Goffman's
models,Pine describes the typical behavior of funeral
directors within their organizational and bureaucratic
settings,their public and private behavior.One would
appreciate still more descriptive and critical incident
material,and a still more critical approach to the data.
Such highly contentious issues as 'grief therapy',the need
for embalming,& the benefits of restorative work & viewing,
are handled gently and disappointingly,without citing much
relevant evidence for or against such practices,rather
than opinions.The results of a study of funeral directors
are reported,which is competent,& provides a good deal of
information (occasionally,as with the "zero-order Product-
-Moment Correlation Coefficients for Eight Variables" on
p.70,uncharacteristically & needlessly obscure &
unexplained).A tranquil,sensible work that will serve us
well until the larger,more detailed & more critical study
that will surely follow.
***

63. CARING FOR THE DYING PATIENT AND HIS FAMILY.ed.A.H.
     Kutscher & M.R.Goldberg. Health Sciences Publications,
     New York. 1973. 72 pp. $ 9.00, $ 3.95 PB

Certainly not the "Model for Medical Education (& Medical
Centre Conferences") it claims to be.A relentlessly complete
transcript of a very nondescript and dull conference that
really did not deserve preservation,except perhaps in
formaldehyde.
*

64. CARING FOR THE WIDOW & HER FAMILY. CRUSE,The
     National Organization for Widows & their Children.
     Richmond. 3rd Edition.1976. PB 40 pence.

Slim,soundly sensible practical booklet that deals
briefly with bereavement,the immediate business & legal
arrangements following death,people to inform,wills,
widows pensions,& matters of health,housing & homes,
income tax,& looking for new occupation.General advice,
& many useful addresses & phone numbers for local
British agencies.
***

65. CASES OF THE REINCARNATION TYPE.Vol.I. Ten Cases in
     India. Ian Stevenson. University Press of Virginia,
     Charlottesville,Va. 1975. 367 pp. $ 20.00

Continuing the studies Dr Stevenson published previously
(2¼ Cases Suggestive of Reincarnation,1974) this is a
painstaking and careful investigation of cases,which
provide more convincing or at least challenging evidence
suggestive of the possibility of reincarnation,than most
previous books in this area.A useful example of how a
scientist can approach unconventional & paranormal subjects.
Lucid,detailed,restrained.
***

66. CATASTROPHIC DISEASES : WHO DECIDES WHAT?A Psychosocial
     & Legal Analysis of the Problems Posed by Hemodialysis
     & Organ Transplantation. Jay Katz & Alexander Morgan
     Capron. Russell Sage Foundation,N.Y. 1975.295pp. $10.00

A highly able explanation of important issues,extending &
complementing both Katz's earlier work (Experimentation with
Human Beings,1972) & Fox & Swazey's recent book (1974).The
authors explore the nature & effects of catastrophic illness,
& such goals & values as the preservation of life,reduction
of suffering,personal integrity & dignity,pursuit of
knowledge,economy & public interest.There's a cogent account
of the development & present status of the technical
procedures;& a study of the characteristics,authority &
capacity of the physician-investigators & patient-subjects,
the functions of informed consent,& limitations of consent.
The stages of decision-making are reviewed,the activities
of professional & public institutions involved;& proposals
for the formulation of policy regarding the allocation of
resources & selection of donors,the administration of such

66 ctd) major medical interventions at local and national
levels,with a review of decisions and consequences. Lucid,
readable,fascinating and challenging.
*****

67. CAUSING DEATH AND SAVING LIVES.Jonathan Glover.
     Pelican Original.Penguin Books,Harmondsworth. 1977.
     328 pp. £ 1.25 ($ 3.95 in Canada).

A clear discussion of the arguments used in prohibiting or
justifying the killing of others,the moral difficulties,&
some of the practical problems.Cool & logical,it deals with
matters relating to: moral theory,autonomy & rights,ends
and means;not striving to keep alive;abortion,infanticide,
suicide,voluntary & involuntary euthanasia, choices
between people in allocating resources,assassination and
war. Mr Glover clearly lacks practical experience of the
matters of which he writes,& is sometimes naïve in such
matters,but in logical discussion he is unusually
competent.
***½

68. CHANGER LA MORT. L.Schwartzenberg & P.Viansson-Ponté.
     Albin-Michel,Paris. 1977.

By a Professor of Cancerology(Oncology) at the Paul
Brousse Hospital,Villejuif,and a journalist of Le Monde;
a review of the current French views of euthanasia,
reporting some cases of active euthanasia.
***

69. CHILDREN AND DYING. An Exploration and a Selective
     Professional Bibliography. S.S.Cook. Health Sciences
     Publishing,New York. 1973.37pp.$1.95(1974 edn,$4.95)

Four short essays (also published elsewhere)on children's
perceptions of death;teenagers & death;& helping children
cope with death.A short bibliography.Rather nondescript.
**

70. CHILDREN AND THE DEATH OF A PRESIDENT.Ed. M.
     Wolfenstein & G.Kliman.Peter Smith,Gloucester,Mass.
     1969. (Orig.Doubleday 1965, Anchor books 1966)
     288 pp. $ 5.00

A unique collection of multi-disciplinary studies emerging
from a 1964 conference,dealing with children's responses to
the Kennedy assassination,and based on a variety of clinical,
observational & survey techniques.Kept interesting by a
liberal use of direct quotations & children's essays.Of
considerable specialist interest.
***

71. CHILDREN'S EXPERIENCE WITH DEATH. Rose Zeligs.
     Charles C.Thomas,Springfield,Ill. 1974.247pp.$10.75.

Absolutely nothing to commend it.Not particularly well-
-informed,nor particularly well-expressed.
*

72. A CHILD'S PARENT DIES:Studies in Childhood Bereavement.
     Erna Furman. Yale University Press,New Haven. 1974
     316 pp. $ 15.00

An excellent,broad,helpful study of grief,loss & mourning
in childhood,based on some detailed studies of bereaved
children & a thorough review of the literature.Of
theoretical & practical use. An uncritical bibliography.
****

73. CHRONIC ILLNESS & THE QUALITY OF LIFE.Anselm L.Strauss.
     C.V.Mosby,St Louis. 1975. 160 pp. PB $ 6.60

A readable,modest and valuable study of how having a chronic
disease affects the quality of life;the psychosocial rather
than medical aspects of living with chronic illness,
focussed on the patient & his family,at home.It covers the
management of crises & treatment regimes,the control of
symptoms & the strategies of the attempts to maintain a
normal life.The middle section has specific studies(by
authors like Jeanne Benoliel) of conditions like rheumatoid
arthritis,ulcerative colitis,childhood diabetes,emphysema,
chronic renal failure,& dying in hospitals.Final chapters on
how to gather information from such patients,to better
understand their needs,& matters of public policy.An
important addition to the literature in an unjustifiably
neglected area.
****

74. THE CITY OF THE GODS. A Study in Myth & Mortality.
     John Dunne. Macmillan,New York.1965/1973 PB.
     243 pp. $ 2.95. (Sheldon Press,London).

A distinguished theologian studies the myths with which man
has tried through the ages to understand the nature of death.
Death in relation to monarchy & democracy;Gilgamesh & Erech;
Sophocles,Homer,Plato,Dante & Shakespeare;Kant,Hegel,
Nietsche & Heidegger.Not easy or elementary reading,but a
unique attempt at a synthesis of theological,philosophical
& historical themes.Choron is more accessible & general;
Dunne has more academic depth in his selected areas.
***

75. CLUES TO SUICIDE. Ed.E.S.Shneidman & N.L.Farberow.
     McGraw-Hill,New York.1957. 228 pp. $ 2.25 PB.

Brilliant & still important early classic of modern
Suicidology,including the famous study of suicide notes
(comparing real & simulated notes);suicide & age,as a
magical act (Wahl),in general hospital,in children,and
its logic. Highly stimulating.
****

76. A COLLECTION OF AMERICAN EPITAPHS AND INSCRIPTIONS
     WITH OCCASIONAL NOTES.Timothy Alden. Arno Press,
     New York. 1976. 5 volumes in 2, 868pp & 584 pp.
     $ 84.00 (1st edition,New York,1814).

Exhaustive and obsessive collection of American epitaphs
with explanatory notes,arranged by states,by city,and
alphabetically within cities by persons.A major source on
early American attitudes to death.
***

77. COMING TO TERMS WITH DEATH (How to Face the Inevitable
     with Wisdom & Dignity).Fred Cutter.Nelson-Hall,Chicago.
     1974. 367 pp. $ 8.95 ; 1977 PB,307 pp. $ 4.95.

A rambling & discursive work,exploring societal attitudes to
death,non-acceptance & phobic denial,& the possibilities of
social acceptance.Cutter develops the distinction between a
personal readiness to die & the suicidal wish to die.Partly
practical,partly a rather vague & pretentious consideration
of the hedonism of youth culture.An idiosyncratic book,
which may stimulate or enervate,according to your personal
tastes.
***

78.   COMMON-SENSE SUICIDE.Doris Portwood. Dodd-Mead & Co.,
      New York. 1978. 142 pp. $ 6.95.

A simple & straight-forward tract in support of "rational"
suicide,especially for the elderly & ailing,calling for its
legalization.An earnest proponent of 'Gray Liberation',she
cites with approval the early feminist Charlotte Perkins
Gilman who killed herself in 1935,saying"the record of a
previously noble life is precisely what makes it sheer
insult to allow death in pitiful degradation.We may not
wish to 'die with our boots on' but we may well prefer to
die with our brains on". She argues persuasively for suicide
as a permitted option & escape from senility for the
victims of 'Catch-65'.
***

79.   COMMUNICATING ISSUES IN THANATOLOGY. Ed.Thomas Fleming,
      A.H.Kutscher,et.al. MSS Information Corp.,New York.
      1976. 343 pp. $ 11.50.

A variable collection of essays.Some dealing with inter-
-personal communication (Cassem & Torpie write well here);
some deal with how the media deal with death;some consider
information exchange/data banks in Thanatology-& some with
death education.Uneven quality.A peculiar Lexicon of Death,
where 9 people (the Foundation of Thanatology always seems
to write in groups like the Mormon Tabernacle Choir) write
about uses and meanings of words in Thanatology,without
managing to be at all helpful.We really don't need that!
***

80.   COMMUNICATION AND AWARENESS IN A CANCER WARD.Jim
      McIntosh. Croom Helm,London. 1977. 208 pp. £ 6.95

Probably the most inadequate and deplorable attempt at a
sociological study of cancer patients yet published.And it
couldn't have been published if the manuscript had been
properly reviewed.Grossly over-simplified account,quite
unrecogniseable by anyone with actual clinical experience
of cancer patients.Contributes absolutely nothing to our
understanding of the patient;its practical advice is
unfounded,naive and immature.Over-priced and without any
redeeming features. Not worth buying;not worth borrowing.
No star.

81.   COMMUNICATION WITH THE FATALLY ILL.Adriaan Verwoerdt.
      C.C.Thomas,Springfield. 1966. 183 pp.

A sound,practical guide,with an especially good study of
the process of informing the patient and the family,
principles and techniques of continued communication,and of
the nature and management of defence mechanisms & emotional
reactions. Basically from the psychiatrist's point of view.
****

82. CONCERNING DEATH : A PRACTICAL GUIDE FOR THE LIVING.
    Ed. Earl A.Grollman. Beacon Press,Boston. 1974.
    365 pp. $ 6.75, PB $ 3.95.

Variable in quality,but thorough.The incessant Question &
Answer format gets monotonous,but it's an unpretentious,
highly competent & helpful work,accessible to the lay reader.
Some excellent contributors,including Cassem,Krant,Jackson,
& Grollman himself.Looks at Protestant,Catholic & Jewish
views of death,the law,insurance,the coroner,the funeral
director,cemetary,memorial maker,cremation,& educator,&
even considers the art of the condolence call or letter.
****

83.   CONFRONTATIONS OF DEATH. A Book of Readings & a
       Suggested Method of Instruction. Ed.F.G.Scott &
       R.M.Brewer. Continuing Education Publications,
       Corvallis,Oregon. 1971. 184 pp. $ 7.65.

Individual selection of original & reprinted articles &
poems,some of considerable interest,some obscure,based on
a local course at the Oregon Center for Gerontology.
Commendable,& useful as an introduction for some courses.
**½

84.   CONFRONTING A DEATH IN THE FAMILY.A Guidebook to
      Crisis Management. Shepard A.Insel. R.T.E.S.Publicns,
      Burlingame,California. 1974. 158 pp. PB

A rather over-hectic,pugnacious & embattled book.Tries
hard to be practical,down to check lists,but doesn't quite
succeed,due to numerous omissions & weak organization.Brief
& obsolete bibliography.
**

85.   A CONSTANT BURDEN.Margaret Voysey. Routledge & Kegan
      Paul,London & Boston. 1975. 240 pp. £ 5.95.

Study of the effects of a mentally or physically disabled
child on the parents,siblings,& family relationships (based
on interviews of 23 parents). They tended to present an
unreal & artificial picture of a 'happy family'with no
problems.Description of the imposition of social,medical,
& religious conventions & expectations,& the reactions &
defences of the parents.
***

86.   A CONSUMER BIBLIOGRAPHY ON FUNERALS.Assembled &
      Annotated by Ruth Mulvey Harmer.Continental Association
      of Funeral & Memorial Societies. 1977. Celo Press,
      Burnsville.NC. 15 pp. $ 1.00.PB.

Brief annotated bibliography of some books,pamphlets and
Government documents & articles,about various aspects of
funerals.Some out of print & not readily obtainable.Useful
more for drawing attention to out-of-the-way chapters &
neglected pieces,than as a guide to mainline literature.
***

87.   CONVERSATIONS WITH ADAM & NATASHA. R.D.Laing.
      Pantheon,New York. 1977. $ 6.95.

Quite simply,conversation between Ronnie & his two
children,about life & death.The children make the wiser
contributions,& express some interesting opinions on death.
***

88.   COPING : A SURVIVAL MANUAL FOR WOMEN ALONE. Martha
      Yates. Spectrum/Prentice-Hall,NJ. 1976. 272 pp.
      $ 4.95 PB ($ 5.75 in Canada).

For "Single,widowed & divorced women"--problems of
aloneness,children,credit,loss,insurance,income tax,etc.,&
how to cope. Section on coping with widowhood & preparing
for it.
**

89.   COPING WITH BREAST CANCER.A Personal History &
      Investigative Report.Rose Kushner.Harcourt,Brace,
      Jovanovich,New York.1975. 448 pp. $ 10.00.

A patient & medical journalist discusses the present state
of mastectomy,its indications,variations and effects.
***

90. COPING WITH PHYSICAL ILLNESS.Ed.R.H.Moos. Plenum Medical
     Book Company,New York. 1977. 440 pp.

An effective collection of reprinted articles,mainly from
the literature of the 70's,dealing with aspects of coping
with serious physical illness.So there are chapters on
chronic grief,stillbirth & birth defects,cancer,infarct,
stroke,burns,hospital environments,transplants,staff
stresses,& terminal care. The quality of the articles
varies greatly,from the practical to the anecdotal,but they
are generally articulate,readily understandable,& useful.
***

91. THE COST OF AGE. Andrew Allentuck.Fitzhenry & Whiteside,
     Toronto,1977. $ 5.95 PB.

A practical guide to the problems,especially financial,of
the elderly in Canada.Chapter 11,Rights of Passage,deals
succinctly & reasonably with death; funerals,burial,memorial
societies;informative & accurate though brief.Other useful
chapters deal with the costs of health care in later life;
Nursing Homes & how to choose them;the problems of returement
homes;food,living expenses;debt & credit;investments;
pensions;& testaments,legacies,insurance & wills. Adequate
journalism,never profound,& often uneasily slick in its
subtitles.But helpful for the elderly in Canada,the
seriously ill,bereaved & incipient bereaved.
***

92. THE COST OF DYING AND WHAT YOU CAN DO ABOUT IT.Raymond
     Paavo Arvio. Harper & Row,New York.1974.159pp.$ 6.95.

Soundly practical book by an experienced consumer activist,
proposing alternatives to the regular expensive funeral
practices.Particularly detailed guidance on how to form &
run a memorial society,& on alternative forms of memorial
service. Neatly produced.
***

93. THE COST OF LIVING LIKE THIS.James Kennaway.Penguin
     Books,Harmondsworth.1972. 170 pp. 35 pence.

'All fatal illnesses are only marginal examples of an ageing
process common to all of us'.A novel about the final weeks
of life of a 38-year-old economist who knows he is dying of
cancer,& his selfish relations with wife & lover.Vivid ,
insightful,compassionate,mercifully unsaccharine; the
novelist was himself killed in a car accident before its
publication.
***

94. COUNSELING OLDER PERSONS : CAREERS,RETIREMENT,DYING.
     Daniel Sinick.(Vol.4.New Vistas in Counseling series).
     Human Sciences Press,New York. 1977. 112 pp. $ 6.95.

Very brief,terse,simplified,outline of couseling older
people with regard to careers,retirement,& death/suicide.
Regrettably spare,but generally sensible;tempers its
presentation of the Kubler-Ross 5,e.g.,with some recognition
of the far greater complexities involved.Appendices list
references on older women,relevant periodicals,& addresses
of organizations concerned with the elderly.Reasonable list
of references.Respectable sentiments,simply expressed,but
very tame,& sadly lacking the fire of a Maggie Kuhn.
**

95. COUNSELING THE DYING.Margaretta Bowers,E.Jackson,J.
     Knight,L.LeShan. Aronson,New York.1975.$ 10.00
     (Nelson,New York, 1964).

Articles by four counselors,each with different approaches
to the problems & techniques of counseling.
**

96. THE COURAGE TO FAIL.A Social View of Organ Transplants
     & Dialysis. Renee C.Fox & Judith P.Swazey. The
     University of Chicago Press,Chicago.1974.395pp.$17.95.

More like excellent journalism than great sociology;a highly
readable & detailed study of aspects of the transplant/
/dialysis situation,including concepts of 'gift-exchange',
& gate-keeping,the experiment/therapy dilemma,patient
selection,the right to'give life' & the right to die,& such
case studies as the development of the artificial heart &
the story of Ernie Crowfeather.Ethical,social,& metaphysical
problems are covered.
****

97. CREMATION.P.E.Irion.Fortress,Philadelphia.1968.$4.00

Explores the history of cremation-its practice,costs &
regulatory controls,with annotated bibliography.
***

98.   THE CRY FOR HELP. ed.N.L.Farberow & E.S.Shneidman.
      McGraw-Hill,New York. 1965. 348 pp. $ 3.45 PB.

A superb & still relevant classic work.Part I-The Community
Response to the cry for help,discusses suicide prevention
centers,research,assessment of risk,studies of death
certification,& equivocal deaths,with a taxonomy of death.
Part II-The Psychotherapeutic Response.Farberow presents
a case which is then discussed from the psycho-analytic
(Hendin),Jungian,Adlerian,Sullivanian,Horney,Personal
Construct(Kelly),& Non-Directive points of view. Part III
is an 1897-1957 Bibliography.
****

D

99.   THE DANCE OF DEATH IN SPAIN AND CATALONIA. Florence
      Whyte. Arno Press,NY.1976.178 pp.$ 14.00.(1st edn.1931)

A study of the meaning of death in 'national character' &
the link between Spanish culture & idiosyncratic & extreme
attitudes to death;the relationship between a person's
social position & his feelings about death;the Dance of
Death and the memento mori traditions.
***

100.   DEALING WITH CRISIS :A Guide to Critical Life
       Problems. Lawrence Calhoun,James Selby & Elizabeth
       King. Prentice-Hall/Spectrum. 1976. $ 4.95.

"A handbook for coping with life's major problems,from
adolescence,sexual dysfunction,abortion & divorce to aging,
illness,retirement & death".A useful attempt to make
relevant information,derived mainly from psychological
research rather than clinical experience,available and
intelligible to the layman;with references to lay and
technical literature.The provision of"Projects & Questions-
(Chastity in adolescents today is its own punishment.Discuss)
makes it sound more like a weak textbook than a self-help
book for adults,& is unnecessary.The discussions of Dying
& Grieving,& Suicide are far more theoretical than practical,
& rather narrow.The emphasis is more on seeking professional
help than on creative dealing with one's own problems.
**

101.   DEALING WITH DEATH.Ed.R.H.Davis & M.Neiswender. Ethel
       Percy Andrus Gerontology Center,University of
       Southern California. 1973. 71 pp. PB $ 2.50.

One of the most interesting slim monographs available,
reprinting short papers presented by distinguished
visiting speakers at the Center.It includes Herman Feifel
on the meaning of dying in American Society;an excellent
essay on psychological treatment of the dying patient by
C.W.Wahl;Ed Shneidman on suicide in the aged;Jeanne Quint
Benoliel on the practitioners' dilemma,problems &
priorities;& Eugenia Waechter on nursing the dying patient.
Brief & thoughtful,an effective appertizer.
***

102.   DEALING WITH DEATH AND DYING.Nursing Skillbook.
       Nursing 77 Books,Intermed Communications,Jenkintown
       (In Britain: Ravenswood Publ.,Beckenham). 192 pp.
       $ 8.95 £ 7.40

We need good books to help nurses deal with the dying;this
one is good in parts.The first section'Dealing with the
Patient' accepts too readily & rigidly the Staging models
(Ruth Gray presents the Kubler-Ross 5 & the Engel 3
simultaneously,in a most muddling fashion.She omitted the
Chicago 7) and is quite directive & prescriptive in
approach.The multiple authors allow more repetition &
omission that one would prefer..The 2nd section,'Dealing
with the Family' discusses family support & bereavement.
Section 3,'Dealing with Yourself & the Staff' helpfully
describes the problems of the caregivers & their needs for
comfort & support.A final section contains four excellent
interviews with patients,a questionnaire seeking opinions
on aspects of death,& the results of over 15,000 responses
from nurses to that questionnaire.There are 3 'Skillchecks'
which pose relevant clinical problems & suggest possible
responses.There's an absence of references or bibliography,
which is a most unfortunate & unnecessary omission.
***

103. Death. Mog Ball. Oxford University Press/Chameleon/
      Ikon. (Standpoints series) 1976.64pp.PB. 60 pence.

The best illustrated resource book for use in teaching
about death with school children & older groups.Profusely
and brilliantly illustrated,broad & irreverent,with an
idiosyncratic & not especially useful text,almost
rendered unnecessary by the pictures.It could hardly fail
to stimulate cogent discussion.
****

104. Death. Maurice Maeterlinck.Arno Press,New York.
      1976. (1st published NY 1912) 106 pp. $ 12.00

Highly controversial when first published in France in
1911,immediately placed on the Index of Forbidden Books by
the religious establishment,& only much later removed.
Discusses the possibilities of annihilation,survival with
individual consciousness,'survival'without consciousness,
and integration into a universal consciousness;and the
yearning of our ego for continuance.Anticipates many later
developments.
***

105. Death. Samuel Eyres Pierce.Sovereign Grace Publishers,
      Grand Rapids,MI. 1971. 46 pp. PB $ 1.00.

A slim,pious,fundamentalist scriptural Christian tract.
*

106. DEATH. Alan Watts. Celestial Arts,California. 1975
      63 pp. $ 3.95.

One of"The Essence of Alan Watts"series.A slim,illustrated
volume;a refreshingly simple expression of Watts' basic,
cheerful philosophy,which deals with a means of acceptance
of death.Avoids the breathy prosiness into which other
attempts at handling this subject tend to sink.
****

107. DEATH,AFTERLIFE AND ESCHATOLOGY.A Thematic Source Book
      of the History of Religions.Mircea Eliade. Harper &
      Row,New York. 1967/1974. 109 pp. PB $ 1.95.

A uniquely broad-ranging collection of original materials
on divergent religions,historical approaches to death--Aztec,
Egyptian,Buddhist,Tibetan,Ishtar & Gilgamesh,Upanishads,
Greece & Rome,Orpheus myths,end of the world & messianic
prophecies.Sioux,New Hebridean,Polynesian,Siberian,Bolivian
& Winnebago rites.
***½

108. DEATH AND ATTITUDES TOWARD DEATH.Symposium Proceedings.
      ed.S.B.Day.Bell Museum of Pathology,University of
      Minnesota Medical School,Minnesota.1972.94pp.$1.00.PB.

Far too precise a transcript of three colloquia looking at
attitudes to death among patients,children,physicians,
relatives,hospital personnal,& a discussion on Death & the
Black.Some original & much unoriginal thought.Rambling,&
bearing no sign of editing.Every inconsequential remark
faithfully recorded,to the detriment of the consequential.
**

109. DEATH AND BEREAVEMENT. Austin H.Kutscher et.al.
      C.C.Thomas,Springfield,IL.1969.392 pp. $ 12.50.

Emphasis on the need for the bereaved to work their way
through the'normal'process of grief,to an 'understanding'
of loss,and a new fruitful life.Somewhat naive,& containing
absolutely no new insights.
*

110. DEATH AND BEYOND IN THE EASTERN PERSPECTIVE.Jung
      Young Lee. An Interface Book;Gordon & Breach,New
      York. 1974. 100 pp. $ 12.50

An articulate attempt to interpret & explain the classical
Eastern view of the existential meaning of death,dying,
after-death states and reincarnation,based mainly on the
Bardo Thodol (Tibetan Book of the Dead) and the I Ching
(Book of Change). An illuminating yin-yang perspective of
life and death.Of more than specialist interest &
application: highly recommended.
****

111. DEATH AND DYING : ATTITUDES OF PATIENT AND DOCTOR.
      Group for the Advancement of Psychiatry,New York.
      Symposium No. 11. 1965/1972. 3rd printing. 78 pp.$2.00.

A useful gathering of five studies on attitudes to death,
including Herman Feifel's classic consideration of the
function of such attitudes.
***

112. DEATH AND DYING : CURRENT ISSUES IN THE TREATMENT OF
      THE DYING PERSON. Ed. L.Pearson. The Press of Case
      Western Reserve University,Cleveland.1969. 235 pp.
      $ 7.30. Paperback edition without Bibliography,$1.95.

Five interesting essays.Bob Kastenbaum on psychological
death;Larry LeShan's perennial'Psychotherapy and the Dying
Patient'again;Cicely Saunders' sound commonsense;Dick
Kalish on death and the family;& Anselm Strauss summarizes
his views on awareness of dying.In the hardcover edition,
a useful annotated selected bibliography.
****

113. DEATH AND DYING EDUCATION.Richard O.Ulin. National
      Education Association,Washington D.C. 1977. 72 pp.
      $ 7.25 ; PB $ 4.00.

An honest attempt at producing a guidebook to Death'nDying
Education,that almost succeeds.Ulin considers the why,where
& what of death education in schools (the world beyond the
school is ignored),& there are also chapters on Aging in
America(not at all relevant,as presented here),cross-
-cultural perspectives,literature & death awareness;the
teacher:preparation & qualifications; a description of a
high-school course he taught;and a very short un-annotated
bibliography of books & films. As with Stanford & Perry,
Ulin's superficial understanding of the subject shows
through;authors like Kubler-Ross are misleadingly
misquoted,& there's an over-reliance on a few sources.Like
Stanford,the best of a drab bunch of first generation
books on Death Ed. : oh,how we long for the second
generation!
***$\frac{1}{2}$

114. DEATH AND EASTERN THOUGHT.Understanding Death in
      Eastern Religions & Philosophies. ed.F.H.Holck.
      Abingdon Press,Nashville. 1974.256 pp.$ 12.95,$4.95 PB.

Seldom stylish,but one of the most thorough studies of
Eastern perspectives on Death.There's a particular
emphasis on the Indian literature,from the Vedas through
the sutras and Puranas to more recent orthodox & heterodox
philosophies;Tagore,Gandhi & Radhakrishnan.There's a study
of Buddha's opinions,of the classical Chinese tradition
(chiefly Confucius) and of Japanese views,from Dogen
to Mishima. Fascinating.
***$\frac{1}{2}$

115.   DEATH AND ETHNICITY:A Psychocultural Study. Richard
       A Kalish & David K.Reynolds. University of Southern
       California Press (Ethel Percy Andrus Gerontology
       Center) 1976. 224 pp. $ 7.50 PB.

At long last an author who admits that death is not a taboo
topic! Probably the most thorough and carefully designed
study of attitudes to death in contemporary Americans,
comparing Black,Japanese,Mexican & Anglo-Americans.Based
mainly on a community interview survey,it is valuable not
only for the data it assembles (well-interpreted without
over-generalizing) but for its discussion of the problems
and realities of planning and carrying out such a project.
Well written up,with the critical attitude and wit one
would expect from the senior author.
****

116.   DEATH AND IDENTITY. Revised Edition. Ed.Robert Fulton.
       Charles Press,Bowie,MD.1976. 448 pp. £ 12.75.
       (original edition,Wiley & Sons,New York, 1965)

The original edition has been out of print for too long,so
the availability of a new edition is very welcome.It does
not contain the same material as the first edition,nor
completely new material,which is a little confusing.With
helpful introductions by the editor.New pieces include
Sudnow's Dead on Arrival;Lifton on the Sense of Immortality;
Blauner's Death & Social Structure;Templer on the Death
Anxiety Scale;the Fulton's on Anticipatory Grief,Van Pine
on the Cost of Dying,Bernardo on Widowhood Status,and Lidz
& others on the Gift of Life & medical ethics.Of the earlier
material retained in this edition,there is Lifton on
Hiroshima,Lindemann,Glaser & Strauss on Awareness Contexts,
and Weisman & Hackett's Predilection to Death.Without
reservation,one of the most competent and valuable
collections of key articles so far available.
****½

117.   DEATH AND ITS MYSTERIES.Ignace Lepp. Macmillan,New
       York, 1969. 191 pp. PB $ 1.95.

Lepp was a French psychotherapist and priest.A windy,
unexciting,dull work.
**

118. DEATH AND MODERN MAN. J.Choron. Collier,NY.1964.
      228 pp. PB. $ 2.95.

What is the purpose and meaning of life if death is total
annihilation? An excellent multidisciplinary study on the
problems of immortality,fear of death,and the meaning of
death.
****

119. DEATH AND NEUROSIS. J.E.Meyer. International
      Universities Press,New York.1975 (originally :
      Vandenhoeck & Ruprecht,Gottingen,1973).147pp.$ 8.50

A distinguished German psychiatrist's review of the
relationship between death anxiety & neurosis.The subject
has been neglected in psychoanalysis;Meyer proposes that
death anxiety is the root of neurotic behavior;& that
separation anxiety,guilt,& castration anxiety are only
transformations of repressed death anxiety.He doesnt quite
succeed in making his case.Awkward translation.This tastes
like the introduction to a much more weighty book yet to
come-but doesn't manage to make us look forward to it.Poor
use of data to support his hypotheses,relying on
generalizations and case histories,choosing a very biased
sample.Assumes a familiarity with German analytical
literature that must be rare.Brief but not always relevant
or adequate excursions into Christianity,existentialism,
and dialectitcal materialism.Many very obvious questions
of practical relevance are ignored.Unusuable with students.
**

120. DEATH AND SENSUALITY: A Study of Eroticism & the
      Taboo. Georges Bataille. Arno Press,NY.1976.
      280 pp. $ 19.00 (1st edition,1962)
      Not available in the British Commonwealth.

Writer,critic & irrational philosopher of the Surrealist
movement,leader of the Macabre group within Surrealism,
writes of the contrasts,contradictions & links between
sensuality & death,including sex & death taboos,sacrifice,
murder & war,& the inherent limits of communication.
Illustrated with a selection from art history.
***

121.   DEATH AND TAXES. Richard E Wagner. American Enterprize
       Press,California. 1973. PB $ 2.50.

Some comments on death,taxes,inheritance,inequality &
progressive taxation.
*

122.   DEATH AND THE COLLEGE STUDENT.Ed. E.S.Shneidman.
       Behavioral Publications,New York.1972. 207 pp.
       $ 9.95 , PB $ 4.95.

A collection of essays by Harvard students on death and
suicide.Includes;combat death,ghetto death,hope & suicide
in the concentration camp,the wake,the James Dean cult,
personal reflections on suicide attempts,death in Sartre,
Unamuno,Elvira Madigan,the Tibetan Book of the Dead,
Hemingway & Agee. Sometimes pretentious.
***

123.   DEATH AND THE DEVIL.Adolf Holl.Seabury Press,New
       York. 1976. 234 pp. $ 9.95.

Eschatology:beliefs on life and death,as well as his own
ecclesiastical life-story.Wierd,meandering,sometimes
surreal,sometimes artificially folksy. Rum.
**

124.   DEATH AND THE FAMILY: The Importance of Mourning.
       Lily Pincus. Pantheon Books,New York.1974 278 pp.
       $ 8.95. Vintage PB,1976,$ 2.95. Faber,London,£4.50.

Written by a social worker with great experience in marital
& family therapy; a brilliant book,sensitive & well-written,
always readable,wise & human.A genuine,fresh & substantial
contribution to the understanding & therapy of bereavement
& the dying family.Highly recommended.
*****

125.   DEATH & THE VISUAL ARTS.Original anthology,Ed.R.
       Kastenbaum,G.Geddes,G.Gruman & M.A.Simpson. Arno Press,
       New York. 1976. 226 pp. $ 17.00 .

Including:The Dance of Death in the Middle Ages & the
Renaissance,JamesM.Clark (1950)exploring the death motif in
art in two epochs-& How the Ancients Represented Death,by
G.E.Lessing,a work which influenced Goethe,describing the
ancient portrayal of death as the brother of sleep,with
peaceful images.
***

126.   DEATH AND WESTERN THOUGHT.J.Choron.Collier,N.Y.
       1963. 320 pp. $ 7.50.   PB $ 2.95.

Classic survey of what the great Western philosophers
thought about death,from pre-Socratic to present day
views. Readable & highly competent.
****

127.   DEATH : AN INTERDISCIPLINARY ANALYSIS. Warren
       Shibles. The Language Press,Whitewater,Wisconsin.
       1974. 558 pp. $ 10.00   PB $ 8.00.

A tour de force that almost makes it,but frustrates where
it does not.Good in parts,annoying prejudiced & limited in
others.Often errs by putting forward personal opinions as
established facts.This is risky,as the author vigorously
over-extends himself into many areas,sometimes beyond his
expertise,sometimes plain wrong.Occasionally challenging,&
even fun. Tends to be incestuous,with inappropriate
dragging in of citations of the author's other works,even
when wholly irrelevant.Interdisciplinary,maybe;but
undisciplined & often very self-indulgent.Sometimes out-of-
-date or ill-informed,often immodest.Often biased by the
author's mildly eccentric philosophical viewpoint,& his
tendency to erupt into squabbles with Sartre or Heidegger.
But it's hard to resent such an over-ambitious,and
grandiloquent attempt,even if its only intermittently
successful.Scampers breathlessly from Lucretuis to
Wittgenstein,Dylan Thomas to Mark Twain,psychic phenomena
to an unashamedly biased book review of Mitford or Kubler-
-Ross,voodoo death to tomb sculpture,the life-span of the
earthworm & the sea-horse to a synopsis of theology.
Unselective,uncritical bibliography. A book to buy &
quarrel with.
***

128.   DEATH ANXIETY: Normal & Pathological Aspects.
       MSS Information Corporation,N.Y.1974.200pp.$17.00.

Odd collection of some very unmemorable papers,many not on
the topic indicated by the title:includes attitudes to aging,
ethical problems in geriatrics,depression in the elderly,
psychiatric views of the life-cycle,etc.One can't imagine
why such a peculiar collection of subjects should be
assembled & printed.Some papers are actually about death
anxiety,but I'm not sure if that's intentional.
*

129.   DEATH:A PART OF LIFE.George G.Otero.Center for
       Teaching International Relations,Denver. 35pp.$4.00.

An experimental teaching unit for use with school-children,
with some materials & exercises to explore fears of death,
funeral notices,death customs (with a cross-cultural
perspective) graveyards,letters of kamikaze pilots,&
eulogies. Reasonably thoughtful & imaginative,& mercifully
lacking the excesses of some other course material.
***

130.   DEATH AS A FACT OF LIFE. D.Hendin. W.W.Norton, N.Y.
       1973. 255 pp. $ 9.95. Warner Books,NY.PB $ 1.95.

Slick,chatty,verbose,very tabloid journalist account of
many aspects of the subject,including criteria of death,
euthanasia,& cryonics(given far more prominence than it
deserves).Compiled from many sources,not always
authorized;often bitty & superficial.
**

131.   DEATH AS AN ENEMY ACCORDING TO ANCIENT EGYPTIAN
       CONCEPTIONS. Jan Zandee. Arno Press,NY.1976
       (1st published 1960) 448 pp. $ 23.00.

Scholarly work on Egyptian attitudes to death,with relevant
material from comparative mythology,symbolism,& psycho-
-linguistics;combined to offer further understanding of
the relationship with death.
*

132.   DEATH AS A SPECULATIVE THEME IN RELIGIOUS,SCIENTIFIC,
       AND SOCIAL THOUGHT. Ed.R Kastenbaum,G.Geddes,G.Gruman,
       & M.A.Simpson. Arno Press,New York.1976. 230pp.$ 19.00.

Includes:George Henry's The Current Theory of Human Progress;
The Central Truth & The Problem of Individual Life(1929);W.W.
Winwood's The Future of the Human Race & the Religion of
Reason & Love(1908);Nicholas Fyodorov's The Question of
Brotherhood;Berdyaev's The Eschatological & Prophetic
Character of Russian Thought(1948) & Death & Immortality
(1937);& Joseph Needham's Science,Religion & Socialism
(1943).Economic,political & social aspects of death,as well
as philosophical,religious & scientific points of view.
***

133. DEATHBED OBSERVATIONS BY PHYSICIANS AND NURSES.
      Karlis Osis. Parapsychology Foundation,New York.
      1961. 114 pp. PB $ 1.75.

Study of the phenomenology of death,based on a questionnaire
survey of 10,000 doctors & nurses,640 of whom responded
(is this a record?).Analyzes their reports of the visions
and hallucinations of the dying,claiming that they
commonly hallucinate,seeing dead persons known to them,
who claim to be there to help them accomplish the transition.
Intriguing findings,with reasonable methodology,though
without essential parapsychological significance.
***

134. DEATH BE NOT PROUD.John Gunther. Harper & Row,1971.
      $ 8.95, Perennial PB 0.95¢.

A father's account of his 17 year-old son's death from a
brain tumour.The first and one of the best of what later
threatened to become a sickly genre.
****

135. DEATH BY CHOICE. Daniel C.Maguire.Doubleday,N.Y. 1973,
      $ 7.95 , Schocken Books,N.Y. 1975 224 pp. PB $ 2.95.

Reasonably thorough review of arguments for and against
euthanasia,mainly in terms of current American experiences.
Heavily studded with citations from secondary rather than
primary sources,and with a few factual errors,from the first
paragraph on. Generally competent,however,without becoming
too repetitious;business-like though rarely moving. Very
regrettably,no index.
***

136. DEATH BY DECISION: The Medical,Moral & Legal Dilemmas
      of Euthanasia. J.B.Wilson. Westminster Press,
      Philadelphia. 1975. 208 pp. $ 7.50.

An efficient and straightforward survey of the medical,
moral and legal aspects of euthanasia,that traces the
development of the problem up to contemporary issues and
examples,and explores the theological and legal arguments,
as well as outlining some guidelines for medical & legal
practice.
***

137.   DEATH COMES HOME.Simon Stephens. Morehouse-Barlow,
       New York. 1973. (A.R.Mowbray,England) 110pp. $ 2.50.

An account by a chaplain,of the sudden death of a child and
its effects on a young family,which develops into an
interdisciplinary consideration of how the various
professionals & friends deal with the bereaved.A reasonable
account of grief & its problems,though less explicit than
it could have been,about how to help,apart from promoting
the services of the Society of Compassionate Friends.
***

138.   DEATH: CURRENT PERSPECTIVES.Ed.E.S.Shneidman.
       Mayfield Publishing Co.,Palo Alto.1976. 547 pp
       $ 12.50, $ 8.95 PB.

A bright and highly personal selection of extracts from
published works on death,selected and arranged with great
skill.A potentially valuable college text.Though some
sources are over-worked,those most highly recommended in
this Bibliography are well represented: Toynbee,Gorer,Aries,
Gil Elliot,Sudnow,Glaser & Strauss,Shneidman,Kubler-Ross,
Hinton,Kastenbaum,Feifel,Saunders and Weisman. A great
smorgasbord.
*****

139.   DEATH CUSTOMS: An Analytical Study of Burial Rites.
       E.Bendann. Gale Research Company,Detroit. 1974. 314 pp.
       $ 12.50. (Originally,Knopf,NY,1930).

Valuable reprint of an early anthropological classic.
Thoroughly documented comparative study of burial rites
especially in Melanesia,Australia,Northeast Siberia &
India. In Part I the similarities in rites and underlying
ideas,are considered-in Part II,the differences are
analysed.A unique work,of substantial theoretical interest.
***½

140.   DEATH,DISEASE & FAMINE IN PRE-INDUSTRIAL ENGLAND.Leslie
       Clarkson. Gill & Macmillan,Dublin.1975.188 pp.£ 8.75.

A curious attempt to write popular & entertaining historical
demography.Looks at the effects of the high & fluctuating
mortality before 1800,on English society;at plague,famine,
early medicine,violent deaths,& burial customs.In 1666 a
law required the use of woollen shrouds,to aid the ailing
woollen cloth industry;so many of Queen Anne's relations

140 ctd) died,keeping the Court in black & crepe mourning
clothes,that black ribbons were at a premium.It's full of
interesting snippets--almost too full:it's a rich source of
anecdotes relating to death in an era that deserves full
study;but it lacks an overall sense of organization or a
general concept of its subject matter.Insubstantial.
**

141. DEATH,DYING AND EUTHANASIA.D.J.Horan & D.Mall.
      University Publications of America,Washington DC.1977.

Undistinguished.Looks at death via several disciplines,such
as law,medicine,philosophy,religion & ethics.Ho-hum....
**

142. DEATH,DYING AND THE BIOLOGICAL REVOLUTION: Our Last
      Quest for Responsibility. Robert M.Veatch. Yale
      University Press,New Haven & London. 1976. 323 pp.

A very readable,rational,discursive discussion of the
ethical and legal aspects of death and dying,proposing
possibilities for formulating a public policy with regard
to the prolongation and termination of life.Theoretical
ethics more than practical clinical realities,but a good
basis for discussion none-the-less.Veatch considers the
morality of death,formal definitions of death,& new options
following the acceptance of Cerebral Death.He distinguishes
such themes as killing versus allowing to die;reasonable
versus unreasonable treatments;allowing to live versus
allowing to die;and discusses the right to refuse treatment
in competent & incompetent adults & in children.There is an
unusually detailed discussion of the patient's right and
obligation to have the truth,& cases are outlined for and
against truth-telling.The closing chapters consider the
newly dead & the use of body organs-& the relation between
natural death & public policy,including the case for death
and against immortality.A useful bibliography of articles
on the ethical aspects of each subject (not even limited,
as Hastings Centre books tend to be,to the Centre's own
publications,an agreeably non-elitist departure.).
****

143.   DEATH EDUCATION : Preparation for Living. B.R.Green
       and D.P.Irish. Schenkman Publishing,Cambridge,Mass.
       1971. 143 pp. $ 3.95 , PB $ 1.95.

Proceedings of a symposium,including essays by Feifel,
Brautner,Dan Leviton (who comes nearest to dealing with
the ostensible subject) & Irish. Brief & unhelpful
summaries of working party discussions,& a vague
bibliography. Has little to do with Death Education.
**

144.   DEATH : EVERYBODY'S HERITAGE. E.Landau. Simon &
       Schuster/Messner,New York.1976.$ 5.95.

An oversimplified general account of death,barely
suitable for high-school children & not suitable for
anyone else. Not recommended.
**

145.   DEATH,GRIEF & BEREAVEMENT : A BIBLIOGRAPHY 1845-1975.
       Compiled by Robert Fulton with others. Arno Press,
       New York. 1976. 253 pp. $ 20.00.

The most comprehensive & reliable bibliography of the
literature on death,grief & bereavement in print.Some
4,000 entries,mainly journal articles,indexed by subject,
with nearly 80 classifications.
*****

146.   DEATH,GRIEF AND MOURNING.Geoffrey Gorer. Arno Press,
       New York. 1976. 205 pp. $ 16.00. (1st publ.NY.1965).
       Not available in the British Commonwealth.

A much-quoted study of the human response to death,with a
survey of the bereaved in Britain,based on a highly
detailed questionnaire study,also reviewing theories of
grief and styles of mourning.Includes Gorer's famous
essay: "The Pornography of Death".
****

147.   DEATH--HERE IS THY STING. Coriolis. McClelland &
       Stewart,Toronto,1967. 150 pp. PB $ 2.50.
       (Available from the Memorial Society Association of
       Canada,Publications Dept.,14 Sinton Court,Downsview,
       Ontario, for $ 1.00).

A Canadian,sub-Mitford,expose of the Funeral Industry,by a
disillusioned funeral director.
***

148.   DEATH IN AMERICA.Ed. D.E.Stannard. University of
       Pennsylvania Press,Philadelphia,1975.159 pp.$ 3.95 PB.

Genuinely contributes something new to our understanding of
death and how it has been treated in American culture.
Scholarly but consistently interesting,the contributors
explore the situation before Gracious Dying became the
routine continuance of Gracious Living.Jack Goody gives a
brief overview of the need to consider death in the
interpretation of a culture.Stannard describes attitudes to
childhood and death in Puritan New England,in a setting of
internally contradictory theological pessimism and terror.
Lewis Saum,from a study of State & local archives,reports
on the popular attitudes to death or pre-Civil War America,
illustrating the precedents of the Great Denial;as does
Ann Douglas' review of schoolbook poetry and popular
consolation literature with its expositions of the
desirability of death,in the Northern States (1830-1880).
Stanley French reviews the cemetary as a cultiral
institution,focussing on the establishment of Mount Auburn
and the "rural cemetary" movement.Patricia Kelly describes
death in Mexican folk culture,its openness and lack of
romanticization.Mary Ann Meyers reviews death in Mormon
thought and practice;and finally there's a translation of
Ariès fine essay "La Mort Inversee" . A valuable,stimulating,
original work,recommended to any serious student.
***$\frac{1}{2}$

149.   DEATH IN AMERICAN EXPERIENCE.Ed. A.Mack. Schocken
       Books,New York. 1973. 201 pp.$ 7.50,PB $ 3.25.

A book of essays on death in modern American culture,from
social,clinical & religious points of view;attitudes to
aging,and death in American poetry. Often unnecessarily
obscure and turgid writing.
***

150.   DEATH IN EARLY AMERICA. Margaret M.Coffin. Thomas
       Nelson,New York. 1976. 252 pp. $ 7.95.

A consistently entertaining study of 'The History and
Folklore of Customs and Superstitions of Early Medicine,
Funerals,Burials,and Mourning",dealing with funeral
customs,coffins & hearses,gravestones & epitaphs,body
snatching,mourning customs,memorials,warnings of imminent
death,cures & remedies. A most valuable collection of
historical material,well illustrated,broad,often amusing
and cheerfully robust,as typified by the Index,from :
"umbrella,warning of dropping",through "Hair,mourning
jewelry",& "cool pantry,use of",to "cakes,dead".
***

151.   DEATH IN MURELAGA. Wiliam A Douglass. University of
       Washington Press, Seattle. 1969.

Death among a Basque community in Northern Spain.What is
known as putting all of one's Basques in one exit.
***

152.   DEATH INSIDE OUT.Ed. P.Steinfels & R.M.Veatch.
       Hastings Center Report. Harper Forum Books.
       Harper & Row,New York. Fitzhenry & Whiteside,
       Canada. 1975. 150 pp. PB $ 7.30

One of the more refreshing books on death.Elegant,clear-
-thinking,critical,thoughtful & stimulating.Principally
concerned with philosophical,ethical & historical issues
rather than practical & personal problems.One of the
comparatively fiew books of genuine intellectual interest
in the field.Includes Aries'Death Inside Out',again,and
Ivan Illich on The Political Uses of Natural Death;Eric
Cassell on Dying in a Technological Society;William May on
the metaphysical plight of the family (the great family
secret:God is dead);Robert Morison on Death:process or
event? Paul Ramsey on the indignity of "death with dignity";
David Smith on Letting Some Babies Die;and other works by
Leon Kass & Tristram Engelhardt.
*****

153.   DEATH : INTERPRETATIONS.Ed. H.M.Ruitenbeek. Delta,
       New York. 1969. 290 pp. PB $ 2.95.

A collection of classical papers on death & mourning,
including Eissler,Jones,Cappon,LeShan,Feifel & Klein;
collected by Ruitenbeek,that busy anthologist. Some
are very dull reading,but it does make some early studies
available again.
***

154.   A DEATH IN THE FAMILY. James Agee. Bantam,New York.
       PB $ 1.50.

Pulitzer Prize-winning novel dealing with the effects of
the sudden death of a young father on a close-knit family.
*****

155.   DEATH IN THE MIDDLE AGES: Mortality,Judgement,&
       Remembrance. T.S. Boase. McGraw-Hill,N.Y.1972.$3.95.PB.

The management of the death system of the middle ages,the
dance of death and burial customs. Not distinguished.
**

156.   DEATH IS ALL RIGHT.Glenn H. Asquith. Abingdon Press,
       Nashville. 1970. 64 pp. $ 2.50.

A thin tract of mini-sermons.Death is all right,because it
is:---an adjournment,the one common experience,a return to
our source,the other end of things,reparation,restoration,
the place of answers,the redemption of promises,the opened
storehouse,a focus,the reason for life preparation,and a
glas encounter with God. A simple presentation of the
positive aspects of death,from the point of view of a
Baptist minister.
**

157. DEATH IS A NOUN : A View of the End of Life.John
     Langone. Little,Brown & Co.,Boston.1972.228pp.$ 5.95.

Much less accomplished than the same author's more recent
work,but a reasonably clear,basic,more-or-less objective
look at death,euthanasia,abortion,capital punishment,murder,
suicide,& concepts of the afterlife.
***
Also a Dell (New York) Paperback,1975, 0.95¢.

158. DEATH: ITS CAUSES & PHENOMENA WITH SPECIAL REFERENCE
      TO IMMORTALITY.Hereward Carrington. Arno Press,New
      York,1976. (1st edn,NY,1921) 307 pp. $ 20.00.

An early classic of formal thanatology,published in the
wake of the First World War,dealing with the experiences
of dying;causes & signs of death;means of preserving or
disposing of the body;biomedical theories;sleep & trance;
death & aging;philosophical & theological views on death
& immortality;& aspects of psychical research.A detailed
early bibliography.
***

159. DEATH OF A MAN.Lael T.Wertenbaker. Beacon Press,
      Boston & Saunders,Toronto. 1974 (1st published NY
      Random House,1957). 190pp. $ 7.50,PB $ 2.95.

One of the first,& in several ways the best,of the books
about a death in the family.Written in part by Charles
Wertenbaker about his last 60 days after he discovered
he had cancer,& completed by his wife;& an account of their
search for a rational & ethical good death,which they
managed to acheive together.A minor classic of its type.
The new edition has an introduction by Charles Fletcher.
****

160. THE DEATH OF IVAN ILLYCH,etc. Leo Tolstoy. New
      American Library,New York. PB $ 1.25. & other
      editions.

Strongly recommended. Brilliant account of the death of a
bourgeois Russian judge,with probably more insight into
the psychology of death than any other major author.
*****

161. DEATH OUT OF THE CLOSET: A Curriculum Guide to Living
      with Dying. Gene Stanford & Deborah Perry. Learning
      Ventures / Bantam Books,New York. 1976. 214pp.$ 1.95.

A generally useful guide to death education in schools (the
authors seem unaware of all that has been happening in
colleges,universities & medical schools).Contains a good
deal of usable advice & suggestions of useable material,
though the authors' judgement is not always impeccable.They
recommend Hendin's very flawed book as the best single
reference for background reading,& Vernick's very imperfect
bibliography;which reveals their great lack of experience &
very limited knowledge of the available literature.There are

161 ctd) handy suggestions for using paperbacks in teaching
(though mainly limited to fellow Bantam stable-mates)with
study & discussion questions on such works as Lynn Caine's
Widow,Agee,Plath,Lewis,Scoppetone,Wolitzer,Levit,Rabin's
Emergency Room Diary,Voltaire's Candide,Lifton & Olson, &
Dostoevsky. We would not all agree that "With no special
training,you can teach death as easily as you teach the
basics",& their insistence that absolutely any teacher can
safely & effectively "teach death".with minimal experience,
preparation or training. Their intentions are honorable;
their optimism isn't justified. We badly need more guides
to Death Education,which is stuck in the "Show & Tell"era,
and this,though far from excellent,is one of the best
available so far.
***$\frac{1}{2}$

162. DEATHS DUELL,OR A CONSOLATION TO THE SOULE AGAINST
      THE DYING LIFE and the Living Death of the Body.
      John Donne. Scloar Press,New York. $ 7.50,PB $ 4.95.

Facsimile edition of Donne's last major sermon in 1631.
***

163. DEATH,SOCIETY & HUMAN EXPERIENCE. Robert J.
      Kastenbaum. C.V.Mosby,St.Louis.(Henry Kimpton,London).
      1977. 328 pp. PB $ 7.95. £ 6.45.

Strongly reminiscent of the same author's Psychology of
Death,though in some ways more interesting,personal,unified,
& thought-provoking.Limited & inaccurate in its comments on
death education(especially in medical school) & on hospices.
Otherwise a literate sequence of essays & meditations on
aspects of death & suicide: on the relations between the
individual & the "death system".Rather like a fruit-cake,
crammed with bits & pieces of various textures & flavours,
some rather tough,some fruitful & nourishing.Likely to be
of interest to thanatologists & those with a theoretical
rather than a practical interest in the subjects;useful
in some contexts as a text for death courses,though it
would have to be supplemented with wider reading.
***

164.   DEATHS OF MAN.Edwin Shneidman. Quadrangle(NYT),New
        York. 1973. 240 pp. $ 8.95. Also Penguin PB.

Characteristically well-expressed study of death by a man
who has introduced many important concepts to the field,
such as the survivor-victims,& help by postvention;equivocal
& subintentioned death,etc. Eloquent & consistently
interesting.
****

165.   DEATH'S SINGLE PRIVACY: Grieving & Personal Growth.
        Joyce Phipps. A Continuum Book.Seabury Press,New
        York. 1974. 143 pp. $ 5.95.

A good example of the current genre of Widowbooks. An
unassuming,down-to-earth & useful account of the experiences
of a woman widowed in her early thirties.Detailed without
losing perspective,positive without losing modesty.
Recommended.
***

166.   DEATH : THE COPING MECHANISM OF THE HEALTH
        PROFESSIONAL. Bernice Catherine Harper. Southeastern
        University Press,Greenville,SC. 1977. 123 pp.

By,about,& mainly for,Social Workers,though some of its
comments will be generally applicable to other health
professionals.It is remarkable how little attention has
usually been paid to the difficulties of the professional
dealing with dying patients & families,& this book is an
important step towards reaching a better understanding of
those problems & the coping mechanisms (there is no
'coping mechanism',Ms Harper) that develop. Ms Harper offers
"A Schematic Comfort-Ability Growth & Development Scale in
Coping with Professional Anxieties on Death & Dying" (an
incredibly clumsy & ugly title!) A closely organized 5 stage
scale,Eriksonian in type,it is certainly interesting though
not adequate. The weaknesses of staging scales & models,
Eriksonian or Rossian,are insufficiently appreciated.But
this first model may encourage us to think more clearly
through this important topic,& develop better models.
***

167.   DEATH : THE FINAL STAGE OF GROWTH.Ed.Elizabeth
        Kubler-Ross. Spectrum/Prentice-Hall,NJ. 1975.
        175 pp. $ 2.95 PB, £ 5.20,£ 1.95 PB.Large-Type
        edition,248 pp. $ 4.95.

An able & personal book,dealing with death in the context
of personal growth.Includes discussions of dying among
Alaskan Indians,& Hindu & Buddhist attitudes. Not
properly referenced.
****

168.   DEATH: THE RIDDLE & THE MYSTERY.Eberhard Jungel.
        Westminster Press,Philadelphia.1975.141pp.$ 6.95;
        Also St.Andrews Press,Edinburgh.

A translation of "Tod" by a European Christian Theologian.
A generally efficient attempt to show how theology can
deal with medical & sociological findings with regard to
death.Especially examines Old Testament & New Testament
attitudes to death. Thoughtful & comprehensible.
**$\frac{1}{2}$

169.   A DEATH WITH DIGNITY.Lois Wheeler Snow. Random
        House,New York. 1974. $ 6.95.

Description of the careful & sensitive care by a Chinese
medical team of a controversial journalist during his
dying.
**

170.   THE DENIAL OF DEATH. Ernest Becker. The Free Press
        (Macmillan) New York.1973. 314 pp. $ 7.95,$ 2.95 PB
        Collier-Macmillan,London, 1976 £ 1.50.

Possibly the most badly-written Pulitzer Prize-winner,from
a literary & literate point of view.A grossly over-valued,
occasionally inaccurate book,that has little of any
practical use for anyone dealing with the dying.Pontificates
shakily on the nature of man,& proposes that his innate
fear of death is the principle source of his activity,
through his efforts to transcend it.Wanders into ill-
-informed comments on mental illness,& reviews the views of
Otto Rank at great length. When an author has the modesty
to die after writing a book on death,though,perhaps some
recognition is due.
**

171.   DEVILS,DEMONS,DEATH & DAMNATION.E.& I.Lerner
       (compilers). Dover Publ.,N.Y. 1971.190pp. $ 3.50.PB.

A collection of medieval & renaissance materials concerning
death,evil.& the afterlife.
**$\frac{1}{2}$

172.   DICTIONARY OF MEDICAL ETHICS.Ed. A.S.Duncan,G.R.
       Dunstan,R.B.Welbourn. Darton,Longman & Todd,U.K.
       1977.   336 pp. PB £ 4.90.

Medical ethics for school-kids."With 116 eminent
contributors" (and,assuredly,some of them are),this book'
aims to provide a definitive reference work on medical
ethics for professionals & lay readers.I hope no-one will
regard it as a definitive reference work.Most of the
contributions are tame,orderly,well-mannered,limited in
imagination,style & scope,bland,prosaic,& often avoid the
really controversial & significant issues.Full of wordy
generalities,but neglecting many major moral & ethical
concepts.Some contributors are well-informed & write well,
like Ronald MacKeith.Others are unfortunately limited in
the extent of their information or erudition.It is almost
entirely biased towards the U.K.,with little understanding
of American & European contributions.Death & Dying issues
are surprisingly limited.Colin Murray Parkes writes well
& succinctly on Bereavement,& Tom West writes sincerely on
Death Attitudes & on Terminal Care (though mainly in airy
generalities,& very hospice-oriented,though some good
terminal care occurs outside them).Euthanasia is only
briefly & superficially discussed by Twycross.Communication
is very inadequately dealt with;Consent is naive & weak;
Counselling & Fringe Medicine weak.Suicide is too Samaritan
biased & often trivial.Sexual topics,especially Homosexuality,
Lesbianism & "Sexual Deviance or Perversions" are appallingly
inadequate,old-fashioned & graceless.Some topics are of
very little ethical relevance.The contributions are too
unreal,too over-simplified,too idealized,too vague,& with
far too little practical guidance. Not a good buy.
Not quite as profound as the Readers' Digest.
*

173. A DICTIONARY OF MEDICAL ETHICS AND PRACTICE.William
      A.R.Thomson. John Wright & Sons,Bristol. 1977.
      264 pp. £ 10.00.

A bad book. It offers to provide doctors with "the guidance
and help which they did not obtain from their teachers"
(judging by this,they were lucky to miss it) and down-to-
-earth practical ethics.It is a moralistic & sometimes
stridently preaching text that rides a stable-full of
hobby-horses.He is anti-abortion,against AID & dubious
about AIH,pro-castration & corporal punishment.What is
totally unjustifiable is that the author's personal views
are presented as fact & as established opinion;special
pleading masquerades as objectivity.The text is heavy with
a mass of quotes,which are unascribed or very vague as to
source,or from very trivial sources.There is far too much
self-proclaimed wisdom.Other people can say that you are
wise,or humble,or virtuous,but you cannot claim these
qualities yourself without proving that you lack them.
His accounts of Bereavement,Moment of Death,Brain Death,
Suicide,& Euthanasia are limited,prosy,amateurish &
unpractical.His item on Care of the Dying is weak and
woolly and over-written.
*

174. THE DILEMMAS OF EUTHANASIA. Ed. J.A.Behnke & S.Bok.
      Anchor Press/Doubleday,New York. 1975.187pp.$2.95.PB.

Based on a series of articles which appeared in Bio Science
in 1973,with three additional chapters;provides a
reasonably efficient but rather lacklustre & dull study of
euthanasia,with a major emphasis on the legal aspects.
***

175. DISASTER: A Psychological Essay.Martha Wolfenstein.
      Arno Press,NY. 1976 (1st edn.1957) 231 pp. $ 17.00.

Possibly the best general study of the impact of disaster &
mass death,threat,impact & aftermath;the expectation of panic
& madness,denial of imminent threat;precautions &
propitiation;sharing danger;the illusion of centrality(I was
the Target);feelings of abandonment;the effects of near-miss;
egoism & altruism;tormenting memories & fears of recurrence.
Competent & interesting.
***½

176.   THE DISCOVERY OF DEATH IN CHILDHOOD & AFTER.Sylvia
       Anthony. Penguin Books,Harmondsworth & Baltimore.
       1973. 280 pp. $ 3.95.

A classic work;an observant & eclectic study of how children
learn and form the concept of death,& how they use this idea,
in a broad cultural perspective. Very readable.
****

177.   DISCUSSING DEATH: A Guide to Death Education. G.Mills,
       R.Reisler,A.Robinson,G.Vermilye. ETC Publications,
       Homewood,Ill. 1976. 140 pp. $ 8.50,PB $ 5.50.

A practical book for death educators,with suggestions for
classroom activities & resources,for students of 5-6,7-9,
10-12,and 13-18 (divided on an over-simplified
developmental concept).Undoubtedly useful though flawed.
Apart from many unfortunate errors in grammar & spelling,
& an over-reliance on unreliable,ephemeral & tertiary
sources (like Hendin's book),its only other major weakness
is a lack of appropriate attention to the difficulties &
casualties that can arise.The "objectives"it lists are not
learning objectives,but much less precise"aims".Some of the
books recommended are long out of print & unobtainable.
***½

178.   THE DISPOSAL OF THE DEAD.3rd Edition.C.J.Polson & T.
       K.Marshall. English Universities Press,London. 1975.
       412 pp. £ 7.50.

The standard British textbook on the subject,dealing with
the legal & practical requirements & techniques relating to
such matters as death certification,dissection,registration
of deaths,cremation,burial,exhumation & embalming,with a
brief account of funeral directing & a short historical
introduction.Authoritative work of reference,enlivened
by the citation of intriguing summaries of relevant
legal test-cases.
***

179.   DISSERTATION ON THE DISORDER OF DEATH : Or,That State
       of the Frame Under the Signs of Death Called
       Suspended Animation. Walter Whiter. Arno Press,N.Y.
       1976. 482 pp. (1st edn.1819) $ 29.00

Forerunner of today's'heroic measures' & 'Cryonics';Whiter
describes instances of resuscitation & considers that
society is failing to revive people through the belief that
death is irremediable.Why be so selective in rescue bids?
A pioneer of life-prolongation & the fears of premature
burial.
***

180.   DRY THOSE TEARS.Robert A.Russell. DeVorss & Co.,Santa
       Monica. 1975 (1st edn.1951) 132 pp. PB $ 2.50.

A highly pious little religious tract offering comfort to
the bereaved.Assures us of Eternal Life (which is achieved
by "A Change in Frequency Vibration" :Oh,so that's how
it's done). Some awful verse called poetry;& a smug tone
that can irritate.Relentlessly positive approach to
grief and "the happy dead".
*

181.   DYING. John Hinton. Pelican Books,Harmondsworth &
       Baltimore. 1967. 2nd edition 1972.220pp.$ 2.95;90 p.

Succinct & highly capable review of existing knowledge on
attitudes to death,what dying is like,terminal care &
mourning,based on a thorough review of the literature up to
the 1960's,& the author's own experience.Compact.
****

182.   DYING AND DEATH: A CLINICAL GUIDE FOR CAREGIVERS.
       Ed. David Barton. Williams & Wilkins,Baltimore.
       1977. 238 pp. $ 14.95, £ 9.90. PB.

A valuable outline of current ideas on clinical terminal
care.Part I,An Approach to Caring for Dying Persons is by
David Barton & a fair summary of recent views. Part II,
Perspectives,is by various authors & varies in quality.
Veatch on ethics,van Eys effective on the dying child,
Peak on the dying elderly person,& both Gattis & Cummings
on 'The Thoughts,Feelings & Reflections of a Person with a
Life-Threatening Illness'.Some loose & frothy chapters,too.
Rich in journal references.
****

183. DEATH AND DIGNITY: The Meaning & Control of a Personal
      Death. Melvin Krant. C.C.Thomas,Springfield,Illinois.
      1974. 154 pp. $ 5.95.

An intelligently & thoughtfully written series of essays
by a noted oncologist,exploring the concepts of
meaningful & slef-controlled dying,& the ways in which
the family,the community,& the hospital staff can
support that search for meaning.
***

184. THE DYING CHILD,THE FAMILY & THE HEALTH PROFESSIONALS.
      An Annotated Professional Bibliography. Ida Marie
      Martinson.(2303 Doswell,St Paul,MN 55108) 1976.
      26 pp. PB $ 2.50.

An annotated listing of some 80 items,mainly concerned with
the death of children,& management of the problems;almost
entirely confined to the American literature,& far from
comprehensive,it's a useful start to meeting an unmet
need in this area.
**

185. DYING IN AN INSTITUTION.Mary Castles. Appleton-
      Century-Crofts,New York. 1979 (in press at time of
      review).

A flawed book,with a redundant & not particularly relevant,
useful nor especially competent review of death;the nature
of institutions,strategies of care-giving,& the rights of
institutionalized dying patients.Its original content is a
section based on interviews with patients & nurses,
exploring their perceptions of themselves,their behaviour,
pain,etc.Over-ambitious,extending itself into too many
areas beyond the author's main expertise or relevance to
the main topic.Needed far more concentration on the
interview study.
**

186. THE DYING PATIENT. Ed.Brim,Freeman,Levine & Scotch.
      Russell Sage Foundation,New York.1970. $ 10.00.

Excellent collection of important studies by major writers
in the field.The best early anthology on the subject,from
a clinical point of view,and a much-quoted work.
****

187.   THE DYING PATIENT.Ed. Ronald W.Raven. Pitman Medical,
       U.K. 1975. 151 pp. PB. £ 3.00.

A mixed bag,with 14 contributors.Some chapters are detailed
& practical,including Lindy Burton on the seriously ill
child,& Michael Simpson on teaching about death & dying.
Ferguson Anderson & D.S.Robbie are soundly helpful on
dealing with pain & other symptom relief.Other contributors
offer the views of social worker,nurse,general practitioner,
and consider pastoral care.Some chapters are prosy and
sanctimonious,with nothing new to say. The index is
inadequate.
***½

188.   THE DYING PATIENT.R.G.Twycross. Christian Medical
       Fellowship,London.1975. 22 pp. PB 20 pence.

Brief pamphlet containing an article by Twycross dealing
shortly with attitudes,isolation,communicating the truth,
fear and pain,relatives,and tramwork.Too brief to do
justice to it's author's knowledge & experience.
**½

189.   THE DYING PATIENT:A NURSING PERSPECTIVE.Ed.M.H.
       Browning & E.P.Lewis.American Journal of Nursing Co.,
       1972.

A compilation of articles selected & reprinted from several
nursing journals.So-so,but nothing outstanding.
**

190.   THE DYING PATIENT: A SUPPORTIVE APPROACH. Ed Rita
       E.Caughill. Little,Brown & Co.,Boston. 1976. 228 pp.
       PB $ 6.95, £ 4.60.

The 7 authors provide a simple,unoriginal,but reasonably
capable account of current opinions on the psychology,
sociology,& elementary nursing,of the dying patient,with
some emphasis on the dying child.Caughill writes well on
coping with death in acute care units-& Green-Epner
emphasizes therapeutic play with dying childrem.Other
chapters,like Hopkins on Death with Dignity,& Elder on
Dying and Society,are more vapid & uninteresting.
**½

191.   THE DYNAMICS OF GRIEF : Its Source,Pain & Healing.
       David K.Switzer. Abingdon Press,Nashville. 1970.
       221 pp. $ 6.50.

An efficient review of the literature on grief & mourning,
principally from a theoretical & non-clinical point of
view.The earlier literature of psychology,psychoanalysis
& pastoral care is quite well covered,as in Anxiety & the
interpersonal nature of self (Freud,Allport,Sullivan);
Separation Anxiety (Klein,Deutsch,surprisingly not Bowlby)
& guilt;Existential Anxiety (not Existentialistic,please,
Dr Switzer!) Heidegger,Tillich,et al.are well reviewed.
The theoretical background to grief is competently
handled,but the final chapter on the healing of grief is
less thorough & helpful than one would have hoped.
***

E

192.   EFFECTS OF EARLY PARENT DEATH.MSS Information Corp.,
       New York. 1974. 176 pp. $ 17.00.

A scrappy collection of papers on the relationships between
early bereavement and adult mental illness.Some technical
papers on statistical correlations,some on children's
responses to bereavement;some of interest,some dull;few
greatly needing to be preserved in hard cover.One really
competent review article would have served most people's
needs much better.
*

193.   THE EGYPTIAN BOOK OF THE DEAD.E.A.Wallis Budge.
       Dover Publ.,N.Y. 1967. 337 pp. $ 4.95.

A splendid reprint of the 1895 edition,with clear colour
illustrations,of this major classic of the anthropology
of death.
***

194.   ELLEN: A SHORT LIFE LONG REMEMBERED. R.Levit.
       Bantam Books, New York. 1975. $ 1.95 PB.

Over-wrought account of a young death;important for the
folk involved directly,but not needing publication.
**

195. EMERGENCY AND DISASTER MANAGEMENT:A Mental Health
      Sourcebook. Ed.H.J.Parad,H.L.P.Resnik,& L.G.Parad.
      Charles Press,Bowie,MD. 1976. 497 pp. £ 20.80.

A unique resource.Part I deals with emergency mental health
services & the design of programs including the mobile
psychiatric emergency team,home treatment of the suicidal
person,the Continuing Relationship Maintenance Program,
Crisis Hostel,etc.;its authors including Klerman & Litman.
Part II deals with modes of Crisis Intervention,including
Farberow on group therapy for the suicidal.Part III deals
with Disaster Aid,with both general & specific studies
including Lifton on Buffalo Creek,& others dealing with
disaster by fire,flood,tornado & earthquake.The final
section deals with preventive programming for effective
crisis coping,including an account of a controlled study
of crisis intervention as primary prevention in acute
bereavement,& a useful & unusual bibliography of 470 items.
The authors include a wide range of health care personnel.
On the whole,the emphasis is on the organization &
implementation of programs of intervention,rather than on
clinical techniques.The book will be of undoubted value
to everyone involved in planning,organizing or implementing
emergency or disaster management programs.
***

196. EMERGENCY PSYCHIATRIC CARE:The Management of Mental
      Health Crises. Ed.H.L.P.Resnik & H.L.Ruben. Charles
      Press,Bowie,MD.1975.175 pp.PB.£ 7.95.

The most valuable practical guide to managing psychiatric
crises.Exceptionally well designed & clearly laid out.Its
chapters deal with general concepts & principles of crisis
intervention,emergencies relating to alcohol,drug abuse,
family crises & environmental disasters.Farberow & Litman
contribute an especially lucid section on suicide prevention,
& Kubler-Ross a helpful chapter on the crisis management of
dying persons & their families. Deserves wide use.
****

197. ENDING. Hilma Wolitzer.Macmillan,N.Y.1975. 232 pp.
      $ 6.95. Bantam,N.Y. 1977. $ 1.95 PB.

A young wife's experience of her husband's dying.Yes,yet
another account of that.
**

198. L'ENFANT ET LA MORT.(Des Enfants Malades Parlent De
      La Mort).G.Raimbault.Editions Privat,Toulouse. 1977
      223 pp. PB.

Ginette Raimbault,a Freudian analyst,has been working with
seriously ill children since 1965.This thoughtful and
sensitive book explores their experiences of death, and
contains many conversations & comments from the children.
The style is relatively lively.
***

199. ERIC.Doris Lund. J.B.Lippincott Co.,Philadelphia &
      McClelland & Stewart,Canada. 1974. 345 pp. $ 7.95.
      Dell PB. $ 2.25.

A mother's account of her 17 year-old son's death from
acute leukemia.Loving,honestly written story of a boy
who lived emphatically & creatively during his illness.
Moving and well-written. In the Paperback edition,don't
be put off by the obscene blurb:"Eric is a star in
Brian Piccolo's league" (sic) (sick,sick).
****

200. ESCAPE FROM PAIN.Paul W.Brand.Christian Medical
     Fellowship,London.1975.15 pp. PB. 15 pence.

A pamphlet dealing rather superficially with the puzzle
of pain.Pain is seen as "a gift from God".Poor work, on
a very important subject,deserving more thought.
**

201. ETHICAL DECISIONS IN MEDICINE.Howard Brodie. Little,
      Brown & Co.,Boston. 1976.340pp. $ 9.95, £ 6.70.

Probably the best available book on medical ethics.Soundly
organized with clearly stated objectives & self-evaluation
components.Proposes a concise method for dealing with
ethical problems,& provides many lucid examples of its use.
It examines key issues including informed consent,
determination of the quality of life,ethical participation,
allocation of scarce resources,euthanasia & allowing to die.
As some recent thanatology research has breached some of
the principles of ethical research in human beings,everyone
involved in this area could benefit from reading this book,
which will also provide a valuable basis for teaching the
subject.
*****

202. EUTHANASIA,Or,Medical Treatment in Aid of An Easy
      Death. William Munk. Arno Press,NY.1976.105 pp.
      $ 12.00. (1st published London,1887)

Advocating good terminal care(rather than the modern use
of euthanasia) with salutory simplicity & sense,& well
worth modern reading. On the phenomena,symptoms & modes of
dying,& the treatment of the dying.Stresses the usual
peacefulness of death;reports early near-death experiences
(130 years before Moody).Sound & useful advice on terminal
care,nutrition & symptom control,with detailed observations
on the uses of opium. It reads very like the present St.
Christophers advice on the management of symptoms.
****

203. EVERYTHING IN ITS PATH.Kai T. Erikson. Simon &
      Schuster,N.Y. 1976. 284 pp. $ 8.95.

A sobre,respectful & moving account of the Buffalo Creek
disaster;an impressive work of sociology & literature.A
valuable study of the death of a community,the phenomena
of collective trauma,the lasting effects of disaster
deaths;of loss of life,communality & the furniture of self.
***½

204. EXAMINATION ON SUICIDOLOGY & CRISIS INTERVENTION.
      Self-Assessment of Knowledge & Attitudes Toward
      Suicide. Charles Press/Robert J Brady,Bowie,MD.
      1970. $ 10.50 / £ 8.35.(Pack of 20).

2 separate examinations in each booklet.Part I tests
factual knowledge,Part II assesses attitudes. A good
idea which could be better done,& too expensive.
**

205. THE EXPERIENCE OF DEATH: The Moral Problem of Suicide.
      Paul-Louis Landsberg. Arno Press,NY.1976. 102 pp.
      $ 12.00. (1st edition,London,1953).

A brilliant young philosopher & devout Catholic who later
died in a concentration camp,explores the relationship
between suicidal dynamics & Christian morality,including
examination of the fact that "man can welcome the idea
of death".
***

206.   THE EXPERIENCE OF DYING. Ed.Norbert Greinacher &
       Alois Muller. Herder & Herder,New York. 1974.
       152 pp. $ 3.95 PB.

Collection of European essays,including Hofmeier;Bloching
on death in contemporary literature-Garrett Borden on the
ritual presentation of death;Jacques-Marie Pollier on
anthropological reflections on the postponement of death;
Giulio Girardi on Marxism & death;& Josef Mayer-Scheur;
Gisbert Greshake;Luciano Cagliotti,& Christopher Kaufer.
***

207.   THE EXPERIENCE OF DYING. Ed.E.Mansell Pattison.
       Spectrum/Prentice-Hall,NJ.1976. 335 pp. PB $4.95;
       £ 8.35, £ 3.45 PB.

Competent reviews of current views of death attitudes,death
& the life cycle,the family,religion,& the will to live.
Additional chapters by other authors on the Malformed &
Burned Child,Childhood leukemia;middle childhood &
Hemophilia,Trauma,Cancer;Adolescence & cardiac pacemakers,
renal transplants,cancer;Young Adults & M.S.,trauma,and
leukemia;Middle Age & the I.C.U.,Cancer,Leukemia,and
Hemodialysis;the Elderly & Euthanasia; and two closing
chapters by Pattison,critically reviewing styles of
dying,& ways of helping. Clinically relevant.
****

208.   EXPERIENCES FACING DEATH.Mary Austin. Arno Press,NY.
       1976. 301 pp. $ 17.00. (1st ed,Indianapolis,1931).

A highly personal,indeed egotistical,account of wavering
defences against death anxiety & attempts to confront it,
by an early feminist & exponent of rugged self-reliance.
**

209.   EXPERIMENT PERILOUS.Renee C.Fox. University of
       Pennsylvania Press,Philadelphia.(1959) 1974
       262 pp. $ 5.95 PB.

A major classic of medical sociology,well researched &
unusually well-written.A study of the patients & doctors in
a small high-risk medical research ward.In its understanding
of the problems & stresses of doctors & patients,& of how
they came to terms with them,& how they jointly confronted
death,it is an unusually perceptive study.
****½

210. EXPLORING THE CRACK IN THE COSMIC EGG.Joseph
      Chilton Pearce. Julian Press,N.Y.1974.173pp.$6.95.

It seems almost a basic rule that the more ecstatic the
comments on the cover,the more abysmal the book between
them.An extraordinarily incoherent book,with much hectic
name-dropping,sloppy use of terminology,& what feels like
a desperate attempt to ride every band-wagon in sight,
trotting between Castaneda's tedious Don Juan,Yuri Geller,
astral travel,misunderstood Zen,garbled Existentialism,
split-brain research,Gurdjief,semi-Maslow,poltergeists and
rabbits. Amongst all this,sections on death anxiety & how
to deal with it,that show no real understanding at all.
*

211. FACING DEATH.R.E.Kavanaugh. Nash Publishing,Los
      Angeles,1972. 226 pp. $ 7.95.Penguin,PB,$ 2.25,
      80 pence,U.K.

Unlike the description on its blurb,this is not a
"startlingly realistic analysis of our outdated attitudes
toward dying",nor does it have "the answers to the myriad
questions"about death. A rambling,muddled,introspective,
egoist,disappointing book.
*

212. FACING DEATH.Bryan Magee. William Kimber,London.
      1977. 447 pp. £ 4.95.

An interesting but very flawed novel.It deals with a young
man's death from Hodgkin's disease during the 1960's,& with
such issues as whether he should be told,& how one searches
for significance in life in the face of death.But Mr Magee
doesn't know terribly much about dying,& his prose style is
clumsy & excessively wordy & self-indulgent.The characters
are wooden & superficial stereotypes,largely glossy
aristocratic "beautiful"people.The situations are idealized
& avoid much of the messy reality of life & death.The
emotional content is arid & unreal,& the action is
constantly interrupted by intense philosophical debates
on the nature of reality & the limitations of the logical
positivists.The driving selfishness of all those who are
supposedly helping the dying man is well portrayed,though.
**$\frac{1}{2}$

213. THE FACTS OF DEATH.Michael A.Simpson. Spectrum/
       Prentice-Hall, 1979. 250 pp. approx.

An eloquent & warm practical book for families & helpers.
reviews succinctly what we know about the nature of death
& dying,patient's rights,how to manage one's own death &
to cope with the dying of another;death & children;suicide:
how to cope with a suicidal person,& with one's own
suicidal impulses; bereavement & grief ; funerals,& how to
plan one's estate & funeral,& how to avoid the Terminal
R.I.P.-off. Maybe they told you the Facts of Life : this is
what they left out.
*****

 214. THE FEAR OF THE DEAD IN PRIMITIVE RELIGION. James
        George Frazer. Arno Press,NY.1976. 3 vols in 1.
        678 pp. $ 43.00. (1st published,1933/34/36).

The author of The Golden Bough describes his view of how
the dead are feared rather than loved,with many examples
from many cultures. Major work of a classical
anthropologist.
***

215. FEARS RELATED TO DEATH AND SUICIDE. MSS Information
       Corp.,New York. 1974. 221 pp. $ 17.00.

A 'selection'of papers on attitudes to death,of very
varied quality & importance,which seems to have been
randomly selected.
**

216. FEDERAL TRADE COMMISSION SURVEY OF FUNERAL PRICES IN
       THE DISTRICT OF COLUMBIA.Federal Trade Commission.
       U.S.Govt.Printing Office,Washington DC. 1974.

An extended price study,showing interesting variations in
price & sales practices.Makes an effective consumer
handbook against exploitation,& explores alternatives.
***

217. FILMS ON DEATH AND DYING. Edward A.Mason. Educational
       Film Library Association,New York. 4 pp. $ 0.75¢

Brief catalogue listing some 40 films.Very incomplete.
**

218. FIRST SNOW. Helen Coutant.Alfred A.Knopf,New York.
      1974. $ 4.50.

An account of the Buddhist view of death,in a book intended
for use with children.
**

219. THE FIRST YEAR OF BEREAVEMENT.Ira Glick,Robert Weiss,
      & Colin Murray Parkes. Wiley & Sons,N.Y.1974.311 pp.

Conceptually sophisticated but rendered highly readable by
incorporating quotations from interviews,this important
book provides a socio-psychological study of the processes
of bereavement.It examines such matters as emotional &
physical reactions,the availability & use of help,the
ceremonies of leave-taking,changes in relationships with
family & friends,& the nature of the recovery process.It
also compares & contrasts the experiences of widows &
widowers (a more neglected group).Combining a larger
statistical sample with case studies,the authors have made
a unique contribution to theoretical & practical
understanding of the processes of grief & its management.
****

220. FORGETTING'S NO EXCUSE.Mary Stott. Faber & Faber,
      London. (Oxford University Press,U.S.A.) 1973
      194 pp. $ 11.75.

Principally a gossipy,scattered,autobiographical rample of
strictly temporary & local interest,with one exception.The
final chapter:An End & A Beginning,is a well-written
account of the author's bereavement & attitudes to
widowhood.If only this section had been extended,the book
would have been of general & lasting interest,for it is
candid & relatively bold.Meanwhile,we'll have to hope it
gets reprinted in better company.
*$\frac{1}{2}$

221. FOR THE BEREAVED.Austin H & Lillian G.Kutscher.
      Frederick Fell Publ.,New York. 1971 157 pp.
      $ 3.95 PB.

Paperback edition of "But Not to Lose"--reviewed separately.
Not impressive.
**

222. <u>FREEDOM TO DIE</u> : Moral & Legal Aspects of Euthanasia.
      O.Ruth Russell.Human Sciences Press,N.Y. 1975.
      352 pp. $ 14.95.

A reasonably thorough study of euthanasia,though polemic
more than dispassionate,& written by an earnest advocate
of its legalization.An interesting review of activities &
opinions in this area from the 1930's to date,& an attempt
to answer all the major arguments of opponents of the
opponents of euthanasia,as well as a description of the
major test cases,legally.There's less attention paid to
moral,ethical & philosophical problems than one might
expect,& a heavy reliance on secondary & tertiary sources
(citing a newspaper report of a claim by Ralph Nader that
"thousands" of Thalidomide babies were born,rather than
quoting readily available authorities on the actual
numbers,for example;& citing Hendin as if he were a major
or original authority on death,a sure sign of naivety).
A commendable attention to both American & British events,
but sometimes seriously biased (2 British conferences in
the 70's,for instance,are very inaccurately cited).A
reasonably thorough bibliography.Not as reliable as is
needed,but useful.
***
222A. <u>FREEDOM TO DIE</u>,etc.Revised Edition,1977.412 pp.$ 14.95,
       Also Laurel (Dell Publ.Co.) 1976, $ 1.95 PB.

A re-issue of the 1975 edition with a 60-page supplement
dealing with five recent cases including Quinlan,van Dusen
& Haemmerli;developments in legislation including a very
brief account of the California Act;Euthanasia Societies &
the policies of various organizations & groups.The
supplement is rather sketchy & reads as if very hastily
patched together,but it is helpful.For all its many faults,
this is probably the most comprehensive general book on
non-clinical aspects of euthanasia.
****
223. <u>FREE FALL</u>. Jo Ann Kelley Smith. Judson Press,Valley
      Forge. 1975.138 pp. $ 5.95 (G.R.Welch,Toronto).

Mrs Smith wrote this account of her experience of death
during the last months of her life.She describes the
encounter as being like the free fall experience in
parachute jumping--an exhilerating sense of freedom with
an increasing sense of separation from what she knows and
loves,leaving the assurance of what she knows for a "leap
of faith". Frank,confident & competent.
***

224. FROM MY WORLD TO YOURS.Jasper Swain. Walker & Co.,NY.
      1977. 102 pp. $ 5.95.

A sad account,far less impressive & convincing than it
strives to be,of a father's attempts to contact his dead
son,& communicate with the world beyond.
**

225. FUNERAL CUSTOMS THE WORLD OVER.Robert W.Habenstein,
      with W.M.Lamers. National Funeral Directors
      Association; Bulfin,Milwaukee. 1963. Revised Edition.
      854 pp. Illustrated. $ 9.00.

Not profound or academic,but a reasonably thorough account
of world-wide funeral customs.
***

226. THE FUNERAL DIRECTOR AND HIS ROLE AS A COUNSELOR.
      Howard C.Raether & Robert C.Slater.National Funeral
      Directors Association;Bulfin,Milwaukee. 1975.
      86 pp. $ 5.00 PB.

Proposes the contentious view that the funeral director
has a significant role as a counselor in helping his
customers deal with their grief,& describes how he should
go about doing this. Perhaps salesmen of bedroom
furniture should also provide sex counselling ?
**

227. THE FUNERAL: VESTIGE OR VALUE? Paul E.Irion. Arno
      Press,New York. 1976. 240pp. $ 16.00 (Originally
      published Abingdon Press,1966).

A professor of pastoral theology considers whether the
conventional funeral meets the needs of society today;
examines the evidence & conflicting claims & arguments.
Decides that it cannot be rejected without emotional harm,
but proposes the development of new & more humane
alternatives.Deals with the function of appropriate ritual
in sanctioning the emergence of the bereaved person's
feelings over a prolonged period of time.Suggests that
authentic new rituals of leave-taking can be developed,in
which a shared religious conviction is not crucial.
Constructive & thoughtful.
***1/2

228. THE GARDEN IS DOING FINE.Carol Farley. Atheneum,New
      York. 1975. 185 pp. $ 6.95.

A novel for children.Corrie Sheldon's father has been ill
in hospital for many months,but neither she nor her mother
will let themselves believe that he's dying.She remembers
what he was like,& tries to find a new way of life without
him,seeking a return of normalcy but not wanting to
acknowledge a permanent loss of him. Finally,she decides
that a part of him will always live in her.Realistic,
slightly repetitive,but likely to be helpful.
***

229. GATHERINGS FROM GRAVEYARDS: Particularly Those of
      London,With a Concise History of the Modes of
      Interment Among Different Nations,From the Earliest
      Periods. G.A.Walker. Arno Press,NY.1976. 258 pp.
      $ 19.00. (1st published,London,1839).

A major reformer,exposing the dangers of the careless
burial methods of his day,& a study of burial and
funeral techniques elsewhere. A 19th Century Mitford.
***

230. GERHARD: A Love Story. Betty Kennedy. Macmillan,
      Canada. 1976. $ 5.95.

In April 1975,Betty Kennedy's husband Gerhard found that he
had cancer.The book is an account of how they and their
children spent the months until his death in December 1975.
The regular story,with nothing special to commend it.
Auto-voyeurism.
**

231. GRAMP. Mark and Dan Jury. Grossman Publishers (Viking
      Press),New York. 1976. 152 pp. Illustrated.$ 5.95. PB.

Simply,superb.A moving,honest & direct account of the dying
of Frank Tugend,as recorded in photographs & words,by a
family who made his death an act of love.Arteriosclerotic
dementia led to a gruelling 3-year deterioration.On February
11,1974,aged 81,he removed his false teeth & announced that
he was no longer going to eat or drink.The family decided to
respect his wishes & not hospitalize him.3 weeks later,he
died at home.Death with dignity? Perhaps,though not how most
people picture it. An invaluable,unromanticized corrective
to the stickily sentimental nature of too much Death Lit.
*****

232.   GRIEF AND HOW TO LIVE WITH IT.D.Morris. Grosset &
       Dunlap,NY.1972.122pp.$ 3.50. George,Allen & Unwin,
       London. £ 1.50.
A genuine,brief,& partly successful attempt at a practical
"How To" book for the widow;quite down to earth.Expensive.
**

233.   GRIEF AND THE MEANING OF THE FUNERAL.MSS Information
       Corp.,N.Y. 1975. 270pp. $ 11.50.
Assembled without much evidence of taste or judgement.There
are many dreadful,amateurish,ill-informed but often
mercifully brief items of significant irrelevance. A couple
of good pieces--Edgar Jackson writes on the management of
grief,with his usual sensitivity,& Schowalter on children
& funerals.An interesting though very naive study of public
experience and attitudes to funeral arrangements by Khlief.
Some peculiar concepts of "Grief Therapy",e.g.--"Organ music
should have a consoling radiance.When playing for a memorial
or funeral service,the organist should produce clean,
uprising sounds". (Sic.I'm not kidding). A paranoid review
of memorial society literature;& an unjustifiably one-sided,
wholly uncritical approach to recent funeral traditions.In
one article,such entirely normal and healthy practices as
closed-casket or limited funerals,or no "visitations",are
described as abnormal "escape mechanisms".This is an abuse
of psychology. Many hearty assertions,apparently regarded
as self-evident,without a shred of supportive evidence.Some
ambitious & rather pretentious chapters on the Funeral
Director's education.The Funeral Home:A Community Resource;
The Funeral Home as a Center of Grief Activity."Where else
do you hear more warm conversations than in and about the
funeral home?" Well,give me a minute;I'm sure I can think of
somewhere. Rhapsodic discussion of colour schemes for the
model mortuary : apparently "muted shades of red,yellow,
yellow-orange...tan,beige and taupe"(taupe?) are IN,though
blue and green can be used as "tiny,vivid accents". Oh
dear,oh dear. O Tempora,O Mortes...
*

234.   A GRIEF OBSERVED.C.S.Lewis. Faber & Faber,London.
       1961/1973. 60pp. PB.45 pence.Seabury Press,NY.$ 4.50.

"No one ever told me that grief felt so much like fear"...
An outstandingly honest,naked observation of a widower's
grief.Begun,without plans for publication,as a means of
self-therapy,written informally in odd notebooks,during
his first weeks alone. Unique,moving,memorable.
*****

235.   GRIEF: SELECTED READINGS.Arthur C.Carr,B.Schoenberg,et.
       al. Health Sciences Publishing Corp.,New York.
       1975. 327 pp. $ 7.50 PB.

A collection of various materials on clinical & religious
views on grief. Not particularly imaginatively selected,and
not including much important material.
**

236.   GUIDE DE LA MORT.Georges Heuse. Masson,Paris. 1975.263pp.

A significant French work;a practical guide to many matters
relating to death and dying,based on a broad understanding
of the European literature on the subject.
***

237.   GUS IN BRONZE. Alexandra Marshall. Alfred A.Knopf,
       New York. 1977. 256 pp. $ 8.95.

A novel about the last 4 weeks in the life of Gus,& how her
family cope.Her husband is memorizing Scarlatti's 555
harpsichord sonatas as a pact with the Gods to keep her alive;
Daphni,15,is sculpting a bronze bust of her mother for the
younger children to remember her by.Sounds just like the
typical American family,doesn't it? Rather far-fetched ; &
have you noticed how far you have to go,these days,to get
something really far-fetched?
**

H

238.   A HANDBOOK FOR THE STUDY OF SUICIDE.Ed.Seymour Perlin.
       Oxford University Press,London & N.Y.1975. 236 pp.
       $ 9.95 , $ 5.95 PB.

Far from comprehensive,but an entertaining look at suicide
from eleven different points of view,including those of the
historian,literary critic (A.Alvarez),moralist,sociologist,
anthropologist,sociologist & biologist.
***

239.   HANDBOOK FOR WIDOWS.National Association of Widows.
        Virago,London. 1978. £ 1.25.

Middling;reasonably useful collection of advice and
addresses for widows;lacking any major familiarity
with the literature or significant perspective.
***

240.   HANGING ON.Hila Colman. Atheneum,New York. 1977.
        215 pp. $ 8.95.

"The intimate journal of a wife's pain-filled year with her
dying husband".Coping with her husband's succession of
strokes.Hospital,rehabilitation center,nursing home,and,
after Medicare stopped caring,coping at home.Frankly dealing
with the real problems,both personal and the injustices of
medical care costs & the daftness of present roles governing
public funds for chronic care.Personal,realistic.Like most
other such books,it is primarily a written self-therapy.It's
less clear in what way it could be of use to others.
**

241.   THE HARVARD GUIDE TO MODERN PSYCHIATRY.Ed.Armand M.
        Nicholi. Harvard University Press,Cambridge,Mass.&
        London, 1978. 690 pp. £ 19.75.

This is an unusually competent review of modern psychiatric
knowledge & practice by a very talented team of Harvard
writers——it may,however,fall between two stools,giving
more than medical students & paraprofessionals need,& not
quite enough for psychiatric residents.Chapter 28 by Ned
Cassem,deals superbly with "Treating the Person Confronting
Death".With a good selection of references,he reviews the
care of the dying with regard to treatment goals,treatment
recommendations,communication,religion,the dying child &
his parents (somewhat out of date)-the care of the suicidal
person,& the bereaved;with due attention to the difficulties
of the caregivers.
****

242.   THE HASTINGS CENTER BIBLIOGRAPHY OF SOCIETY,ETHICS &
        THE LIFE SCIENCES.1976-77. Compiled by Sharman Sollitto
        & Robert M.Veatch.Revised Nancy K.Taylor. Institute of
        Society,Ethics & the Life Sciences,Hastings-on-Hudson.
        82 pp. PB. $ 4.00.

A selected & partially annotated bibliography,covering a
wide range of subjects,sometimes valuably & thoroughly,but
sometimes rather superficially.Often insufficiently critical

242 ctd.) or selective.Topics covered include ethical
theory,behavior control(psychosurgery,psychotherapy,
institutions,commitments & the right to treatment)
experimentation & consent,genetic counseling,genetic
engineering,health care delivery,patients rights,birth
control,abortion,& allocation of scarce medical resources.
With regard to death & dying,it is more limited,more
clearly incomplete & less specially useful.Understandable
but unhelpful bias towards the Hastings Center Report & its
own authors. Especially weak in the psychological,
sociological & clinical areas;stronger in ethical & legal
issues.
***

243.   HELP FOR THE BEREAVED.What the Family of the Deceased
       Should Know. Curtis A Smith. Adams Press,Chicago.
       1972. 23 pp. PB. $ 1.50.

A difficult project,not very well done.Laws & procedures
differ so much between countries & states,that such books
are either too specific or too general.Discusses funerals,
death certificates,financial affairs & benefits,& includes
some sample letters. Reasonably handy.
***

244.   HELP FOR YOUR GRIEF: TURNING EMOTIONAL LOSS INTO
       GROWTH. Arthur S.Freese.Schocken Books,New York.
       1977. 207 pp. $ 9.95.

Summarizes some of what is known about grief & mourning,
& offers some guidelines about how to deal with it.
Discusses physical & psychological effects of grief; past,
present & future funeral & grief responses; grieving by &
for children;& the place of religion in these processes.
Probably well-meaning,but not at all special,not very
good,journalism.
*

245.   HELPING CANCER PATIENTS--EFFECTIVELY.Nursing Skillbook,
       Nursing 77 Books,Intermed Communicns,PA & Ravenswood,UK.
       1977. 187 pp. £ 7.40 $ 8.95.

A very helpful guide to the nature of cancer,the problems of
cancer patients,& how they may best be helped & informed.
Provides a general intriduction to cancer surgery,radiation,
chemotherapy & immunotherapy,& then specific sections on
cancer of the lungs,breast,colorectum,stomach,female

245 ctd.) reproductive organs,prostate,bladder,head & neck,
& on leukemia & Hodgkins Disease.Practical & reasonably up-
-to-date,with a commendable emphasis on patient education.
This book would be very useful to all non-medical
thanatologists dealing clinically or in counselling,with
cancer patients.
***½

246. HELPING CHILDREN COPE WITH DEATH & SEPARATION:
      RESOURCES FOR TEACHERS.Joanne Bernstein. 1976.
      ICBD,Urbana,Ill. $ 1.85. PB.

A brief guide to some books,films & general references,usable
by teachers working with children.Lists some books for
children,dealing with death & separation;some references on
bibliotherapy;a very limited list of films,filmstrips &
cassettes,some totally irrelevant to either subject;& some
additional references.Far from comprehensive,useful only
for the teacher lacking any other guidance.
**½

247. HELPING CHILDREN WITH THE MYSTERY OF DEATH.E.L.Reed.
      Abingdon Press,Nashville. 1970. 143 pp. $ 3.50.

Sickly."A Book of religious substance",& sticky substance
at that;with kiddie's verses,stories & games,and also some
"enriching materials for adults" (sic).Pious in the worst
sense;pompous,unrealistic & so very much less helpful than
it claims to be. I wouldn't let my kids read it under any
circumstances.
*

248. HELPING YOUR CHILDREN TO UNDERSTAND DEATH.Anna M.Wolf.
      Revised edn.1973. Child Study Press,NY.64pp.$ 1.50.PB.

Possibly the best book available to help parents & children
talk about death.Simple but not simplistic,wise but not
know-all,& soundly practical.Well grounded in child
development & family dynamics,it deals sensibly with the
common questions of children & parents.Issues of faith,
inescapable in this area,are considered from the viewpoint
of the major faiths;other matters covered include suicide,
assassination & war,& hypocrisy.Very highly recommended to
all who deal with children,have children,or have been
children.
*****

249. HELPLESSNESS : On Depression,Development & Death.
      Martin Seligman. W.H.Freeman,San Francisco. 1975.
      250 pp. £ 6.20; PB ₤ 3.20, $ 4.95.

There's a growing body of research showing that helplessness
is a learned behaviour.After experiences of being powerless
to affect the outcome of significant situations,the
individual gives up,ceases responding,& the helplessness
becomes a self-fulfilling prophecy.Seligman argues cogently
that these phenomena are important in understanding anxiety
& depression,sudden psychosomatic death,& the causes &
effects of fatal illness.He raises many intriguing questions,
& makes useful therapeutic suggestions.Reviews a very wide
range of research.More original & thought-provoking than
many books in this area.
****

250. HERE COMES IMMORTALITY.Jerome Tuccille. Stein & Day,
      New York. 1973. 191 pp. $ 6.95.

A cheerful & reliably superficial study of "life-extension
techniques".The first part scampers through cryonics,cloning,
& other even more dated innovations,arguing that physical
immortality is attainable & we're not far from achieving
this dubious blessing."Incredibly",he chirrups,"there are
those who object to even the prospect of death's demise.
Theologians,doctors,undertakers,ecologists...(who)...would
have a great deal to lose if people could live forever";but
he boasts of "showing them up for the obstructionists they
are".In the second part,a science fantasy,he describes the
sort of society immortality could produce,after the first
re-animation (Walt Disney,he expects :but then Walt always
was interested in animation,I suppose).Wholly uncritical,
naive & determinedly trendy,this might have made an
entertaining & deservedly evanescent magazine article,rather
than literary froth in hard covers.
*

251. THE HIGH COST OF DYING.R.M.Harmer.Collier,NY.1963.
      263 pp.PB 0.95 ₵.(Now out of print,but some copies
      still available from the Continental Association of
      Funeral & Memorial Societies at $ 1.00.)

Another attack on the American funeral industry.Competent &
reasonably well-documented despite the cover(Rips away the
shroud cloaking rackets...).Less entertaining than Mitford.
Emphasizes the non-profit burial society approach.
***

252.   THE HISTORIE OF LIFE & DEATH WITH OBSERVATIONS
       NATURALL & EXPERIMENTALL FOR THE PROLONGING OF LIFE.
       Francis Bacon. Arno Press,NY.1976 .323 pp. $ 22.00.

1st edition,London,1638. Longevity & death fascinated Bacon,
but this is his only extended treatise on death,prolongation
of life,euthanasia,transfusion & transplantation.It
constituted a radical break with the traditions of Galen &
Aristotle,& contains many extraordinary precursors of
modern techniques & thinking in these subject areas.
***

253.   HISTORY OF AMERICAN FUNERAL DIRECTING.Robert W.
       Habenstein & W.M.Lamers. National Funeral Directors
       Association;Bulfin,Milwaukee. 1962. 654pp.$6.50.PB.

The standard history of the American funeral directing
industry.While hardly a critical study of such funeral
practices,it's a reasonably thorough account of their
development.
***

254.   A HISTORY OF IDEAS ABOUT THE PROLONGATION OF LIFE:
       The Evolution of Prolongevity Hypotheses to 1800.
       Gerald J.Gruman. Arno Press,NY.1976.102pp. $ 12.00.

The belief that it is both possible & desirable to
significantly extend the length of life has existed since
ancient times,in scientific & cultural expressions.An
opposing tradition has insisted that life cannot &/or
should not be prolonged by human agency.A significant
historical basis for current discussions of attitudes.
***

255.   HOME CARE FOR THE DYING CHILD:Professional & Family
       Perspectives. Ed.Ida Marie Martinson.Appleton-Century-
       Crofts,New York. 1976. 352 pp. PB.$ 9.75. £ 7.80.

Arising from a 3-year study of the home as an alternative
site,& the parents as alternative care-givers,in caring for
the dying child.Describes the Home Care Project,& the
experiences of the parents & professionals involved.It would
have benefitted from fewer but longer chapters,fewer
sentimental anecdotes,& more rigorous evaluation of the
results of the project.The detailed clinical account of
acute leukemia & its haematology is unnecessary to the

255. ctd.) theme of the book.Some chapters,such as Reese on
staff support systems,& Anglim on re-integration of the
family after the death,are especially effective.
***½

256.   THE HOSPICE MOVEMENT : A Better Way of Caring for the
       Dying. Sandol Stoddart. Stein & Day,New York.
       1978. 266 pp. $ 8.95.

The most comprehensive account yet of the "Hospice
Movement".It describes the history of the hospices and
hospitals (not always making any clear distinction between
them) & conveys something of the atmosphere & processes of
hospice care.The story is at times over-dramatized,yet
'faction'is hardly needed when the facts speak so eloquently
for themselves.A nice book,but not really a wise book. It
reflects a far too common tendency to confuse issues:hospices
are one good way in which to care well for the dying,but
they are not the only appropriate place,& it is highly
unlikely that they will ever care for a majority of dying
patients.Some "hospices",or clinics using that title,provide
extremely bad terminal care;some hospitals,& some family
doctors/general practitioners provide excellent terminal
care.The modern movement back to better care for the dying
was only partially related to the hospices,& still involves
a great number of people not working in a hospice. Beware
the Edifice Complex; don't mistake the building for what
should go on inside it.
***

257.   THE HOUR OF OUR DEATH.(A Record of a Conference on
       the Care of the Dying). Ed. Sylvia Lack & Richard
       Lamerton. Geoffrey Chapman,London (Collier-Macmillan,
       Canada) 1974. 60 pp. £ 1.95 , $ 7.15.

In the guise of a book about the care of the dying,here is a
report of the conference which,in the guise of a discussion
of terminal care,was an anti-euthanasia crusade.The one item
on topic is a gentle presentation by Cicely Saunders,
illustrated by some of the Hospice photographs.Donald Macrae
gives a moderately interesting essay on"A Sociologist's
View of Euthanasia,& Ferguson Anderson comments on "The
Elderly at the End of Life". There are some woolly summaries
of conference "discussion"on euthanasia,one-sided and hardly
an accurate reflection of what occurred in the groups,and
often with an embattled "How do we fight off euthanasia

257 ctd.) legislation?" approach.There is an appallingly
limited and just sloppy bibliography,nearly half of which
is,for no justifiable reason (it wasn't even discussed at
the conference) devoted to the homeopathic "therapy" of
cancer. This book may be of interest to friends of the
authors and editors.
*

258.   HOUSES FOR THE DEAD. A.W.Turner. David McKay,N.Y.
       1976. 144 pp. $ 7.95.

Explores burial customs of other cultures through short
narratives depicting the reactions of someone in that
place & time,speaking didactically.Stresses the functional
aspects of such customs,sometimes usefully.Doesn't deal with
modern customs,& has strange concepts of what "modern" and
"scientific" mean. Not recommended.
*

259.   HOW COULD I NOT BE AMONG YOU? Ted Rosenthal.
       Braziller,N.Y.1973. 77 pp. PB $ 2.95. Avon Books,NY,
       1975. PB. 95 pp. $ 1.50.

At the age of 30,Ted found that he was dying of acute
leukemia.In some of his last months,he built a log cabin &
wrote poetry,singing of death and of life.Some of this was
filmed,to make a prize-winning documentary. This book
contains the poems,comments,& stills. Profoundly moving
piece of work. Though the poet subsequently led a far less
authentic life in his final months,doesn't spoil the
freshness & immediacy of these poems.
****$\frac{1}{2}$

260.   HOW TO AVOID PROBATE.Norman F.Dacey. Crown Publishers,
       New York. 1965 (48th printing 1978) 360pp.$ 7.95.

A highly valuable book of consumer self-defence.It discusses
the absurd difficulties & expenses of probate & settling
estates,& then clearly discusses ways of avoiding unnecessary
expenses.Includes details of dealing with the Inter Vivos
(Living)Trust,home,checking & savings accounts,mutual fund
shares,securities,the close corporation,life insurance, the
"Dacey Trust",Wife'sTrust,leaving money to charities,making
gifts to a minor,reversionary trusts,personal effects,small
unincorporated businesses & automobiles;how to change your
mind and alter such plans;& how to make a will.It includes

260 ctd.) clear,duplicate copies,on perforated pages,of
the necessary legal instruments,ready for you to complete.
(Additional copies available from the National Estate
Planning Council,180 Church St.,Naugatuck,Conn.06770) .
Delightfully subversive,its even written in plain English!
(except for the legal forms,for the Law always strives to
be incomprehensible.For most people,legal documents are like
a foreign movie;but Dacey mercifully provides English
sub-titles.).
****

261.   HOW TO PROBATE AN ESTATE.William J.Moody.New Revised
       edition,1977. Cornerstone Library,N.Y. 95pp. $ 2.30.

Though partly outdated by the introduction of the Uniform
Probate Code,this slim volume gives clear guidance on
probate;a simple,step-by-step explanation of its processes,
& the administration of an estate,with a checklist of the
duties of executors.Basic advice on estate planning,with a
sample Will; & a useful glossary of terms.
***

262.   HOW TO SURVIVE THE LOSS OF A LOVE.Melba Colgrove,
       Harold Bloomfield,Peter McWilliams. Bantam Books,New
       York. 1977. 120 pp. $ 1.95 PB.

The Joy of Grief? Or How to Get Away With Publishing a Very
Slim book with Very Few Words on Each Page.
Some people
seem to think that anything
is poetry
if you print it this way.
It isnt.
Promises to be a guide to overcoming all your emotional
hurts & survive any of a list of 30 losses from death to
loss of teeth. Sparse,but over-written,it gushes in a
mercifully fitful stream.Too self-consciously clever. Oh no,
find another way to survive if you can.
*

263.   THE HUMAN ENCOUNTER WITH DEATH.Stanislav Grof & Joan
       Halifax. E.P.Dutton,NY. 1978. 240pp.$8.95,$ 3.95 PB.

The first substantive product of the group using psychedelic
drugs with the dying.An interesting review of this field,
and its relevances and correspondences with the practices
of other cultures.Still very little evidence that such
therapy works,but intriguing claims.
***

264.   HUMAN HOPE AND THE DEATH INSTINCT.David Holbrook.
       Pergamon Press,Oxford. 316 pp. 1971.

Probably Holbrook's major work.It carries further his
earlier concern with the way a mechanistic civilization
distorts the natural growth of humans,forcing on them a
way of life split between thought & feeling,& lacking in
organic unity.Here he explores the consequences of this
situation,& the sources of human integration &
fulfillment.
***

265.   HUMAN LIFE AND HUMAN WORTH.Douglas M.Jackson.
       Christian Medical Fellowship. 1970. 16pp.15 pence.

A surgeon's consideration of definitions of life & death,&
the assessment of the worth of human life.Heavily &
excessively dependent on quotations;a too-brief though
worthwhile attempt to relate medical realities to ethical
ideas.
**

266.   HYDROTAPHIA,URNE-BURIALL,Or,A Discourse of the
       Sepulchrall Urnes Lately Found in Norfolk.Together
       with the Garden of Cyrus,or the Quincunciall,Lozenge,
       or Network Plantations of the Ancients,Artificially,
       Naturally,Mystically Considered. Thomas Browne.
       Arno Press,New York. 1976. 207 pp. $ 12.00.

Facsimile of the London,1658 edition. A literary,
philosophical & anthropological classic,inspired by the
discovery of ancient burial urns. Apart from the catchy
title,it is vigorously written; seeing man as a noble and
sacred being,while also recognising his self-deceptions and
defensive strategies.
***

I
267.   IF YOU WILL LIFT THE LOAD... A Guide to the Creation
       of Widowed to Widowed Programs in Your Community.
       Phyllis R.Silverman,with A.Musicant & S.Richter.
       Jewish Funeral Directors Association,or Gutterman-
       -Musicant-Kreitzman,Inc. 1976.125pp. $ 8.95.

A practical manual,useful for community group leaders,about
founding Widowed-to-Widowed Programs,with case studies.
***

268. I HAD THIS LITTLE CANCER... A Personal Story of
      Survival. Jean Pradeau. Abelard-Schuman,New York ;
      Fitzhenry & Whiteside,Canada. 1976.147pp. $ 9.50.

A jaunty,individual,realistic account of living with cancer;
a salivary gland carcinoma,surgery,radiotherapy and
chemotherapy. Originally published in France in 1975 as
"Un petit truc de rien du tout".Observant of his own
reactions as well as those of his family,doctors,friends,&
other patients.The author,a journalist,forms a relationship
of some pride with his very own cancer;belligerant,Gallic,
rambling,frank,determined.
**½

269. I HEARD THE OWL CALL MY NAME. Margaret Craven.
      Doubleday,NY. 1973. $ 4.95. Dell,NY. $ 1.25. PB.

A bishop sends a young priest,terminally ill but not
knowing this,to work in a small North American Indian
community,to learn "enough about life to be ready to die".
***

270. THE INABILITY TO MOURN:PRINCIPLES OF COLLECTIVE
      BEHAVIOR. Alexander & Margarete Mitscherlich.
      Grove Press,N.Y. 1975. 332 pp. $ 12.50.

The first European work of Freudian psychohistory,seeking
to build relationships between individual case-histories
& national development.The original German edition(Die
Unfahigkeit zu Trauern,Piper,Munich,1967) was a best seller.
It considers the illusions in German thought & behavior
before,during & after the Nazi period,the response to
defeat,avoiding mass melancholia by derealization of the
past,identification with the victors,& manic physical
reconstruction.Also broader issues of collective behavior,
tolerance & authority.Relevant to Thanatology in regard to
the ways in which societies collectively respond to
defeat,death & disaster.
**½

271. IN AFTER DAYS: Thoughts on the Future Life. W.D.
      Howells,et al. Arno Press,NY.1976.233 pp. $ 18.00.

1st published in 1910,essays by 9 figures of the late 19th
Century,late in their lives;notably Henry James "Is There A
Life After Death?", William Dean Howells,Julia Ward Howe,and
others.
***

272. <u>INFORMED CONSENT.</u> Jane Cowles. Coward,McCann &
     Geoghegan,New York.(Longman,Canada).1976.224pp.$ 9.50.

A good idea,not awfully well done."Breast cancer is the
disease women fear most in the bosom oriented society...
450,000 women will confront a Breast Cancer Crisis This
Year"says the blurb,& "This Revolutionary Book is Vital" to
them.Well,not quite.It's thesis one can applaud:that a
woman & her family should be able to know enough about the
illness & the treatment options to participate in the
treatment decision.Written with all the objectivity,
sensitivity & style of a Soap Opera,with dialogue that might
seem clumsy in a B-Movie,it's not so good. The author tends
to exhort us towards a new orthodoxy,rather than an open
exploration of options : 2-stage procedures,local biopsy,
modified radical mastectomy with breast reconstruction,
mammagraphy & xerography are IN;1-stage procedures,lumpectomy
& thermography are OUT. The existing evidence on the subject
is not thoroughly or objectively reviewed,all alternatives
are not explored,& the nitty-gritty details of coping with
a mastectomy & living with the results,are neglected. Ill-
-balanced & shrill,unfortunately.
**

273. <u>IN NECESSITY & SORROW: Life & Death in an Abortion</u>
      Hospital. Magda Denes. Basic Books,NY.1976.
      247 pp. $ 10.00. Penguin Books,NY.1977. $ 2.95 PB.

A very subjective & biased mass of material on abortion,
organized around the author's own very ambivalent
experiences.Sometimes moving & disturbing.Unfortunate that
it seems to claim to be also a social & scientific study,
for it is not objective enough to claim to be that.The
experiences described are not especially typical;the data
on which her conclusions are based is not fully revealed.
Yet one of the few books attending at all to the griefs
of abortion.
**

274. <u>IN THE MATTER OF KAREN QUINLAN.</u> (Vol.I.) University
      Publications of America,Inc.Washington DC. 1977.

The complete legal briefs,court proceedings & decision in
the Superior Court of New Jersey.
***

275. INTIMATIONS OF MORTALITY. Violet Weingarten. Alfred
      A.Knopf,N.Y. 1978. 256 pp. $ 8.95.

A memoir. Ms Weingarten died in summer 1976,just after the
publication of her fourth novel.She began this journal after
her 1st operation for cancer,& continued it through her last
two years.A wryly observant account of her experiences,
including the unhelpfulness,to her,of so much of Death Lit.
***

276. IS LIFE REALLY SACRED? Paul W.Brand. Christian Medical
      Fellowship. 1974. 14 pp. PB 15 pence.

A pamphlet recording a rather weak sermon that wanders
around life & death and gets nowhere especially interesting.
More deservedly ephemeral than any in this CMF series.
*

277. IS THERE AN ANSWER TO DEATH? Peter Koestenbaum.
      Spectrum/Prentice-Hall. 1976.212 pp. PB £ 2.70,
      $ 3.75 (Canada $ 4.25).

One of a series of Spectrum books on Humanistic Psychology.
Koestenbaum,a Professor of Philosophy,practices a variety
of existential psychotherapy.He explores the theme of the
positive confrontation with death being an experience of
personal liberation,important in developing an authentic
sense of meaning in an alienating world.Not consistently
oriented towards the theme of death,as he also seeks to
advance his personal Cause:that the philosophical approach
to mental health is a bona fide science,academic discipline,
& profession. Less professional axe-grinding would improve
the book greatly. Nonetheless,comprehensible without being
too condescending,sober,& positive without being over-hearty.
***

278. IS THERE LIFE AFTER DEATH? Compiled David H.Scott.
      Bantam Books,New York.1977. 88 pp. $ 1.00. PB.

The Afterlife Bandwagon whirls again."A Book of Testimony",
with pieces by Billy Graham,Norman Vincent Peale,& a reprint
of Kubler-Ross's forward to Moody's book. This is almost
literary incest.
*

279. JEAN'S WAY. Derek Humphrey.Quartet Books,London.
      1978. £ 4.95.

An over-emotional & unobjective account of the author's
wife's death & the issue of mercy-killing.Widely
publicized in Britain because the author is a journalist,
but not a particularly memorable or original or helpful
contribution to the debate on euthanasia.
**

280. JEWISH REFLECTIONS ON DEATH.Jack Riemer. Schocken
      Books,NY. 1974. 184 pp. $ 7.95,$ 3.45 PB.

An eloquent anthology of great interest & value to Jew and
non-Jew alike.The laws of Judaism,especially with regard to
bereavement,show great psychological & spiritual wisdom,
giving a structure to grief that relates to death firmly
and realistically as a normal part of life.These essays
give a clear account of the beauty & insight of the
traditional procedures for the business of mourning;& also
explore the modern problems relating to death,from the
Jewish experience,of suffering & solace.An unusually
interesting book.A short glossary of Hebrew terms used would
aid the comprehension of non-Jewish readers.
*****

281. THE JEWISH WAY IN DEATH & MOURNING. Maurice Lamm.
      Jonathan David Publ.,Flushing,NY.1969. 265 pp.
      $ 7.95, $ 3.50 PB.

A reasonably thorough account of the Jewish tradition in
dealing with death & grief,with a detailed glossary of
transliterated Hebrew terms. Usable in conjunction with 280.
****

282. JOB'S ILLNESS--LOSS,GRIEF & INTEGRATION.:A
      Psychological Interpretation.J.H.Kahn.1975.166 pp.
      Pergamon Press,Oxford,NY. $ 14.00, £ 7.00.

Idiosyncratic exploration of an idée fixe.Rambling,meandering
repetitive & leaden;less a work of scholarship than
variations on a theme--the Bible story of Job,who is seen
as ranking with other archetypal myths like Oedipus &
Prometheus.As an effort to diagnose & explain Job's situation
psychologically rather than ideologically,it is rather
trivial.In its occasional confrontation of the meaning of
suffering & grief & their functions,it is promising.
*

283.   JOHNNY GOT HIS GUN.Dalton Trumbo. Bantam,NY. $ 1.50.

A powerful anti-war novel;a 19-year-old World War I veteran
has been left,after multiple injuries;blind,speechless,&
limbless.He beats out messages on his pillow with his head,
begging to be taken out of his hospital room,to show the
world a survivor of Every War.
*****

284.   A JOURNAL OF THE PLAGUE YEAR.Daniel Defoe. New
       American Library,New York. PB 0.95 ¢.

An account of London during the 1665 Great Plague,& the
responses to epidemic death.
***

285.   JOURNEY TO THE OTHER SIDE.David R.Wheeler. Ace Books,
       New York. 1976-77. 183 pp. $ 1.95 PB.

"Life After Death--Startling New Evidence from people who
have died & lived to tell about it!" In an introduction,
Kubler-Ross writes "I'm totally convinced there's life
after death....it's so beautiful."
*
K

286.   KAREN ANN QUINLAN: DYING IN THE AGE OF ETERNAL LIFE.
       B.D.Colen. Nash Publ.,N.Y. 1976. $ 7.95.

By a Washington Post reporter,this book considers the moral,
theological,sociological & philosophical dilemmas
exemplified by the Quinlan case.Interviews & cases illustrate
the problems of those making life-&-death decisions.Not
especially ambitious or scholarly,but readable.
**½

287.   KINFLICKS.Lisa Alther. Chatto & Windus,London,1976.
       Penguin 1977.PB 95 pence.A.A.Knopf,NY (Random House
       Canada)1975.Signet.NY 1977 $ 2.25. Also 'Haut-Kontakte'
       Ullstein Verlag,Berlin.1977. DM 34.

"My family has always been into death",it begins.At long
last someone who had something new to say about Death in
America,& a sparkling style to say it in.The story of Ginny
Babcock is not merely brilliantly funny & poignant as a
novel (it's a cliche for a reviewer to admit to laughing
aloud,but the occurrence is still rare enough to be worth
recording). It is also a fine account of varying responses

287 ctd.) to death;and of the dying,from idiopathic thrombocytopenic purpura,of Ginny's mother,for whom Death was a demon lover for whose assignation one must be ready. "The trick was in being both willing to die and able to do so at the same time.Dying properly was like achieving simultaneous orgasm".
*****

L

288. THE LAST DAY OF APRIL.Nancy Roach. American Cancer Society,California Division. 1974. 40pp. PB.

Intended to help parents of children with malignant and possibly fatal disease;a simple,honest,practical account of how one family coped with the situation.Without excessive self-pity or theorizing beyond their experiences,it is accurate & useful.
****

289. THE LAST ENEMY : A Christian Understanding of Death. Richard W.Doss. Harper & Row,NY.1974. 104 pp.$ 4.95.

Somewhat over-valuing itself,this book scampers through some very well-worn areas of current thinking on death, pretty superficially.It is more competent in its exploration of traditional & radical theology,& of Christian approaches to the understanding of death.
**

290. LAST RIGHTS: A Case for the Good Death. Marya Mannes. William Morrow & Co,NY 1973 $ 5.95; Signet,NY 1975 PB. 166 pp. $ 1.50.

Vastly overpraised,replete with grossly hyperbolic blurbs, but a reasonably effective look at the search for "death with dignity" & euthanasia.Not at all profound,indeed rather light-weight,but a handy glance at the subject.
***

291. THE LAST WORD.Melvin G.Williams.Oldstone Enterprizes, Boston. 1973. 41pp. $ 2.00. PB.

Subtitled "The Lure & Lore of Early New England Graveyards". A pleasant,unassuming little book about gravestones,their art, their inscriptions(from the basic'MA DYED'to the elaborate) & how to make rubbings from the stones.Well illustrated,if stylistically a little over-blown at times.
***

292. LEARNING TO LIVE WITH CANCER.Kelly M.Sveinson.
      Clarke,Irwin, Toronto. 1974. 122 pp. $ 1.95 PB.

Written by a man with Hodgkin's Disease.Low key & frank,it
offers advice to other cancer patients on how to live
positive & fruitful lives,despite their illness;with some
advice to doctors & to families.
**

293. LEARNING TO SAY GOODBYE WHEN A PARENT DIES.Eda
      LeShan. Macmillan,NY. 1976. 85 pp. $ 5.95.

Choppy,jumpy style.Believes a child can deal with anything
if told the truth.Anecdotes.Grades 5-9.Moving from the
general to the particular. Breathless.Who would use it ?
For what? Trite.
**

294. LIFE AFTER DEATH.Elizabeth Hanley. Leisure Books
      (Nordon Publications)NY. 1977.206 pp. $ 1.50. PB.

"One of the most astounding books ever written...it contains
hard,clear evidence that there is indeed life after death...
a major breakthrough...at last--positive proof that life
exists after death...astounding new facts that will forever
alter human existence".And if Ms Hanley had a fault,which
of course she doesn't,it might be modesty. Post blurb est
omne animalem triste. The terminal rip-off strikes again.
A collection of reincarnation anecdotes which reads very
much like pulp fiction,with awkward dialogue & a committed
naivety (such naivety can't come easily,it must need
practice).
*

295. LIFE AFTER DEATH. Arnold Toynbee,Arthur Koestler,et
      al. Weidenfeld & Nocolson,London.1976. 272 pp. £ 4.95.

Quite a literate account of possibilities & consequences
of belief in life after death. Curiously,a book that the
publisher has almost kept secret.
****

296.   LIFE AFTER LIFE.Raymond A.Moody. Mockingbird Books,
       Georgia. 1975. 128 pp. $ 2.95. Bantam,NY.1976. 185pp,
       PB $ 1.95. Corgi,London,1977. 65 pence.

The results of an unscientific,anecdotal,but thoughtful
study of people who had experienced "clinical death" &
been revived,& their accounts of the experience.It provides
an interesting & useful confirmation of the existing
clinical literature (which Dr Moody doesn't seem to have
read) on the phenomenology of near-death experiences; it
extends previous studies by describing some striking
similarities in the survivors reports beyond those already
recognized. Naive,especially in some of its conclusions and
interpretations.Despite its claims,it provides no"evidence"
whatsoever of "the survival of the human spirit beyond
death",or of "life after death";for these survivors,by
definition,have not been dead,as currently defined.May
stilulate properly structured research in this important
area. Appallingly misleading blurbs,"Actual case histories"
(are there any other sort?)"that reveal there is life after
death" (his qualifying & modifying statements are well
hidden in the book)."May change mankind's view of life,death
& spiritual survival forever". Richard Bach (author of
Jonathan Livingstone Seagull,that well-known authority on
avian thanatology) calls this straight honest research.But
there is no research in this book.Ignores significant
negative data. He is congratulated on his "courage"in
publishing this book.I don't see what courage it took.
**

297.   LIFE AFTER LIFE : The Investigation of a Phenomenon:
       Survival of Bodily Death. Raymond A.Moody. Stackpole
       Books,Harrisburg. 1976. 125 pp. $ 5.95,$ 1.95 PB.

Life after life after life after life,book after book after
books. Are there Literary Agents after death, I ask?
The basic Moody collection of stories.
*

298.   LIFE AND DEATH.H.S.Zim & S.Bleeker. Morrow,New York.
       1970. $ 4.85.

A book for children,describing what happens to the human
body when it dies,how death is dealt with,& what burial
customs are followed.
**

299. LIFE AT ITS CLOSE.C.Gordon Scorer.Christian Medical
     Fellowship. 1973. 15 pp. PB 12 pence.

A slim pamphlet looking at such themes as the quality of
life,life as God-given,immortality,& paradoxical
attitudes to death.
**

300. LIFE BEFORE DEATH. Ann Cartwright,Hockey & Anderson.
     Routledge & Kegan Paul,London.1973.280pp.$18.95.

The best & most competent study yet made of the last year
of life.Who dies?Of what? Where? With what restrictions
and symptoms? Needing & getting what help? Looks at the
care provided by doctors,nurses,community services,friends
& relatives;the extent of awareness of death;& sources of
information.Methodologically sound;a significant source.
***

301. LIFE BEGINS AT DEATH. Leslie D.Weatherhead.Abingdon
     Press,Nashville.1969. 80pp. PB $ 1.95.

In response to a series of questions,Dr Weatherhead,a
priest,discusses such matters as:Can we prove there is life
after death? What is it like? (Yes,even:Is there sex after
death? Probably,he thinks,though how the etheric body
manages it,is unclear.). What of those who die without
belief? Is reincarnation a reasonable belief? Concise &
clear account of a general Christian point of view,with
some personal oddities.
**½

302. LIFE IS FOREVER: Evidence for Survival After Death.
     S.Smith. G.P.Putnam's Sons,New York. 1974.

A psychic's account of "beyond-the-grave communications",
which she proposes as evidence for survival after death.
If you like this sort of thing,you may believe it.
*

303. LIFE IS VICTORIOUS! HOW TO GROW THROUGH GRIEF.
     Diane Kennedy Pike. Simon & Schuster,New York. 1976.
     Pocket Books, New York,1977.PB. 238pp. $ 1.95.

A relentlessly cheerful & positive approach.
The Joy of Grief.
**

304. LIFE-LINES. Lynn Caine. Doubleday,N.Y. 1977. $ 8.50.

Coping with loneliness as a woman alone; managing money and
business transactions,love affairs,disciplining the children,
and developing trust in other women.
***

305. LIFE OR DEATH--WHO CONTROLS? Ed. Nancy C. & John M.
      Ostheimer. Springer Publishing Company,NY. 1976.
      308 pp. $ 12.50, $ 7.95 PB.

An odd book,edited by a specialist in African
sociopolitics and his wife.Apart from 2 apparently original
essays,the other 22 chapters are reprints of articles 1st
published in journals in the early 1970's.Some are written
by recognizable experts,some are trivial products of
newspaper reporters & columnists. It deals with important
issues,however: Eugenics,abortion on demand,compulsory
sterilization, & euthanasia. The section on How to Die
includes a scrap of early Kubler-Ross & Mannes,& some
very light journalism. An irregular,mainly frothy,
unoriginal & unremarkable book.
**

306. LIFE-SPAN DEVELOPMENTAL PSYCHOLOGY (NORMATIVE LIFE
      Crises). Ed. Nancy Datan & Leon Ginsberg. Academic
      Press,New York. 1975. 314 pp.

Includes Kastenbaum on "Is Death a Life Crisis? (on the
confrontation with death in theory & practice);Lopata on
Widowhood, & Harshbarger on Death & Public Policy.
***

307. A LITTLE BOOK OF COMFORT. Ruth C.Ikerman. Abingdon,
      Nashville. 1976. 79 pp. $ 4.50.

A simple & practical book for the bereaved & their
companions,suggesting more constructive responses to
grief,within the Christian tradition.Some may find it
mawkish & sentimental;certainly some will find it helpful.
Better than one might have anticipated from the author of
"Meditations for Bird Lovers",prayers inspired by bird
watching.
**

308.   THE LITTLE BOOK OF LIFE AFTER DEATH.Gustav Theodor
       Fechner. Arno Press,NY. 1976. 108 pp. $ 12.00.

1st edition,Boston,1904. Translated from the German by
M.C.Wadsworth,with an introduction by William James.
Combining oriental & occidental concepts,Fechner outlines
possibly the first developmental approach to human identity
& death,& self-fulfillment.An oddly contemporary approach
in many respects.
***

309.   LIVING AND DYING. Robert Jay Lifton & Eric Olson.
       Praeger,NY 1974. $ 6.50,Bantam PB 1975.143pp.$1.95.

Intended as"part of a series for young readers", "an essay..
...as an introductory statement of our ideas for our
university students & colleagues".An attempt,in simple and
spare prose,to explore,in psychological and historical
perspective,why"death & life are painfully out of joint in
our time". Especially effective brief reviews of Lifton's
views on Symbolic Immortality & the impact of the nuclear
age on attitudes to death.Sometimes a mite over-inclusive
in its arguments.
****

310.   LIVING AND DYING AT MURRAY MANOR. Jaber E Gubrium.
       St Martin's Press,New York.1976. 221 pp. $ 8.95 PB.

Participant observation study of a nursing home,with
comments on aging,death & institutional care.Not special.
*

311.   LIVING POOR WITH STYLE.Ernest Callenbach.Bantam,NY.
       1972. 600pp. $ 1.95 PB.

Captioned "The Encyclopedia for Survival in the Seventies",
& "How to Live a Rich,Full Life--Cheap",this aimiable
book addresses itself to the management of a rational,simple,
alternative lifestyle,cheaply & economically,for the
deliberately or unwillingly poor.The final chapter deals
with Dying & Death,& such matters as "What must be done
when a death occurs",& "How to take on the Undertaker",
advocating simple burial. Succinct,practical & sensible .
***

312. LIVING—WHEN A LOVED ONE HAS DIED.Earl A.Grollman.
      Beacon Press,Boston. 1977. 114 pp. $ 9.60.

Somewhat disappointing,but a good try.Brief,verse-form
comments on grief--shock,suffering,recovery & a new life.
Awfully dull photo illustrations.But with Grollman's
usual insight & empathy.
***

313. LIVING WITH A MAN WHO IS DYING.Jocelyn Evans.
      Taplinger Publishing Co.,NY.1971. 143 pp. $ 5.95.

An observant & matter-of-fact account of the last months
of the life of Aron Evans,(a pseudonym),who died at 33 of
abdominal cancer.Though handled clumsily by the medical
profession,the Evans" managed to achieve a relatively
dignified & ultimately peaceful death at home. An example
of how badly even well-meaning doctors can handle the
problems of terminal illness,& how a loving family can in
part ameliorate this.
***

314. LIVING WITH CANCER.Ernest H.Rosenbaum. Praeger,NY.
      1975. 214 pp. $ 10.00.

A graceful,humane book,consisting mainly of eleven
detailed case-histories of cancer patients of differing
personalities & lifestyles;& interviews with nurses,social
workers,volunteers & clergymen.Though repetitive at times,
it deals straight-forwardly with the problems of life with
cancer. While describing dying,it emphasizes the positive
aspects of terminal living.
****

315. LIVING WITH DEATH. Osborn Sederberg. Dutton,NY.
      1976. 132 pp. $ 7.50.

Discussion of psychological problems of death for younger
readers---very general,not very interesting.Nothing new.
It's not clear what age-group it is best meant for,if any.
**

316.   <u>LIVING YOUR DYING</u>.Stanley Keleman. Random House /
       Bookworks,San Francisco. 1974/75. 158 pp. PB. $ 3.95.

Jacketed in excessive praise ; this frothy,repetitious,light,
vague & wandering volume offers an unremittently jolly
approach to death."Sexuality is almost a training for dying"
..."Every act of sex is like an act of dying---its converse
should also,could also,be true"..."Is there a person alive
who would not like their dying full of excitement?" Well,
I for one would appreciate a more peaceful end.Unlearned,
unreal,a very Sixties book,published well after its time;
the epitome of the plastic & tinsel fluorescence of
sloppy pop psychology. However,the friends & reviewers
cited by the publishers insist that it is required reading
for all philosophers,all physicians,all patients,& anyone
else you can lay your hands on. He has"achieved the
unimaginable:he has given us back dying" (well,thanks Stan);
if enough people lived by it,"it could change the world" ;
"perhaps the most important work of its kind in our
generation". Even Gods are usually more modest than this.
*

317.   <u>LONELINESS: THE EXPERIENCE OF EMOTIONAL & SOCIAL</u>
       <u>ISOLATION</u>. Robert S.Reiss. M.I.T.Press,Cambridge,
       Mass. 1973. 250 pp. $ 8.95, $ 6.95 PB.

Considers both emotional loneliness caused by the absence
of a specific loved person,& social isolation resulting
from severance from a group.
***

318.   <u>LONG-TERM CARE OF OLDER PEOPLE: A Practical Guide</u>.
       Elaine M.Brody. Human Sciences Press,NY.1977.402 pp.

A generally competent & practical guide to many aspects of
long-term care of the elderly,dealing with the development
& planning of long-term facilities,& the provision of social
work services for such facilities.Incredibly,there are less
than 5 pages dealing with dying & death,in a very wishy-
-washy fashion;& bereavement is neglected completely.These
are major & inexcusable omissions,& fail to reflect much
important & relevant work that has been done in this area.
*

319. LOSS AND CHANGE. Peter Marris. Pantheon Books,New York
      Random House,NY. 1974. 190 pp. $ 7.95. Routledge &
      Kegan Paul,London. Doubleday-Anchor PB 1975. $ 2.95.

An imaginative,original & significant study by a highly
competent sociologist (author of the earlier "Widows &
their Families").It deals with the effects of loss in the
context of serious personal & social change.He describes the
"conservative impulse",a need to maintain continuity in goals
& relationships.Includes a study of widows;the effects of
urban redevelopment,destroying familiar environments,tribal
problems in Nigeria,& other examples.
***

320. LOSS AND GRIEF : PSYCHOLOGICAL MANAGEMENT IN MEDICAL
      PRACTICE. Ed.B.Schoenberg,A.C.Carr,D.Peretz,& A.H.
      Kutscher. Columbia University Press,NY. 1970.
      PB 400 pp. $ 4.95. £ 5.80.

Strongly recommended.Deals with the broader issues of
reactions to loss of different kinds,including loss of
limb,organ,sensory loss orloss of sexual function;also
with the reactions to death in the patient,family,& the
health care team. A very high standard of contributions from
a distinguished group of authors. A 45-item annotated
bibliography.
*****

321. THE LOSS OF A LOVED ONE.D.M.Moriarty. C.C.Thomas,
      Springfield. 1967. $ 8.50.

Psychoanalytic in orientation,& concerned with the
traumatic effect of a death in the family on the surviving
children,& on personality development,with case histories.
Not recommended.
*

322. LOVE...AND DEATH.Abraham Kaplan. University of Michigan
      Press,Ann Arbor. 1973.(Longman,Canada).100pp.$ 5.95.

Eleven 'Talks on Contemporary & Perennial Themes"--love,
women,religion,morals,technology,free speech,unreason,
loneliness,mental health,aging,& death--by Dr Kaplan.Gentle,
humane,wise,acute & perceptive;originally a series of talks
on television,they have an unusually high titre of sense &
simple style. Many of them are relevant to thanatology.
***½

323. THE LOVED ONE. Evelyn Waugh. Dell,NY. PB $ 0.75.
      & other editions.

Brilliant,macabre,ferocious novel on Hollywood burial
customs;Mr.Joyboy,Mortuary Hostesses,& Whispering Glades.
Almost as sickly as the real thing can be.
****

324. LOVE MUST NOT BE WASTED.Isabella Taves. Thomas Crowell,
      New York.Fitzhenry & Whiteside,Canada.1974/75.214 pp.
      $ 8.00.

Another of the too rapidly growing genre of literate woman
writer's personal accounts of bereavement & widowhood,even
if a relatively good specimen.A"Woman's book" in the non-
-pejorative sense.Sincere,a little circuitous & repetitious
at times. These books,by the nature of their authors,tend to
deal with the experiences of rather unusual,highly capable
career women rather than being typical of the needs of all
women.
***½

325. MAKE TODAY COUNT.Orville E.Kelly. Delacorte Press,NY.
      1975. 203 pp. $ 7.95.

In 1973,Orville learned he had a lymphoma.He ultimately came
to terms with his illness,& founded Make Today Count, an
organization for dying patients & their families.Here he
tells his own story.Sincere & sentimental,sometimes
simplistic,sometimes self-indulgent.Would be more impressive
if the blurb were less absurdly hyperbolic,e.g."For as many
generations as are left upon the earth,this book will alter
attitudes". Does any book merit that puffery? Really?
**½

326. MAMA'S GHOSTS. Carol Lee Lorenzo. (illustrated by
      E.Keith. Harper & Row,New York. 1974. $ 4.95.

Fiction,for 4 to 6 year-olds. Ellie's much loved
grandmother is dying,but able to help her learn to
relinquish even someone she loves.
***

327. MAN AGAINST HIMSELF. Karl Menninger. (Harcourt,Brace
     & World,1938) Harvest Books,1966. 430 pp. $ 1.95 PB.

A great classic survey of Eros & Thanatos--death,suicide,
chronic suicide (asceticism & martyrdom,neurotic invalidism,
alcoholism,anti-social behavior & psychosis);focal suicide
(self-mutilation,malingering,polysurgery,purposive accidents,
impotence & frigidity) & organic suicide(psychological
factors in organic disease). Brilliantly integrative,
fascinatingly chatty & anecdotal.Highly influential.
****

328. THE MANAGEMENT OF MALIGNANT DISEASE. Ed. Cicely
     Saunders. Edward Arnold,London. 1978. 200 pp.

Contributions include Cicely Saunders on Appropriate
Treatment,Appropriate Death; chapters on pathological,
psychological & physical aspects of malignant disease.
Murray Parkes on the psychology involved,Twycross on Relief
of Pain,& Robbie on Nerve Blocks;control of other symptoms;
radiotherapy & cytotoxic & hormone palliation;& palliative
surgery.Tom West describes inpatient management in a
hospice,& Barbara McNulty describes outpatient & domiciliary
management based on a hospice.Other sections deal with the
General Practitioner,terminal care in the National Health
Service,& moral & legal issues. Dr.Saunders' closing
chapter discusses her philosophy of care. Undoubtedly a
major & valuable contribution to the clinical management of
cancer,which should complement other books. This book
deals with cancer,& not the problems of other terminal
illnesses,which is perhaps a pity-& it deals with the
British scene & National Health Service alone.
****

329. MANAGEMENT OF THE DYING PATIENT & HIS FAMILY.
     MSS Information Corp.,NY.1974. 198pp. $ 17.00.

An almost random assortment of reprints.Some good--Feifel,
Verwoerdt;many weak & repetitious & unoriginal. Despite
the title,it almost entirely neglects the family point of
view. Some of Maddison & Quint's work is included.
**

330. MAN AND LIFE:A Sesquicentennial Symposium. Ed.Charles
      D.Aring. University of Cincinnati Press, 1969. 92 pp.

If only reports of symposia & the like represented an
organized synthesis of what was said,bravely omitting the
minutiae of discussion! An able & well above average
collection including Jacques Barzun on the Quality of Life,
Rene Dubos on Biological Limitations of Freedom & ethical
issues, David Bazelon on legal aspects,& Michael DeBakey on
his own point of view.
***

331. MAN DOES SURVIVE DEATH: THE WELCOMING SILENCE.
      D.Scott Pego. Citadel Press (Lyle Stuart Inc).
      191 pp. $ 3.95 . PB. (1973 1st published as The
      Welcoming Silence).

There's really not enough substance in this wispy,frail
book to comment upon. Not recommended for any purpose.
The welcome it deserves....is silence?
*

332. MAN'S CONCERN WITH DEATH.Arnold Toynbee & others.
      Hodder & Stoughton,London. 1968. 280 pp. £ 2.25.

One of the early & persisting classics of the Death Lit.
Among its competent chapters are several by Ninian Smart on
philosophical & religious concepts,Keith Mant on the medical
definition of death,Simon Yudkin on death & the young,& Eric
Rhode on death in 20th century fiction.But best of all are
the splendid chapters by Arnold Toynbee,erudite & elegant
& superbly literate.The Epilogue,a moving account of
Toynbee's personal experiences & his feelings about the
imminent prospect of death,is especially poignant reading.
*****

333. A MANUAL OF DEATH EDUCATION & SIMPLE BURIAL.Ernest
      Morgan. Celo Press,Burnsville,NC. 1977.8th edition.
      PB. 64 pp. $ 2.00.

Still good.Maybe a bit more sensible & better organized; a
succinct guide & aperitif.Includes sections on coping with
the dying,& grief,ground rules for self-termination(I
wonder why they can't say Suicide?),& some teaching tips
for death education & role-play;details of funeral &
memorial societies with a directory of addresses;simple
burial & cremation & how to do it;& how the dead can help
the living,with organ donations. The Death Ed.section
needs improvement.
***

334. MASTECTOMY: A PATIENT'S GUIDE TO COPING WITH BREAST
      SURGERY. Nancy Robinson & Ian Smith. Thorsons.
      1977. 128 pp. £ 3.95 ; £ 2.50 PB.

Subtitled:"What to expect & how to adapt to life afterwards,
from a practical & psychological point of view". What to
expect in hospital;surgery or radiation;prostheses,clothes,
physiotherapy;reactions of family; with case histories.
***

335. THE MATTHEW TREE. H.T.Wright. Pantheon Books,NY.
      1975. 115 pp. $ 5.95.

An American 'A Very Easy Death'.Mrs. Wright(a pseudonym)
writes movingly of her father's last seven years of death
& multiple strokes.Not morbid,self-pitying of sentimental,
but honest,good-humoured & graceful. "Why?",the father keeps
asking; and,later, "Please".
****½

336. THE MEANING OF DEATH. Ed. H.Feifel. McGraw-Hill,NY.
      1959 / 1965. 350pp. PB. $ 2.95.

Good selection of classical articles on death---Jung,Tillich,
Marcuse; death & literature,art & religion;& clinical &
experimental studies. Representative & useful,influential
& significant. The book which played a large part in
arousing the current interest in death.
****

337. MEDIA GUIDE ON DEATH & DYING. Anonymous.
      Biomedical Communications,NY.1978. $ 6.00.

A briefly descriptive bibliography of some 200 films,tapes,
& slide programs.
***

338. THE MEDICAL ANNUAL,1976. Ed.R.B.Scott & J.Fraser.
      John Wright & Sons,Bristol. 1976. 492 pp.£ 11.00.

The 94th issue of an annual Year-book of Treatment.Its
chapters contain competent reviews of advances in therapy
in all areas of medicine including oncology,not always as
up-to-date as one would wish (too many 1973 &'74 references
for a late 1976 book).The editing is sub-standard & many
sections contain sloppy grammar & sheer bad English.There's
a reasonable review of recent advances in the chemotherapy
of cancer by J.M.A.Whitehouse,& a useful chapter on Care of
Patients with Terminal Malignant Disease by Albertine

338 ctd.) Winner & Cicely Saunders.This is unfortunately
brief,but includes the useful appendix on the drugs used
at St Christopher's for symptom control.A good chapter in
an uneven book.
***

339. MEDICAL HUBRIS ; A REPLY TO IVAN ILLICH. David F.
      Horrobin. Eden Press,Montreal. 1977. 146 pp. $ 9.00.

An uncompromising response to Illich's Medical Nemesis,
accepting most of his criticisms of the state of medicine,
but challenging his understanding of the causes & his
proposals for change.Able argument,convincingly displaying
the weaknesses & striking inconsistencies of Illich's
claims.He includes a chapter on "Death against Death",
dealing with Illich's fascination for death.He identifies
the oddities of historical perspective used,& the emptiness
of some of the rhetorical flourishes.Elsewhere,he demolishes
the curiously sadistic view of pain which Illich advanced,
so lacking in compassion.If pain is really so beneficial
as Illich says,we should share it out more democratically;
and not let the poor have more than their fair share.
***

340. MEDICAL NEMESIS :The Expropriation of Health.Ivan
      Illich. Pantheon Books,NY.1976.275 pp. $ 8.95. Also
      Bantam,New York, 1977. PB. $ 2.50.

A new edition of the Malleus Maleficarum of Medicine,as
prepared by a small & well-equipped Mexican inquisition;
the work of many Inquisitors,presented under the name of
the Savanarola of the Seventies (or maybe the Machiavelli?)
It includes a fine chapter on death in a historical
perspective by Valentina Borreman.While lacking a really
comprehensive understanding of the area,her familiarity
with some of the historical & European literature is good.
***

341. MODERN TRENDS IN PSYCHOSOMATIC MEDICINE -3. Ed.Oscar
      W.Hill. Butterworths,London. 1976. 520pp. £ 14.00.

A collection of detailed reviews of areas of psychosomatic
medicine,some very relevant to clinical thanatology.John
Hinton provides a very perceptive chapter on "Approaching
Death",dealing with psychiatric symptoms,awareness,adjustment,
coping & maladjustment.Raphael & Maddison write an uncommonly
helpful chapter on The Care of Bereaved Adults.Other useful
sections deal with Autohypnosis,Birley & Connolly on Life

341 ctd.) Events & Physical Illness (competent but limited)
and Merskey on the nature of pain (though disappointing in
ignoring its treatment). Other chapters show a great lack
of balance,often excessively beating the author's own drum,
rather than genuinely reviewing the field.Often over-long
& very idiosyncratic such as Lum on anxiety as
hyperventilation & Carroll on psychendocrine aspects of
affective illness (obsessed with his own work on Cortisol).
Two sections are of questionable value to the book:Gower's
excellent but misplaced review of Pheromones (of minimal
relevance),& a wierd piece on health beliefs in rural
Guatemala. A thoughtlessly edited book with a few valuable
chapters.
**$\frac{1}{2}$

342.   MORAL DILEMMAS IN MEDICINE.A Coursebook in Ethics for
       Doctors & Nurses. A.V.Campbell. 2nd Edition.
       Churchill Livingstone. 1975. 210pp. £ 1.95.

A straight-forward,readable account of basic ethics,with
an agreeable balance between theoretical & practical issues.
Discusses issues like the individual conscience & the common
good,the concepts of happiness & justice,laws,rules and
situations;natural & unnatural;applying rules to cases;
freedom of choice,responsibility & determinism;self-interest
& benevolence— all issues of general clinical significance
which few doctors understand adequately.Current problems
considered include priorities of health care (too briefly),
abortion,resuscitation & euthanasia,human experimentation,
& transplantation. There is a limited bibliography.
***$\frac{1}{2}$

343.   MORE THAN YOU DARE ASK. The first year of living with
       Cancer. McN.& Anne Shaw Turnage. John Knox Press,
       Atlanta. 1976. 114 pp. $ 6.95.

An unusual & idiosyncratic account of the first year of
living with cancer by Ann & her minister husband.A sort of
inspirational diary & collage,with scraps of narrative,
correspondence,prayers,leditations,attractively presented.
Sometimes rather cloying & over-sweet,usually realistically
questioning,as a guide to practical faith.In some respects
too zealously stresses the miracle-seeking rather than the
simple acceptance of what is happening.
***

344. THE MOTHER,ANXIETY & DEATH: The Catastrophic Death
      Complex. J.C.Rheingold. Little,Brown,Boston.1967.271pp.

Three interrelated subjects are considered: the mother-child
relationship,the meaning of anxiety,& the psychology of
death.Rheingold describes the Catastrophic Death Complex (a
primary fear of mutilation & annihilation) with wide
possible relevance to the pathology & therapy of the
neuroses,to understanding the roots of basic anxiety,& of
maternal fantasies & acts of filicide.A broad & relatively
non-doctrinaire synthesis of wide interest to specialists
in thanatology,psychiatry & psychology.
***$\frac{1}{2}$

345. MURDER IN SPACE CITY: A Cultural Analysis of Houston
      Homicide Patterns. Henry P.Lundsgaarde.Oxford
      University Press,Oxford & NY. 1977.226 pp. £ 8.00.

In 1969 nearly 300 people in Houston,Texas,were victims of
homicide,yet less than half of the killers received any
substantial official punishment.This book trys to understand
why,using techniques of cultural anthropology to study
homicide in the modern urban community;exploring the social
context of such violent deaths;& the police,medical,
political & judicial procedures for handling such cases.
***

346. MY BROTHER DEATH.Cyrus Sulzberger. Arno Press,NY.
      1976. (1st Publ.Harpers,NY,1961).226 pp. $ 16.00.

A bizarre assembly of personal meditations on themes of
death;rather like a forerunner of the 20th Century Book of
the Dead--often macabre & chillingly matter-of-fact.There
are reviews of cultural implications of death-;of Saints &
their martyrdoms from Benjamin the impaled to Mary of Egypt
who ate only lentils;the deaths of Kings;religious
persecutions;death in battle,or by starvation.It concerns
itself with the recent constitutional problems attending
the eating of a Senator by his constituents,& with runic
symbols. Wierdly memorable.
****

347. THE MYTH OF SISYPHUS. Albert Camus. Vintage/Random
      House,NY. 1961. 150pp. $ 1.50 PB. (1955 edition,
      Alfred A.Knopf.Originally Le Mythe de Sisyphe.
      Librairie Gallimard,Paris,1942).

On absurdity & suicide,philosophical suicide & absurd
freedom,absurd man & creation.A keywork on the philosophy
of suicide & death. "There is but one truly serious
philosophical problem,& that is suicide.Judging whether
life is or is not worth living amounts to answering the
fundamental question of philosophy.".
***

N
348. NATIONAL DIRECTORY OF THE FOUNDATION OF THANATOLOGY.
      Foundation of Thanatology,New York. $ 7.50.

A very expensive listing of 164 "thanatology-oriented"
people from various disciplines,in 35 U.S.States & Canada.
Only relatively few are recognized experts or leaders in the
field.I cannot imagine for what purpose this Directory might
be useful to anyone.
*

349. NATURAL SALVATION: The Message of Science,Outlining
      the First Principles of Immortal Life on the Earth.
      Charles Asbury Stephens. Arno Press,NY. 1976.
      184 pp. $ 14.00. (1st published 1905).

An American physician who argued that the Christian promise
of salvation from death might be accomplished in secular
form by scientific progress.An early pioneer of Gerontology,
this was his final work.Includes 2 biographical essays,
setting his work into personal & historical context.
**

350. THE NATURE OF MAN: Studies in Optimistic Philosophy.
      Elie Metchnikoff. Arno Press,NY.1976.343 pp. $ 21.00.

Lst published 1910.The book in which Metchnikoff introduced
the modern usage of the terms Thanatology & Gerontology.His
essays on the scientific study of aging & death,& methods of
ameliorating the suffering & fear of death,are basically
optimistic & positive in outlook.
***

351.   NEW ENGLAND CEMETARIES.Andrew Kull. Stephen Greene
       Press,Brattleboro,Vermont.1975.224pp.$ 9.95,$ 5.95 PB.

A guidebook to 262 New England cemetaries,how to find them
& what to look for in them,with regard to old cemetary art.
With detailed maps.
**

352.   NEW MEANINGS OF DEATH .Ed. Herman Feifel. McGraw-Hill,
       N.Y., 1977. 367 pp. $ 11.95.Also in PB.

A splendid volume---even more interesting & accessible than
Feifel's 1959 classic.Includes Feifel on Death in
contemporary America;Kastenbaum on death & development
through the life-span; Bluebond-Langner on meanings of
death to children; Shneidman on death & the college student;
Weisman on the Psychiatrist & the Inexorable;Garfield on the
personal impact of death on the clinician; Saunders on St.
Christophers again;Kelly on Make Today Count;Kalish on death
& the family;Leviton on death education;Lifton on immortality,
Simpson on death & poetry;Gutman on death & power;Shaffer &
Rodes on death & the law.Also Raether & Slater on "Immediate
Postdeath activities in the U.S.',offering us 5 stages of
funeralization (oh dear,oh dear),& make some unsubstantiated
claims. The weakest chapter by far,but forgiveable amidst
such riches.
*****

353.   NIGHT SEASON.Christiaan Barnard & Sigfried Stander.
       Hutchinson,London. 1977. £ 4.95.

As a novelist,Barnard is a great surgeon.Somewhat overblown
story of Charles de la Porte who diagnoses inoperable cancer
in a young woman doctor he had once loved.He decides she
will be happier left in ignorance of her approaching death,
but she finds out & her husband sues him for malpractice.He
dabbles in a guerilla group,& explores a little of the
problem of the white South African would-be liberal,as
well as issues of dying & euthanasia. The pen is not
mightier than the scalpel.
**

354.   NO MORE DYING:The Conquest of Aging & The Extension of
       Human Life. J.Kurtzman & Phillip Gordon.Tarcher,LA.1976
       188 pp. $ 7.95. Dell Publ.,NY.1976.250pp. $ 1.95,PB.

The announcement of the death of death is a mite premature.
A breathless rush through trends & fancies.
*

355. NORMAL & PATHOLOGICAL RESPONSES TO BEREAVEMENT.
     MSS Publ.Corp.,NY. 1974. 238 pp. $ 19.50.

One of the most useful volumes in this weak series.Papers
include Volkan on pathological grief & linking objects,the
mourning responses of parents on the death of a newborn
infant;anniversary responses to sibling death in childhood;
psychiatric sequelae of the Sudden Infant Death Syndrome
& spontaneous abortion-& 3 very overlapping papers by
Maddison on conjugal bereavement.Many major omissions.
***

356. NOT ALONE WITH CANCER.A Guide for Those who Care;
     What to Expect,What to Do. Ruth D.Abrams. Charles C.
     Thomas,Springfield.1974.2nd printing 1976.128pp.$4.95.

Written by a psychiatric social worker with some 25 years
experience of working with cancer patients & their families.
In a conversational style,& based in good part on her
previous publications,it discusses means of coping and
communicating among patients with cancer at different
stages (localized,regional involvement,& advanced).A
compassionate monograph.
***

357. NOT DYING: A Psychoanalysit's Memoir of his Wife's
     Death. F.Robert Rodman. Random House,NY.1977.216pp.
$ 7.95.

Very disappointing book with no advantages over the many
others of precisely this type.
**

358. THE NURSE & THE DYING PATIENT.Jeanne C.Quint.
     Macmillan & Co.,NY.1967. 307 pp. $ 3.15. PB.

Paperback re-issue of this soundly practical & observant
book which focusses on what happens to the student nurse
when she encounters dying patients,& how she can be prepared
to cope more effectively with the problems that arise.Many
references to the nursing literature;practical advice on
patient management & on the implications for schools of
nursing.Profusely illustrated with comments of nurses and
patients.
****

359.   THE NURSE AS CAREGIVER FOR THE TERMINAL PATIENT & HIS
       FAMILY.Ed.A.M.Earle,N.T.Argondizzo & A.H.Kutscher.
       Foundation of Thanatology,NY;Columbia University Press
       N.Y. 1976. $ 17.50.

Based on the proceedings of a Symposium,including a course
outline & a reading list,proposed as models for adoption.
By no means are they suitable models.Mildly interesting
at best.
**

360.   NURSING CARE OF THE CHILD WITH LONG-TERM ILLNESS.
       Ed.Shirley Steele. 2nd.edition. Appleton-Century-
       Crofts,New York. 1977.560pp. $ 23.50, £ 14.80.

A popular text,dealing with chronic respiratory,kidney,skin,
cardiac & endocrine problems.The new edition includes better
discussions of sexuality & the disabled,medical ethics,and
an expanded & revised section on cancer in childhood.
Chapter 13 deals reasonably competently with the nursing
care of the child with a fatal prognosis.
***

361.   NURSING THE DYING PATIENT.(Learning Processes for
       Interaction).Charlotte Epstein.Teston Publ.Co.,
       (Prentice-Hall) NY. 1975. 210 pp. £ 5.55.

This book says practically nothing about Nursing the Dying
Patient.Throughout,it is guilty of the stereotyped,
sentimental,uncritical & grossly oversimplified thinking it
theoretically condemns in others.Steeped in jargon,it
claims that the dying patient suffers "an enormous injustice"
if cared for "by those who have not been compelled to
contemplate their own deaths".(Ve haf vays off making you
contemplate!) Clinical care is totally ignored.The entire
emphasis is on interaction ("find the dying person down the
street...and interact with them" Yeeeugghh!) The author
seems to have read no further than Kavanaugh,Kubler-Ross,and
Glaser 'n Strauss,despite a 'Selected Bibliography' which
lists numerous unavailable works; she appears to believe
that there are only"two or three well-known names in the
field" who are "natural teachers"— and that there is no
other successful teaching in medical faculties— an
incredibly ignorant point of view,showing very negligent
preparation for a book of this nature.Horrifyingly
simplistic in its interpretation of this field of

361 ctd.) understanding,it applies its limited ideas with
extremist rigidity.Thou shalt go through 5 stages; Thou
shalt talk about thy death ("Sit for a moment & think about
all this,trying to feel the sense of shock that fills you")
"It is undeniably true that being with a dying person makes
it more difficult for us to deny our own mortality" : a
sort of Holiness by Osmosis.The nursing ideal portrayed
(the correct answer,indeed,to one of the Multiple Choice
Questions,is"Come back again & again,each time saying only
'I'm available when you want me'") is oddly unpractical.
Totally uncritical & unacademic,it makes Totems of Kubler-
Ross' stages of dying and Kavanaugh's(whose?) stages of
Grieving (which are thoroughly unoriginal).There is absurd
reification ,speaking of"Kavanaugh's guilt"(he may well be
guilty,but that's his business),and Kavanaugh's fifth stage
of loss & loneliness" (never speak for yourself,when you
can stand on the fine clay feet of another).The Dying
Trajectory is misunderstood,& its brief discussion
illustrated by erroneous & irrelevant examples. In general,
the book gives incredibly brief accounts of a few aspects
of the vast field of current knowledge of dying,then proposes
a repetitive series of games,role-play & pseudo-simulation
exercises,discussing possible outcomes & responses to the
games (except nausea).It relies on group work,and is
inapplicable to individual study. A very disappointing book,
which revels with onanistic glee in rolling about in one's
own true feelings ("Wrap yourself around the thought of
your own dying");it quite ignores the disadvantages & even
risks of "compelling"students to confront issues they may
not be ready or able to handle.There is no consideration of
the personal difficulties that such emotional and
sentimental orgies can arouse.This is unhelpful &
irresponsible.
*

0
362. ON BECOMING A WIDOW.Clarissa Start. Family Library,NY.
      1968/1973. 124 pp. $ 0.95 ¢.

Another widowed journalist's book.Brief,frank,& mildly
helpful,to a point.
***

363. ON DEATH AND DYING. Elizabeth Kubler-Ross. Macmillan,
      NY. 1968.$ 7.95,$ 2.25 PB.250pp. Tavistock,London,
      1973 paperback edition £ 1.30.

Strongly recommended.A classic & highly influential work,in
which Dr Ross advanced her model of the"5 Stages" in the
progress of the dying patient.Interesting & humane,with
sound practical advice & transcripts of some interviews.
*****

364. ON DYING AND DENYING.Avery Weisman. Behavioral Publ.,
      New York. 1972. $ 12.95.

A very significant study of "terminality",concentrating on
the central role of denial.Very competent & illustrated
with many clinical examples. Of the highest quality both
intellectually & practically.
*****

365. ON DYING WELL: An Anglican Contribution to the
      Debate on Euthanasia. Lord Amulree,et al. Church
      Information Office,London. 1975. 76 pp.   85 pence.

A consideration of euthanasia from the point of view of the
Anglican Church,rejecting the case for voluntary euthanasia,
arguing that there should be other means of "exercising care
& compassion towards a person in his dying & of relieving
his ultimate distress",& focussing concern more on the
quality of terminal care.Produced by a distinguished Working
Party from medicine & theology,it considers moral,theological
& legal aspects of the question,& some case histories.
***

366. ON THE THEOLOGY OF DEATH. Karl Rahner. Seabury Press,
      New York. 1961. 119 pp. $ 2.95 PB.

An explanation of Catholic theological research and theory
on various aspects of death. This is not *the* theology of
death,by the way,Dr Rahner, but *a* theology of death.
**$\frac{1}{2}$

367. ORAL CARE OF THE AGING & DYING PATIENT.Ed. A.H.
      Kutscher & I.K.Goldberg. American Lecture Series.
      C.C.Thomas,Springfield,Illinois. 1973.

Incredible thanatokitsch. "With the Dentist At The Gates",
and "Use of an Electrically Driven Toothbrush in the
Management of Oral Hygiene in the Dying Patient". If one
didn't know better,one might suspect that this was a work
of brilliantly witty satire. But it isn't.
*

368. THE ORIGIN OF DEATH :Studies in African Mythology.
      Hans Abrahamsson. Arno Press,NY. 1976. 178 pp. $ 15.00.

1st edition Uppsala,1951. A comprehensive,detailed and
competent study of death myths,in the tradition of Baumann
& Frazer;the life-and-death myths in African culture.Avoids
the ethnocentrism of European value systems & ideologies.
Classifies the myths with which man seeks to explain the
origin of death,into such general types as "The message
that failed",& personifications of death,examining their
distribution,similarities and differences.Death is often
seen as due to a mistake,or a punishment; but is sometimes
seen as desirable & sought-after.
***

369. OVERCOMING THE FEAR OF DEATH.D.C.Gordon. Pelican PB,
      Penguin Books,Harmondsworth & Baltimore. 1972.
      115 pp. $ 1.25.

Analyses a cluster of other fears composing the fear of
death—— including fear of losing time,of decay, the
unknown,& irreversibility;fear of life,loss of self,loss of
pleasure,cessation of thought. He argues that human
behavior is aimed at attaining "peak experiences" in which
man is unified with himself,others & the world—— and
death should be welcomed as the ultimate fulfilling
experience.
**

370. OVER THEIR DEAD BODIES: Yankee Epitaphs & History.
      Thomas C.Mann & Janet Greene. Stephen Greene Press,
      Brattleboro,Vermont. Illus. 1962.116 pp. & 4.95.

A collection of interesting epitaphs & tombstones,in some
sort of historical perspective.
**

P

371.   PARASUICIDE.Ed. N.Kreitman. John Wiley & Sons.NY.
        1978. 193 pp. $ 21.95, £ 8.90.

The problem of parasuicide;the clinical,psychological and
social circumstances of parasuicide patients,with some
recommendations for prevention and care. Has received
several unfavourable reviews,& is disappointing.Not very
helpful about management.
***

372.   PASSING ON : The Social Organization of Dying.David
        Sudnow. Prentice-Hall,Englewood Cliffs,NJ. 1967
        176 pp. $ 4.20 PB.

Excellent sociological study of death in a county hospital
& its management by the staff;including counting of deaths
& their visibility,social death,preparing & moving bodies,
how we announce death & bad news;uses of a corpse,etc.
Fascinating reading,introducing a new way of looking at
what we do. Strongly recommended.
*****

373.   PASTORAL CARE OF THE DYING & BEREAVED:SELECTED
        READINGS. Ed. R.B.Reeves,R.E.Neale,& A.H.Kutscher.
        Health Sciences Publ.,NY. 1973. 160pp. $ 3.95.

A generally useful collection of 19 reprinted articles,
mainly from Pastoral Psychology & the Journal of Religion
& Health. Not always clearly or legibly printed.
***

374.   THE PASTOR'S IDEAL FUNERAL MANUAL.Ed. Nolan B.Harmon.
        Abingdon Press,Nashville. 1970. 224 pp. $ 2.95.

Prayers & the order of service for Episcopal,Presbyterian
& Methodist funerals,with Biblical reference list.
**

375.   THE PATIENT,DEATH & THE FAMILY.Ed. S.B.Troup and
        W.A.Greene. Charles Scribner's Sons,NY. 1974.
        172 pp. $ 9.25.

A collection of essays emerging from a 1971 Rochester
conference.Includes Robert Jay Lifton on Symbolic
Immortality ; George Engel on Signs of Giving Up;Avery
Weisman succinctly practical on Care & Comfort for the

375 ctd.) Dying; Anselm Strauss summarising his views on
trajectories of dying; & the playwright Robert Anderson's
Notes of a Survivor,telling of the pain of deception in
dealing with his dying wife. An unusually un-hackneyed book.
Brief & stimulating,though with out profound depth.
***

376. PATIENTS : LIFE & DEATH in the Modern Hospital.
     Polly Toynbee.(Published in Britain as'Hospital')
     Harcourt,Brace,Jovanovich,N.Y.1977.278pp. $ 8.95.

After'Airport',& 'Wheels',comes'Patient'. Plain reporting of
some of the events in a reasonably typical Teaching Hospital
--in the Maternity & Paediatric Wards,a general surgical
clinic,a general medical ward,Emergency Ward,Orthopaedic
Clinic,Nephrology Unit,& Geriatric dept.Cinema verite in
words.Occasional unnecessary errors;frequent unneeded
romanticising (these events don't need emotional or
dramatic tarting up);& too much recourse to cliches (
especially of the noble,heroic,nurse-angel).But it still
effectively portrays the hospital experience of life and
death,& exposes some of the gritty realities(as in regard
to artificial kidneys & transplants,& the grimness of
geriatric life) that are often ignored by the rarified
ethicists. A patient asks how long her kidney transplant
will last.The doctor pats her arm:"Don't worry.It'll last
the rest of your life". Well yes,but... A patient on renal
dialysis speaks about how easily he could give up & let
himself "accidentally"bleed to death. Not especially well-
-written,but the patients themselves are memorable.
***

377. P.D.A.(PERSONAL DEATH AWARENESS).Breaking Free of Fear
     to Live a Better Life NOW. J.William Worden & William
     Proctor. Prentice-Hall,N.J. 1976. 196 pp. $ 7.95.

How disappointing! A breathless,hectoring.exclamatory gallop
through Thanatology.PDA is an unhappy invention,an unreal
phenomenon that is poorly defined & conceptualized,and
awfully unhelpful.Prescriptive & directive—your PDA must
not be too high or too low— while promising you freedom
"immediately & in the future".Indeed,the reader is assured
of "an entirely new insight into life",which will "help
make your future years even more meaningful & rewarding.
You can gain"freedom to recycle yourself" (I am looking
forward to that one!) and "freedom to choose where". Full

377. ctd.) of conversations & extraordinarily unmemorable
quotes from nonentities,with rather tedious little
exercises & games.This really does not do justice to the
qualities of the senior author.
*

378. PERSISTENT PAIN: MODERN METHODS OF TREATMENT. Vol.1.
     Ed. Sampson Lipton. Academic Press,NY. 1977.
     272 pp. £ 10.50.

None chapters on practical aspects of the treatment of
various types of chronic pain:percutaneous cordotomy by
Ganz & Mullan;spinal(intrathecal) & extradural analgesia
by Maher & Mehta;Acupuncture by Mann;psychiatric
management by Merskey;Surgery by Miles;Pituitary
Neuroadenolysis by Moricca;peripheral nerve blocks by
Swerdlow;& drug therapy by Williams. Less emphasis than
one would wish on the rwlative merits of the different
therapiesor on the rationale of choice of methods.
***

379. PERSPECTIVES ON DEATH.Ed.L.O.Mills. Abingdon Press,
     Nashville. 1969. 288pp. $ 6.50,PB $ 4.95.

Heavy & exceedingly dull.Covers important areas including
death in the Hebrew bible & Apocalyptic literature,New
Testament,& the Early Church;death & transcendance in
contemporary literature;psychiatric,social,pastoral &
ethical perspectives. But very verbose and unnecessarily
dull.
**

380. THE PHENOMENON OF DEATH :Faces of Mortality.Ed. E.
     Wyschogrod. Harper Colphon Books,NY.1973.235pp.$3.45.

Valuable collection of papers.Some good (LeShan,Kubler-Ross,
Lifton),some ordinary;& some pretentious & forced,like
Wyschogrod herself in"Sport,Death & the Elemental",and
Lamont on the "Double Apprenticeship".They're awful.
**½

381. THE PHYSICIAN & THE DANCE OF DEATH.A Historical Study
     of the Evolution of the Dance of Death Mythus in Art.
     Aldred Scott Warthin. Arno Press,NY. 1976.142pp.$12.00.

A richly illustrated & fascinating book,examining such
themes as Death and hubris (death claiming the doctor
himself),death as egalitarian leveller,& familiarity with

381 ctd.) death providing freedom from anxiety.Illustrated
from the great early murals,pre-Holbein manuscripts, block
books & incunabula, Holbein & the great Renaissance Dance,
his imitators in the Rococo period, Durer & Rethal,the 18th
& 19th century caricatures,& the impact of World War I on
the modern Dance of Death. A competent but highly
specialized bibliography.
****

382.   PHYSIOLOGICAL RESEARCHES ON LIFE AND DEATH. M.F.
        Xavier Bichat. Arno Press,NY.1976.334 pp. $22.00.
Written by the young French prodigy of scientific medicine
2 years before his own early death;seeing Life as "the sum
of all those functions which resist death". Emerging from
the romanticism & rationalism of the French Revolution,this
book constituted a major challenge to existing thinking on
death,applying the methods of the new scientific approach
to medicine,including early experiments.First edn.1800.
***

383.   THE PRACTICE OF DEATH.Eike-Henner Kluge. Yale
        University Press,New Haven. 1975.269 pp.$ 10.00.
A rather boring philosophical discussion of ethical decision-
-making about euthanasia,suicide,abortion,infanticide and
senicide.The usual stuff,in a wordy & cold analysis. Not
recommended at all.
*

384.   THE PREDICTION OF SUICIDE.Ed.A.T.Beck,H.L.P.Resnik,
        & D.J.Lettieri. Charles Press,Bowie,MD. 1974.
        249 pp. $ 12.95. £ 11.95.
A series of papers presented at a 1971 Conference.Not a
handbook for the assessment of suicide risk,but a reflection
of the state of the art,such as it is (or as it was in 1971).
Authoritative & sophisticated,but competing nosologies and
categories are confusing.More emphasis on the generation of
data and probabilities than on its use.So,this man has a
probability of later suicide of one in 100: what do I do
about it? Lester on demographic versus clinical prediction
of suicide behaviors,Litman on prediction models,Motto on
refinement of variables,are especially interesting.Other
contributors include Diggory,Beck,Farberow,Worden & Zung.
***

385.   PRENEED BURIAL SERVICE. Hearings Before the
        Subcommittee on Frauds & Misrepresentations
        Affecting the Elderly of the Special Committee on
        Aging,U.S.Senate.88th Congress,Second Session.
        U.S. Government Printing Office,Washington DC.1964.

Useful reading for wary consumers,about the bilking of
senior citizens,& preneed mortuary & cemetary purchases.
***

386.   PROBLEMS OF DEATH: OPPOSING VIEWPOINTS. Ed.
        David L.Bender. Greenhaven Press,Anoka,Minnesota.
        1974. 153 pp. $ 7.95, PB $ 2.65.

A good book for classroom use,in stimulating discussion and
critical thinking in areas related to death.Includes short
selections of statements of divergent opinions on the topics
of Abortion,Euthanasia,Capital Punishment,Suicide,and
American Funeral Practices.The items are succinct and
challenging,& there are useful exercises,stressing the need
to distinguish between facts & opinions,between statements
which are probable and those which aren't.Readily
understandable without being condascending;challenging
without being shrill.
****

387.   THE PROFIT AND LOSS OF DYING. Clyde Irion.DeVorss
        & Co.,Santa Monica. 1969. 152 pp. $ 3.95.

Death from the other side.There are those,we are assured,
"who have passed through the veil of transition",who still
strive to be of service to mankind.Indeed,a vast network
of spiritual teachers from the "other side",known as the
Imperator Groups.One such group,under the direction of a
"spiritual personality known as Aramias",has brought this
book to us,"speaking through Mrs.Grace Ulrich Grause,
a trained channel". I can't go on.
*

388.   THE PROLONGATION OF LIFE:OPTIMISTIC STUDIES.Elie
        Metchnikoff. Arno Press,NY. 1976. 343 pp. $ 23.00.

In the year of his Nobel Prize in Medicine,Metchnikoff
wrote this discussion of'natural death'& the possibility of
longer life. 1st published 1908.
***

389.   PROPOSALS FOR LEGISLATIVE REFORM AIDING THE CONSUMER
        OF FUNERAL INDUSTRY PRODUCTS AND SERVICES.W.A.
        Neilson & C.G.Watkins. Celo Press,Burnsville,N.C.
        1973. 150 pp. $ 5.00.

Apart from the catchy title (in this context,'consumer' is
not a pleasant term,it smacks of anthropophagy),this is a
study commissioned by North American Funeral & Memorial
Societies of the funeral industry,relevant existing
legislation,& detailed proposals for law reform and an
optimal Funeral Service Industry Act. Earnest,dry,deserves
attention,but hard to read.
**

390.   PSYCHE AND DEATH (Archaic Myths & Modern Dreams in
        Analytical Psychology).Edgar Herzog. Hodder and
        Stoughton,London. 1966. 224 pp. £ 1.50.

An erudite study,from a predominantly Jungian and
anthopological point of view,of the origins & transformations
of the image of death,& archetypal concepts of a being which
brings about death,in popular rites & mythologies.Herzog
then compares & contrasts these themes with the dreams of
patients he has analyzed.Of highly specialized interest,but
can be read by a wider audience,for its cultural and
psychological insights.
***

391.   THE PSYCHIATRIST & THE DYING PATIENT. K.R.Eissler.
        International Universities Press,NY.1955 (reprinted
        1973). 388 pp. $ 3.45.

Some essays of variable interest on theoretical aspects of
death from a Freudian point of view,& three case-histories
of analyses unto death.Of specialist interest,little
practical value.
***

392.   THE PSYCHOLOGICAL AUTOPSY.A.Weisman & R.Kastenbaum.
        Behavioral Publications,NY. (Community Health
        Journal Monograph 4). 1968. 59 pp. PB $ 3.50.

A study of the terminal phase of life,describing and
exemplifying the techniques of the Psychological Autopsy,
a valuable and under-used method of studying death.
***

393.   THE PSYCHOLOGY OF DEATH. Robert Kastenbaum and Ruth
       Aisenberg.   Springer Publishing Co.NY. 1972. 500pp.
       $ 11.95. Duckworth,London.1974.£ 8.95. Concise
       Edition,Springer,NY. 1976. 434 pp. PB. $ 9.95.

Quite simply the very best book on the psychology of death,
& one that is unlikely to be improved on for some time.Very
well organized & highly useful to any professional or
scholar involved in work related to death.A truly critical
review; stimulating,eclectic & honest. Looks at concepts
of & attitudes towards death,developmentally & clinically,
& the relevant cultural milieu;also thanatomimesis,longevity,
suicide,murder,accidents & illness. Stylish,yet straight-
-forward & not self-conscious. Strongly recommended.
*****

394.   PSYCHOPHARMACOLOGICAL AGENTS FOR THE TERMINALLY ILL
       AND BEREAVED. Ed.Goldberg,Malitz & Kutscher.
       Columbia University Press,NY. 1973.340pp. $ 12.50.

An effectivebut over-long study of the uses of drugs in the
care of the dying & bereaved.Apart from some quite
irrelevant inclusions,there are some good reviews,for
example,of the uses of Chlorpromazine,Heroin & LSD,and some
discussion of the nature of grief and of pain. Poorly edited.
***

395.   PSYCHOSOCIAL ASPECTS OF CYSTIC FIBROSIS.Ed. Patterson,
       Denning & Kutscher. Columbia University Press,NY.
       1973. 230pp. $ 12.50.

Contains some excellent material on death in children and
adolescents,& death from chronic disease;along with some
very unnecessary articles.Poorly edited.
***

396.   PSYCHOSOCIAL ASPECTS OF TERMINAL CARE.Ed.Schoenberg,
       Carr,Peretz & Kutscher. Columbia University Press,NY.
       1972. 388 pp. $ 17.50. £ 16.00.

One of the most useful of the long and sometimes dismal
Columbia U.P. series,with some excellent review articles
by Schoenberg & Carr,Kastenbaum,Weisman,Abrams,Krant,Rees,
and Cicely Saunders. (Not really worth £ 16.00,though!)
****

397. PSYCHOSOCIAL ASPECTS OF TERMINAL PATIENT CARE. Ed.
      Charles A.Garfield. McGraw-Hill,New York. 1978.&

Though somewhat variable in quality of contributions,this
contains an outstanding piece by Shneidman on aspects of
therapeutic communication with the dying.
****

398. PUTTING THE ILL AT EASE.Evelyn Wilde Mayerson.
      Harper & Row,New York & London. 1976. 315 pp.
      PB. £ 7.45.

A detailed & well-written textbook of doctor-patient
communication (though what an awful title!),clearly based
on a sound understanding of clinical communication,even if
not of all the practicalities of daily medical practice.
76 illustrations,neatly drawn,but seldom apposite,& not
labelled or linked with the text. There are good chapters
on the aged patient & on pediatrics;& a chapter on Death &
Dying.Though the author has not read very widely in this
field,her advice on communication with the dying & grieving
are realistic & give down-to-earth suggestions.One of the
best resources available on clinical communication skills.
****

Q

399. QUESTIONS AND ANSWERS ON DEATH AND DYING.Elizabeth
      Kubler-Ross. Collier/Macmillan,NY.1974. 177pp.$ 1.65.

Elizabeth Kubler-Ross hasn't yet produced a book that was
not warm,caring and insightful.Alas,in this one poor
editing sometimes obscures these qualities as repetition
numbs them.Worth persevering with for some of its comments.
**

R

400. RACHEL. Arthur A.Smith. Morehouse-Barlow,NY. 1975.
      PB. 55 pp. $ 2.25.

Rachel,the author's daughter of 10,died suddenly at school.
In this modest,honest book,sensible & sensitive,Rev.Smith
describes his family's responses & offers helpful and
ultimately hopeful advice,without excess sentimentality,
and without preaching sweet platitudes."Written to,for,&
about parents of children who have died & for those who seek
to guide them".
***½

401.   THE REALIZATION OF DEATH. Avery Weisman. Jacob
       Aronson,NY. 1974. 207 pp. $ 12.50.

A detailed exploration of the origins,varieties and the
procedures of the Psychological Autopsy,a technique for
systematically gathering information,reconstructing and
synthesizing the events of the terminal phase of life.Well-
-written,but more useful for the professional thantologist
than for the average health care worker.
***

402.   REFLECTIONS ON LIFE AFTER LIFE.Raymond A.Moody.
       Bantam/Mockingbird,NY.1977. 118 pp. $ 3.95.
       Corgi,London. 1978. 150pp. 85 pence. Bantam,NY
       1978. $ 1.95.

Following sales of over 2,750,000 copies of "Life after Life",
here comes "Son of Life After Life".A useful supplement to
the original work,covering some of it's omissions.Still it
is misleadingly presented as dealing with the "survival of
life after bodily death",which is not the same topic at all.
Let us be absolutely clear: the fact that brain &
psychological function survives for a variable but short
period after the heart &/or respiration stops,has been known
by very many people for many years.There would be utterly
no point in attempting resuscitation if this were not so.
As we have recognized brain-death & the non-return on brain
function as the ultimate definition of death,death lies well
beyond the point from which people come back to chat to
Dr Moody. He has no evidence for"life"after death,unless one
plays silly games with obsolete definitions.Similar
experiences occur in the absence of any variety of"death".
Though Near-Death experiences say something significant
about Man,they may not be about Death at all.
In this book,Moody describes some new,less common features
of Near-Death Experiences.There's a brief & trivial chapter
on suicide;some historical examples(not complete,he still
doesn't seem to have done much homework). An appendix on
"Methodological Consideration",his reflections on how one
might investigate these phenomena.Shows a surprisingly
limited & naive concept of scientific method.Evasive about
major & readily avoidable weaknesses in his methds of
inquiry,he does not answer his critics.One hopes Dr Moody
will take advantage of the enormous success (financial &
popular)of these books,to investigate properly these
fascinating phenomena---this side of death.
***

403. REHABILITATION OF MASTECTOMY PATIENTS.June Marchant.
      William Heinemann,London. 1978. 112 pp. £ 2.75.

Discussions of dealing with the physical & psychological
problems of mastectomy;intended for doctors,nurses,
ancillaries,& perhaps patients.
***

404. RELIGION & BEREAVEMENT.Ed.A.& L.G.Kutscher. Health
      Sciences Publishing Co.,1972.224 pp. $ 12.50.

Dreadfully low standard of contributions,very badly edited.
Many quite awesomely unhelpful contributions.Banal,banal.
*

405. REPORT OF THE PILOT PROJECT,JANUARY 1975-1977,
      PALLIATIVE CARE SERVICE,ROYAL VICTORIA HOSPITAL
      McGILL UNIVERSITY. October 1976. 520pp. $ 18.00.
      From: Palliative Care Service,Royal Victoria Hospital,
      687 Pine Avenue West, Montreal, Canada H3A 1A1.

Catchy title. A bulky & useful collection of items assembled
to summarize the activities & evaluation of the 2-year pilot
project which established the Royal Vic's PCS,a multi-
disciplinary team dealing with the needs of dying patients
& their families,within a general hospital setting.It
includes details of the unit's functions & techniques,
selection & training of staff,& the results of research &
evaluation,as well as reprints of articles by PCS staff,
and the ethically controversial & evaluatively trivial
Buckingham study. Of considerable interest to anyone
developing terminal care & related services.
***½

406. RESPONDING TO HUMAN PAIN : For Persons Who Help.
      J.B.Ashbrook. Judson Press,Valley Forge. 1975.
      192 pp. $ 10.00.

A readable,very simplified,trandy introduction to the
helping process;sometwhat over-dramatized at times,but
reasonably competent.Attends to the use of community
resources & referrals;& has separate chapters on the
problems of dependency,aging & death.Could be a useful
introductory work for those who want to become involved
in volunteer work with seriously ill patients.
***

407. THE RESURRECTION OF THE DEAD. Karl Barth. Arno Press,
      N.Y. 1976.213 pp. $ 15.00.

A highly important analysis of early Christian views of the
Resurrection of the dead,& St Paul's Epistle to the
Corinthians,separating analogy from core meaning,and that,
in turn,from historical or supposed fact.
***

408. RETURN TO LIFE: TWO IMAGININGS OF THE LAZARUS THEME.
      Original Anthology. Ed.R.Kastenbaum,G.Geddes,G.Gruman
      & M.A.Simpson. Arno Press,N.Y. 1976. 128 pp. $ 14.00.

Includes the Preface from JOHN,XI,1,44; Leonid Andreyev's
Lazarus,and Eugene O'Neill's Lazarus Laughed. It has often
been regretted that Lazarus was not properly interviewed
about his experiences of death.Andreyev considers what we
might have learned,as does O"Neill in what he once called
by far his best play,since much neglected. Not available
in the British Commonwealth.
***

409. THE RIGHT TO DIE. Milton Heifetz & Charles Mangel.
      G.P.Putnam's Sons,N.Y. (Longman Canada) 1975. 234 pp.
      $ 10.50. Berkeley Medallion PB 1976,245pp. $ 1.95.

Dr Heifetz,a neurosurgeon,argues cogently that the patient
has a right to refuse life-saving treatment and,in some
circumstances,to doctor-assisted suicide.He proposes an
"airtight" (?) Living Will,& that physicians should cease
treatment of the hopelessly ill & withhold it from deformed
children.Emphatic & terse,the book is readable if not
stylish.The positive aspects of better terminal care rather
than quicker termination are not much stressed though
present,& the Bibliography is similarly biased.None the less
its unequivocating statements will fuel more appropriate
discussions of the topic.
***½

410. THE RIGHT TO DIE;DECISION & DECISION MAKERS.Group for
      the Advancement of Psychiatry,NY. Symposium No.12,
      1973.80pp. $ 3.50.

An oddly evasive collection of essays dealing with the
ostensible topic somewhat tangentially;little disciplined
debate,but some interesting ideas & examples.
**

411. THE RITES OF PASSAGE.A.van Gennep. University of
      Chicago Press,Chicago. 1961.

Classic study of the rites & ceremonies attending changes
of status; Chapter 8 discusses funerals & death.
***

412. THE RULE & EXERCISES OF HOLY DYING:In Which Are
      Described the Means & Instruments of Preparing
      Ourselves & Others Respectively for a Blessed Death.
      Jeremy Taylor. Arno Press, N.Y.1976. 288pp. $ 19.00.

A classic work of the Ars Moriendi,by the Chaplain to King
Charles the First;urging death education & daily preparation
for the death-bed;proposing techniques for assisting the
dying.A work of significant historical & contemporary
significance.
***½

413. THE SANCTITY OF SOCIAL LIFE:Physicians' Treatment of
      Critically Ill Patients. Diana Crane. Russell Sage
      Foundation,N.Y. 1975. 286 pp. $ 13.50.

A uniquely valuable study based on extensive interviews,
observations,hospital record audit & detailed questionnaires.
Rather than pontificating on what ought to be done,Crane
describes what doctors actually do for the criticallly ill.
She shows that while withdrawal of treatment is widespread
in some types of case,positive euthanasia is rare.Both
adults & children seem to be regarded as 'treatable'while
they retain the potential for interacting in some meaningful
way with others.A much-needed antidote to the usual
speculative literature on this subject,with commendable
detail & objectivity.
*****

414. THE SAVAGE GOD.A.Alvarez. Weidenfeld & Nicolson,London
      1972.250pp. £ 3.50. Bantam,NY. PB $ 1.95.

A study of attitudes towards suicide & death through history
& literature,& the fascination this theme has had for
writers at all times. Includes an account of his relations
with Sylvia Plath,& her suicide,& his own suicide attempt.
*****

415. SCAPEGOAT: THE IMPACT OF DEATH-FEAR ON AN AMERICAN
      FAMILY. E.Bermann.University of Michigan Press,
      1973. 357 pp. $ 10.00.

Study in depth of a family faced with overwhelming death-
-fear in response to the father's precarious health,in
which the young son became the scapegoat for the family's
problems,& presented as unmanageably aggressive at school.
Excellent,detailed & imaginative study of considerable
specialist interest.
***

416. SCIENCE AND IMMORTALITY. William Osler. Arno Press,
      N.Y., 1976. 54 pp. $ 10.00. (1st published 1904).

The text of Osler's first Ingersoll lecture "On the
Immortality of Man",at Harvard.Rich in his usual classical
allusions;includes Osler's data on the death-bed
behavior of 500 patients;his discussion of how science was
breaking the foundations of traditional beliefs,& of his
own faith. Osler as pompous and wordy as ever.
***

417. A SECOND CHANCE TO LIVE: THE SUICIDE SYNDROME.Text
      by Ernie Leogrande,Photographs by George Alpert.
      Dacapo Press,N.Y. 1975. $ 15.00, $ 6.95 PB.

The personal story of 7 people who attempted suicide but
later decided to live.Oddly morbid,& it's very hard to
understand what purpose is served by this book.
**

418. SELECTED BIBLIOGRAPHY ON DEATH & DYING.Ed.J.Vernick.
      N.I.H./U.S.Govt.Printing Office. 60pp. 65¢.

Handy for sporadic use,but a poor bibliography,with about
one-third inappropriate references,either highly
inaccessible papers in foreign languages or obscure
journals,or reference to large works on wholly different
subjects!
**

419. SELF-DESTRUCTIVE BEHAVIOR.Ed.A.R.Roberts. C.C.Thomas,
      Springfield,Illinois. 1975. 215 pp. $ 17.50.

Smorgasbord publishing.8 chapters on various aspects of
self-destructive behavior.Barely & badly edited,very variable
in scope,depth & quality.No integration or organization.A
bizarre chapter denying a self-destructive component in

419 ctd.)   obesity.Poor presentation,poor discussion,little
recognition of the major difficulties in the field,barely
critical.Oh dear,what a self-destructive book! Epidemiology
& taxonomy not well handled;statistics & prevention:very
elementary stuff;Ferrence et al. on self-injury:generally
good work in a neglected area;Pokorny on automobile
accidents:chatty & rather superficial; Herzman on the
problems of research:quite good.
**

420.   SEPARATION: ANXIETY & ANGER.Vol.2. of Attachment &
       Loss. John Bowlby. Basic Books,NY.1977 (original
       1973),456 pp. $ 4.95 reprint PB. Also Penguin PB
       re-issue,1978. £ 1.50.

Examines the effects of separation on the child's
development,& the psychopathology that can result.Proposes
a genetic theory of fear & anxiety.Bowlby has too negative
a conception of dependency,but provides a basic theoretical
model for separation anxiety.
***

421.   THE SEXUALLY OPPRESSED. Harvey Gochros & Jean Gochros,
       Editors. Association Press,NY. 1977. 296 pp. $ 14.95.

A collection of 21 original papers.Beginning with studies
of the historical roots of sexual oppression & of social &
sexual deviance-it then presents discussions of groups whose
sexual needs have been largely overlooked or suppressed by
the general public & by many in the helping professions—
such as aging male homosexuals,black widows,prisoners,
adolescents,the handicapped,the aged,& the terminally ill.
Most of the essays consider the constraints & problems of
the group,the myths & stereotypes,& strategies for improving
the situation.A very important subject,& a reasonably
helpful book.
***

422.   SHOULD TREATMENT BE TERMINATED? T.C.Oden. Harper &
       Row,NY. 1976. 100pp. $ 2.95 PB.

"Moral Guidelines for Christian Families & Pastors". A simple
succinct,lucid guide,within the Christian tradition,
discussing dilemmas of life-support:who decides? by what
guidelines?; and respect for life & acceptance of death.
Seriously flawed by a lack of proper references for its
citations.
***

423. SIMONE DE BEAUVOIR : ENCOUNTERS WITH DEATH.Elaine
      Marks. Rutgers University Press,New Brunswick,NJ.
      1973. 184 pp. $ 9.00.

Though an awareness of mortality & fear of death is a
pervasive theme in literature,there are few if any such
intelligent & intelligible studies of this theme as this
book.Highly literate & readable.Examines the theme of death
in the writings of the arch priestess of existentialist
authors with grace & commendable psychological insight.As
a results,this work is not merely of literary importance,
but also uncommonly interesting as a contribution to
studies of the psychology of death.
****

424. SISTER DEATH. O'Kelley Whitaker. Morehouse-Barlow,NY.
      1974. 110 pp. $ 4.50.

A short study of a Christian approach to death,optimistic
& positive.Simplistic in some ways,& with an erratic brief
bibliography.
**½

425. Socio-Cultural Expressions & Implications of DEATH,
      MOURNING & BEREAVEMENT IN ISRAEL,arising out of the
      War Situation.Phyllis Palgi. Jerusalem Academic
      Press. (P.O.B.2390 Jerusalem) 1974. 47 pp. $ 3.50.
      PB. (Order from:Sales Publication Dept.,Research
      Authority, Tel Aviv University ,Israel.)

A slim volume reprinting a long article from the Israel
Annals of Psychiatry by the Chief Anthropologist to the
Ministry of Health.She discusses the impact of war deaths
on Israeli society,in relation to traditional mourning
rituals,the major cultural differences in the population,
& other factors influencing outcome.One of the few
competent comments on the unique experiences in Israel;
tantalizingly brief.
***

426. SOCIOLOGY OF DEATH An Analysis of Death-Related
      Behavior. G.M.Vernon. Ronald Press,NY. 1970.
      357 pp. $ 9.50.

Detailed summary of many different studies,often
derivatively. Not great sociology,but can be useful.
***

427.   SOMEONE YOU LOVE IS DYING. Martin Shepard. Harmony
       Books, New York. 1975. 220pp. $ 7.95.

By the author of 'The Love Treatment','Beyond Sex Therapy',
and 'Sexual Marathon'.An over-dramatized & superficial
series of conversations between 'Marty'and friends,with
quotations & anecdotes.Nothing new or novel,but a general
representation of the most trendy current views on coping
with death & grief. Sometimes useful,often shallow,with
self-conscious'contemplations'. If the author took himself
a lot less seriously,it would be helpful.The terminal
R.I.P.-off strikes again.
**

428.   A SORROW BEYOND DREAMS :A Life Story.Peter Handke.
       Farrar,Strauss & Giroux,NY.1974. 70pp. Souvenir
       Press,London.1976. £ 2.75.

A distinguished Austrian author writes about his mother's
despair,her life without living,& her suicide.Confronts
the facts of her life,to try to comprehend what she did,
and why,eventually,she did it.
**½

429.   STAY OF EXECUTION. Stewart Alsop. Lippincott. 1973.
       312 pp. $ 8.95.

An autobiographical account of living with death.In July
1971 Alsop,a journalist,was told he had leukemia,likely to
kill him in a year.He lived longer,& described his varied
experiences after the diagnosis was made,& his conclusions:
"A dying man needs to die,as a sleepy man needs sleep,&
there comes a time when it is wrong,as well as useless,to
resist."
***

430.   STRAIGHT TALK ABOUT DEATH WITH YOUNG PEOPLE.Richard
       G.Watts. Westminster Press,Philadelphia. 1975
       92 pp. PB. $ 2.95.

Based on the author's work with junior high school students
& intended as a resource & basis for dialogue;this mild &
disappointing,rather wishy-washy book leaves too many
matters inexplicit & unclear.Deals with fears of death,
grief,funerals,& religious beliefs about life after death.
The totally irrelevant illustrations are typical of its
tendency,despite its promises,to avoid confronting the
stark reality of death,& to stick to cosy generalizations.
*

431. STRANGER STOP AND CAST AN EYE.A Guide to Gravestones
      & Rubbings. C.Walker Jacobs.Stephen Greene Press,
      Brattleboro,Vermont. 1973. 128 pp. $ 4.95.

Cemetary browsing & tombstone rubbings: why to do it and
how to do it.
**

432. SUDDEN & AWFUL.American Epitaphs & the Finger of God.
      Thomas C.Mann & Janet Greene. Stephen Greene Press,
      Brattleboro,Vermont. 1968. 112 pp. $ 4.95.

Epitaphs & tombstones of early America,demonstrating the
hazards of life & death those days.Illustrated.
**

433. SUDDEN UNEXPECTED DEATH IN INFANTS.MSS Publ.Corp.,NY.
      1974. 218 pp. $ 17.00.

Some useful review & research papers on S.I.D.S.,though,as
usual in this series,some major omissions.A few odd,
aberrant papers— one on sudden death in adults,one on
varicella myocarditis,for instance.A few studies on parental
reactions to S.I.D.S. Not up-to-date or comprehensive,
**½

434. THE SUICIDAL PATIENT: RECOGNITION & MANAGEMENT. Ari
      Kiev. Nelson-Hall,Chicago. 1977. 157 pp. $ 12.00.

Very short(just over 100pp of text) & very disappointing.
Attempts a philosophical & historical review of suicidal
behavior (brief,inadequate,& so much better done in other
books).Then he presents the results of his study of a "self-
-selected"group of suicidal patients,with clinical vignettes
& descriptions of 7 profile types based on a cluster
analysis of correlational patterns among various demographic
& personal historical elements.However,it's hard to
evaluate the relevance or significance of these findings,as
the "self-selected"nature of the group studied may bear
little relation to the patients we meet elsewhere.
"Management" is more thoroughly dealt with in the title
than in the text. It's advice is too brief,trite,& vague to
be of help to any active clinician.Never successfully
coherent or useful.
*

435. SUICIDE. Jacques Choron. Scribner,N.Y.1973.$2.95.PB.

A history of suicide from ancient days to recently,mainly
from a philosophical point of view,but also considering
the prediction and prevention of suicide.
**

436. SUICIDE.E.Durckheim. Free Press,NY. 1951.405pp.$3.95.

Paperback edition of the old classic sociological study of
suicide;parts of which are obviously out-dated,parts of
which are still most apposite.
***

437. SUICIDE & ATTEMPTED SUICIDE. Erwin Stengel. Pelican/
      Penguin Books,Harmondsworth.1964. 135 pp. 65 pence.

An early and popular work,not significantly up-dated since
publication.Considers the statistics,methods,motives and
causes of suicide,its psychodynamics & prophylaxis,reviewing
the data available up to the early 1960's. Sadly out of
date now.
***

438. SUICIDE AND HOMICIDE:Some Economic,Sociological and
      Psychological Aspects of Aggression. A.F.Henry & J.F.
      Short. Arno Press,N.Y. 1976 214 pp. $ 15.00.

A provocative study of suicide,suggesting that people of
high social status are more likely to kill themselves,&
people of low social status,more likely to kill others,
during hard times;that suicide & homicide rates are
related to business cycles. 1st published 1954.
***

439. SUICIDE:A Social & Historical Study.H.R.Fedden.
      Benjamin Bloom,NY(Arno Press),1972. 350pp. $ 17.50.

Discusses the suicide horror of tribal custom,the ancient
world's concept of the individual's liberty to die,suicide
in early Christian times,the Renaissance & the Enlightenment.
Replete with intriguing anecdotes and illustrations.
****

440. SUICIDE: ASSESSMENT & INTERVENTION. Ed.Corinne Hatton,
      Sharon Valente & Alice Rink. Appleton-Century-Crofts,
      N.Y. 1977. 220pp. £ 7.80, $ 9.75.

A book which aspires to be the Suicidology Desk Reference,
"an indispensible manual for practitioners in suicide

440 ctd.) prevention"—— and very nearly achieves this
ambitious aim.Soundly practical,sensible,accessible &
clearly written,consistently interesting & useable.The
contributors,mostly based at the L.A.Suicide Prevention
Center,include Wold,Pretzel,Peck & Litman.Regrettably
uses a clumsy style of references.It genuinely belongs on
the desk,rather than the shelf,of everyone involved in
suicide prevention or emergency psychiatric services.
****

441.   SUICIDE IN DIFFERENT CULTURES.Ed.Norman Farberow.
       University Park Press,Baltimore. 1975.286pp.$19.50.

Gathers the experience of experts in 14 countries,on suicide
as a social phenomenon,from Finland to Taiwan,among
Bulgarians & American Indians.Relatively well-organized &
integrated,though it might have been conceptually bolder.
Includes individual studies of political & other individual
suicides,including Mishima & Schauman.A starting-point
rather than an end-point.
***

442.   SUICIDE: INSIDE AND OUT.David K.Reynolds & Norman L.
       Farberow. University of California Press,Berkeley &
       London.1976. 226 pp. $ 10.95 £ 8.75.

A detailed & responsible account of an Experiential Research
(Participant Observation) study of the situation and
experiences of the suicidal patient in a psychiatric
hospital.The most competent account of this research
technique (though with an inadequate consideration of the
ethical dimensions)and a review of previous similar studies.
A unique account of the interaction between hospital staff
and suicidal patients;the suicidal identity;what solutions
or advice the suicidal patient is offered;& the real
ineffectiveness of security measures & suicide prevention
precautions. Lively and readable.
***½

443.   SUICIDE: THE GAMBLE WITH DEATH.Gene & David Lester.
       Spectrum(Prentice-Hall) 1971. 176 pp. $ 2.75. PB.

A very simple & straightforward review of the results of
the 1960's work on suicide;now partly out of date.
uncommonly lucid and well organized.
****

444. SUICIDOLOGY: CONTEMPORARY DEVELOPMENTS. Ed. E.S. Shneidman. Grune & Stratton,NY.1976. 57 pp. £ 15.95.

The great standard contemporary work on suicide.Each chapter is introduced by extracts from early classics such as David Hume on Suicide in 1777.Part I-Demography,includes trends in the U.S.rate & Black suicide;Part II-Methodology,includes Worden on lethality factors,Motto on developing & validating scales for estimating risk-Part III deals with logical and cognitive aspects including Shneidman on reasoning patterns in suicide notes.Part IV on Clinical Correlates,includes Simpson on self-mutilation,Hendin on student suicide,and Shneidman on the gifted.Part V,Philosophical & Legal Aspects,includes Kastenbaum's challenging:'Suicide as the Preferred Way of Death'.Part VI,on responding to suicide, includes Kiev,Fox,Litman et al,on intervention & prevention.
****

445. SUNSHINE.Norma Klein. Avon Books,NY.1974.$ 1.95.

The story of 2o-year-old Jacqueline Helton who died of bone cancer in 1971,keeping a tape-recorded diary during her last 18 months of life,for her young daughter.Later made into a film.
***

446. SUPPORT SYSTEMS AND MUTUAL HELP:Multidisciplinary Explorations. Ed.. Gerald Caplan & Marie Killilea. Grune & Stratton,NY. 1976. 325 pp. £ 13.85,$ 19.50.

An important contribution to the understanding of support & care,with particular relevance to care of the dying & bereaved.Five theoretical chapters develop models of support systems & mutual help,self-help & family support; empirical studies of Parents Without Partners,& Recovery, Inc.;the five chapters from the Laboratory of Community Psychiatry,including Seminars for the Separated,the Widow--to-Widow program,peer consultation among clergy,& Caplan's experiences of the organization of support systems for civil populations in Israel in time of war.Of interest to thanatology,though of only the most peculiar & forced relevance to the subject of the book,is Ruth Caplan's chapter on death-bed scenes & graveyard poetry in 18th Century English literature.A good chapter in the wrong book.
***$\frac{1}{2}$

447.   THE SURVIVOR: An Anatomy of the Death Camps. Terrence
       Des Pres. Oxford University Press,N.Y. 1976. 218pp.
       $ 10.00. Pocket PB,1977, 257 pp. $ 1.95.

Another of the works seeking to understand the holocaust.
Des Pres gathers material from many personal accounts &
other studies,& writes with some passion about the capacity
to live under prolonged crisis & threat of death,sustaining
damage to mind & body,yet still survive alive & human.He
sees the survivor as the new hero of our time,he who turns
away from death(succeeding the tragic hero who defied death
for the sake of his cause).He affirms life by what he
endures.Des Pres is sceptical about traditional
interpretations of the experience,of concepts like survivor
guilt & identification with the aggressor,stressing the
adaptive rather than the symbolic functions of the behavior.
Survival,he believes,depends on the inmate's self-conscious
choice of life at all costs rather than surrender to apathy
and death.
****

448. SYLVIA PORTER'S MONEY BOOK.Sylvia Porter. Doubleday,NY.
     1975. 1105 pp.$ 16.95.Also Avon,NY.1976(up-dated)
     1105 pp, $ 5.95 PB.

A large & comprehensive volume on living cheaply and
economically.Good advice on Wills,estates,& funeral planning.
The book as a whole will be valuable to the newly widowed
and wodowered,facing the need to cope with new financial
problems.
**

449.   SYMBOLIC WOUNDS. Bruno Bettelheim. Collier,NY.1962/
       1971. 194pp. $ 1.50 PB.

"Puberty rites & the envious male";"How Pre-literate man
masters fear by trying to make woman's power his own".
Considers the rituals of puberty such as circumcision.
Integrative & imaginative overlap between ego psychology
and anthropology.Not a great example of either,but
a useful example of the results of exploring their common
grounds. Aids understanding self-destructive behavior.
***

T
450. TALKING ABOUT DEATH.E.A.Grollman Beacon Press,Boston,
      1970. 30 pp. $ 1.95 PB.

Strongly recommended.A beautiful book,probably the best
available for use in discussing death with children.Well-
-illustrated & constructed;simple,direct,honest.
*****

451. TALKING ABOUT DEATH:A Dialogue Between Parent & Child.
      Earl A.Grollman. Beacon Press,Boston.1976. 98pp.$3.95.

Simply,excellent.A new edition of the excellent earlier
version,with a greatly expanded guide to parents on how to
use it & to discuss death with children.Lists some resources
such as organizations,cassettes,films,books. Explicit and
observant.
*****

452. TEACHING OUTLINES IN SUICIDE STUDIES & CRISIS
      INTERVENTION.Ed.H.L.P.Resnik & B.C.Hawthorne. PB
      Charles Press,Bowie,MD. 1974. 169pp. $ 7.50 (£ 7.20)

To help instructors in selecting course material &
references; outlines of various topics with bibliographies.
**

453. TELL ME ABOUT DEATH,TELL ME ABOUT FUNERALS.Elizabeth
      Adam Corley. Grammatical Sciences,Santa Clara,Cal.
      1973. 35 pp. $ 2.00. PB.

Intended for elementary schoolchildren.A little girl's
Grandpa has died,& Papa (a doctor) answers her questions.
There's an attempt to deal with several of the principle
concerns of children who encounter death,sometimes much
over-simplified.The author,a licensed Embalmer/Funeral
Director,deals mainly with funerals,explaining briefly
embalming (which is not,of course,"to stop the body from
carrying bad germs"),caskets("the inside is usually very
pretty".Well,that's something to look forward to);funeral
ceremonies;pall bearers (confised by the child with
Polar-bears,so "I think Grandpa's funeral will be funny",
a rather forced joke);hearses,cemetaries,mausoleums,
cremation & columbaria. There's a reasonable emphasis on
the availability & value of wide & free choice.
**½

454. THE TERMINAL PATIENT— ORAL CARE. Ed.Kutscher,
     Schoenberg & Carr. Columbia University Press.1973.
     275 pp. $ 12.50.

For those who thought that even in the age of over-
-specialization,you couldn't publish a large book about
dying teeth— confirmation.A very rum book indeed.
Repetitious & obsessively comprehensive,including "Oral
Care of the Dying Patient:A Social Worker's Point of
View",& the pastoral care of patients with oral cancer.
One doesn't want to mock,but this book desparately needs
some sense of proportion. One breathlessly awaits its
sequels— Podiatry & Dying Feet,perhaps,and the Dying
Person's Cook Book ?
*

455. TERMINALVÅRD. Loma Feigenberg. Liber Läromedel,Lund.
     1977. 231 pp.

A significant book by a distinguished Scandinavian
thanatologist describing his clinical experience and his
individualist,distinctive & personal way of working with
the dying patient.
***

456. THE THANATOLOGY LIBRARY.Roberta Halporn. Highly
     Specialized Promotions,NY. 1976.33pp. $ 2.00.

A very briefly & tersely annotated catalogue of some books
on Thanatology.Well-meaning but seriously ill-informed.
Completely mistaken about the origins of thanatology.
Pretends to be"the first annotated listing of books in
print"on thanatology,when it is perhaps the 30th.Its claims
are not reliably true,its advice is unreliable & at times
oddly inaccurate.Its evaluation of the books it lists is
hard to understand: for examply,it automatically bestows
a 'star'to denote a'classic',on every publication by any
member of the Foundation of Thanatology--even,in some cases,
before the book has been published or available for review!
Not usable & impossible to recommend. *
Also offers a"Basic Collection in Thanatology",which Ms
Halporn considers "the absolute minimum" of books needed
by a library.A librarian would do very much better to buy
a far superior selection of books independently and
individually.Definately not recommended. 39 books totalling
$ 221.35,variously priced in different pages of the

456 ctd.) catalogue at $ 216.38 or $ 186.60;or the books
plus some filmstrips worth $ 30235,at $ 285 or $ 255.45.
All I can recommend from Highly Specialized Promotions
are their pleasantly simple Thanatology gummed Book
Plates (either 'Ex Libris',or'Donated to the Library By')
at $ 2.50 for 50. ***

457. THE BOOK (On the Taboo Against Knowing Who You Are).
    Alan Watts. Vintage Books,NY. 1972. 146 pp. $ 1.65.PB.

A classic,elegantly,lucidly & wittily written book.Dealing
with the delusion of the lonely separate ego alienated
from the universe,with his usual skillful understanding of
Eastern & Western religions & philosophies.Offers a
coherent philosophical style which genuinely deals with
fear of death & a manner of coming to terms with life.
Highly recommended.
*****

458. THEORY OF SUICIDE.Maurice L.Farber. Arno Press,NY.
    1976.115 pp. $ 12.00. (1st edn.1968).

A student of Kurt Lewin,Farber considers suicide as a
"disease of hope",& offers a general theory of suicide
supported by a variety of evidence;identifying the kind of
person especially vulnerable,& the stresses in society that
impel him to suicide.A study also of the phenomenology
of hope.
***

459. THE THREAT OF IMPENDING DISASTER. Ed. Grosser,
    Wechsler & Greenblatt. M.I.T.Press,1964/71. 335 pp.
    $ 3.50. PB.

The psychology of stress,including major chapters on
cultural variations in attitudes toward death & disease,
reactions to imminence of death;& some of Lifton's work on
the psychological effects of the Atom Bomb in Hiroshima.
***

460. THE TIBETAN BOOK OF THE DEAD.Ed. W.E.Evans-Wentz,
    Oxford University Press,NY.(1927) 1960.250pp.PB.
    $ 2.25.

The After-Death Experiences on the Bardo Plane,according to
Lama Kazi Dawa Samdup's English Rendering. The great ancient
work of instruction on how to manage the experience of death
& what follows.Good explanatory material by Dr Evans-Wentz.
***

461.   THE TIBETAN BOOK OF THE DEAD.Transl.F.Fremantle and
        C.Trungpa. Shambala (Random House)NY. 1975.$3.95.PB.
An alternative edition.
***

462.   A TIME FOR DYING. B.Glaser & A.Strauss.Aldine.1968.
        270pp. $ 11.95.

Based on intensive field work in hospitals,this book
advances the model of Dying Trajectories—the course and
progress of a death. Looks at sudden death (expected and
unexpected) & lingering trajectories;death in hospital &
at home,& the ways in which we socially structure death
$ the events surrounding it. Rather too long.This & the
previous book by the two authors are essential reading
for anyone doing detailed studies in this field.
****

463.   A TIME TO LIVE. Jane Seskin.Spectrum(Prentice-Hall),
        Englewood Cliffs,NJ. 1977. $ 4.95.

Another book from the author of"Young Widow".I'm not
sure why.
**

464.   TO DIE WITH STYLE.M.J.McCoy. Abingdon Press,
        Nashville. 1974. 175 pp. $ 5.95.

Avid,breathlessly enthusiastic.Attempts to develop a
cheerful guide to dying stylishly,with awareness."This",
she claims"is a central task of living that offers a
glorious possibility....the experience that final creative
surge. I can achieve my death". Sounds like simultaneous
orgasm.
**

465.   TO LIVE & TO DIE: WHEN,WHY & HOW.Ed.P.Williams.
        Springer-Verlag,NY. 1973. 346 pp. $ 12.95.

Odd,wide-ranging book;sometimes superficial,usually
interesting.Topics include genetic engineering,contraception,
abortion,euthanasia,transplant ethics,marriage,& covers
some issues poorly dealt with elsewhere.
***

466.   TOLSTOI'S "IVAN ILYCH" & A COMMENTARY.A.C.Carr.Health
        Sciences Publ.Corp.NY.1973. 65pp. $ 1.25. PB.

Reprint of the Tolstoy short story with weedy commentary.
**

467.   TOO YOUNG TO DIE.(Youth & Suicide).Francine Klagsbrun.
       Houghton Mifflin Co.,Boston. 1976. 201pp. $ 6.95.
       Pocket Books,NY. 1977. 192 pp. $ 1.25 PB.

A relatively non-sensational presentation of the facts and
current opinions about adolescent & young adult suicide,
including some interviews with young attempters,friends and
families,& a competent survey of the theoretical issues
involved.One of the few books for the intelligent lay
person that can be recommended.
***½

468.   TOWARDS A SOCIOLOGY OF DEATH & DYING.Sage Publ.,
       Beverly Hills, California.1976. $ 3.95.

Seven articles dealing with current trends in D & D in
contemporary America.Keep travelling,we're nowhere near
a sociology of death yet.
**

469.   TWENTIETH CENTURY BOOK OF THE DEAD.Gil Elliot.Allen
       Lane,Penguin Press,London,1972.£ 2175. Random House/
       Scribner,NY. 1972 $ 7.95. Penguin 1973,242 pp.$ 1.65.
       Ballentine Books,NY.1973. $ 1.65 PB.

A disturbing work,which coolly provides a new necrology.It
studies the one hundred million man-made deaths in the
20th century;the wars,the tecnologies of macro-violence-
& the effects on our society & our understanding of the
nature of man.A unique account of this century's most
populous nation— the nation of the dead.
****

U
470.   UNDERSTANDING & COUNSELLING THE SUICIDAL PERSON.
       Paul W.Pretzel. Abingdon,Nashville.1972. 250pp.

A summary of suicidology,its statistics & theories,from
Durkheim to Shneidman.Illustrated with case-histories.Good
emphasis on the aftermath of suicide,& care for the victims.
Philosophical & religious attitudes to suicide are reviewed
in the closing chapters.Directed to the clergyman,but more
widely useful,too.
***

471.   UNDERSTANDING GRIEF:Its Roots,Dynamics & Treatment.
       Edgar N.Jackson. Abingdon Press,Nashville. 1957.255pp.

One of the major early works in the field,with examples
from the parish ministry & advice for the pastoral
counsellor.Explores the dynamics of grief & guilt,normal
& pathological responses to bereavement,& the functions of
religion in dealing with the experience of grief.Integrates
material from a wide variety of sources.
***

472.   UP FROM GRIEF: Patterns of Recovery. Bernadine Kreis
       & Alice Pattie. Seabury Press,NY. 1969.146pp. $ 6.95.

A vivid,brisk & soundly practical book about grief,full of
conversations & chat.Discusses stages of shock,suffering &
recovery;how to help a friend in grief;how to help
yourself;& how ministers help.A good,commonsense chapter
on"Grief,loneliness & sex".
***½

V
473.   A VERY EASY DEATH. Simone de Beauvoir. Penguin Books,
       Harmondsworth.1969.92 pp. 85¢.Celo Press,NC.1965.139pp
       $ 1.25. Warner PB,NY.1973.$ 1.25. 65 pence,U.K.

Unreservedly recommended.A brilliant & unforgettable
account of her mother's death in France,a death that was
anything but easy. Deeply moving description of a proud
woman's clinical humiliation & the conflicting love and
hostility her daughter experienced in confronting the death.
*****

474.   THE VESTIBULE.Ed.Jess E.Weiss. Ashley Books,Port
       Washington,NY. 1972. 128pp. $ 5.95.

An early specimen of the genre,with short essays & extracts
about near-death experiences,&"return"from "death". Authors
include Rickenbacker,Swedenborg,Helen Keller & Kobler-Ross.
**

475.   THE VIEW FROM A HEARSE.Joseph Bayly.David Cook Publ.
       Co.,Elgin,Illinois. Revised Edn.1973.122pp.$1.25.PB.

Bitty & jerky in style,sincere but exaggerated,panting &
trite,& not much help.Expresses a traditional Christian
viewpoint,but with assertion rather than explanation.
Relies heavily on quotations from standard thanatology
sources,but adds nothing new or necessary to an
overburdened literature.
*

476. VITAL SIGNS (The Way We Die in America). John Langone.
      Little,Brown, Boston.1974. 363 pp. $ 8.95.

An excellent & entertaining piece of expert journalism.With
interviews & apt quotations from a variety of works;it looks
directly at what happens to the dying & those who take care
of them,with a minimum of theorizing & preaching.
****

477. VOLUNTARY EUTHANASIA: Is there an Alternative? Duncan
      W.Vere. Christian Medical Fellowship,London.1970.
      61 pp. PB. 20 pence.

A short booklet proposing a case against euthanasia from a
Christian & medical angle.Limited in its attention to the
definitions of death,& the problems of those incapable of
voluntary assent.Light & chatty.
**$\frac{1}{2}$
W

478. THE WAITING WORLD:What Happens After Death. Archie
      Matson. Harper & Row,NY.1975. 160pp. $ 6.95.

Yet more dear-death experiences & parapsychology,but not
even of the usual unimpressive standard.
*

479. WARD 402. Ronald Glasser. Braziller,NY.1973.232pp.$6.95.

A novel closely based on fact,about an intern on the
Pediatric Ward & his involvement with an 11 year old girl
with leukemia,dealing eloquently with the difficulties of
not always doing some of the things we can do,when they
shouldn't be done;with doctors who can't stop treating.
Are they still treating the child...or themselves?
****

480. THE WAY WE DIE:An Investigation of Death & Dying in
      America Today. David Dempsey. Macmillan,NY.1975.276
      pp. $ 9.95, 1977 PB $ 3.95.

Though classified by the publisher as"Sociology",this is
competent journalism more than bad sociology.Chatty,
anecdotal,entertaining but neither especially well-
-informed nor showing more than a superficial understanding
of its subject-matter,it wanders through death,transplants,
longevity,the right to die,the experience of dying,mourning
& burial;like a good Cub-Scout leader taking the patrol on
a nature ramble.Sections of the book appeared before in the

480 ctd.) New York Times Magazine, & the Kutschers were
special advisers. It shows.
**

481. WE ARE BUT A MOMENT'S SUNLIGHT: UNDERSTANDING DEATH.
       Ed.C.S.Adler,G.Stanford,S.M.Adler. Pocket Books,N.Y.
       1976.

Selections from literary works showing different
perspectives on death.Not very good.Generally simplistic &
not appearing to be based on very much understanding of
the subject.
**

482. WE LIVED WITH DYING. Margaret Woods Johnson. Word
       Books,Waco,Texas.1975. 128 pp. $ 4.95.

Alas,another published self-therapy.Wayne Woods,a Lutheran
minister,died within 7 months of diagnosis of cancer.While
it may be very helpful for a widow to record her experiences
& her love,in most instances this should not be published.
But there is very little humility in bereavement,it seems;
we are all,in print at least,unique mourners of unique dead.
Mrs Johnson seems too self-concious of her "fragile gift of
writing" (how very fragile,my dear) and its "gentle
beauty unaware",using these Gifts of God "as He so nudges".
Oh God. Disquietingly cutesy.
*

483. WESTERN ATTITUDES TOWARD DEATH:From the Middle Ages
       to the Present. Philippe Aries. Johns Hopkins
       University Press,Baltimore.1974.111pp.$ 6.50,$ 2.25 PB.

A unique & highly accomplished historical perspective,
looking at attitudes to death in the West as reflected in
public & private ceremonies & customs,literature & art.
Ingenious social history,spare but consistently interesting.
****

484. THE WHEEL OF DEATH. Ed.Philip Kapleau.Harper & Row,NY.
       1971.Harper Colophon 1974 PB.110pp.$ 2.25.

An unusual & finely crafted anthology,not merely assembling
selections from Zen Buddhist & related sources,but balanced
& ably composed;exploring death,karma,re-birth & dying,the
deaths of Zen masters,& Kapleau's own practical instructions
to the dying,the bereaved,& those who accompany them.
Useful notes & glossary.
***½

485. WHY DID HE DIE? Audrey Harris. Lerner Publications,
      Minneapolis (J.M.Dent & Sons,Canada).1965.32pp.$4.25.

A childrens book about death.A good idea,disappointing in
its quality.It is written in very bad verse,to which
children should never be exposed.It's simplistic,& doesn't
attend to children's real fears about death.There's a great
emphasis on death as happening to "old,old"people,when
their hearts are "very tired,and could no longer tick".It
is admitted that some children die,very rarely,if their
hearts are weak.More attention to reality,more accuracy,
& simple prose are urgently needed.Of no use;a grim fairy
tale— stick to Grimm's.
*

486. WHY ME? WHY MINE? Clear Thinking About Suffering.
      Paul F.Adams. Abingdon Press,Nashville. 1974.$2.95.

A compassionate & sensible Christian response to the bitter
questions raised by human suffering,proposing some
alternative views & responses.
**½

487. WIDOW. Lynn Caine. William Morrow,NY.1974;Bantam PB
      1975. 182 pp. $ 1.75. McDonald & Jane's,London.
      1975. £ 2.95.

An honest autobiographical account of widowhood.A typical
specimen of the new genre of widowbooks,& perhaps the most
successful if not the most insightful.
***½

488. WILLS:A DEAD GIVEAWAY.Millie Considine & Ruth Pool.
      Doubleday & Co.,Garden City,NY.1974.

"Wills of some of the world's most interesting testators".
Tries far too hard,& it shows.
*

489. THE WOMAN SAID YES:Encounters with Life & Death.
      Jessamyn West. Harcourt,Brace,Jovanovich,NY. 1976.
      180pp. $ 7.95. Fawcett,NY PB.$ 1.95. Victor
      Gollancz,London.

"What the hell do I care about death with dignity? Others
might like to be spared the sight of something undignified.
If I don't feel it,what do I care?" said Carmen.This is the
story of 3 women:the mother,Grace,who died gracefully;
Jessamyn who in her 2o's was expected to die of advanced TB

489 ctd.) but didn't;and her sister Carmen who she nursed through her final illness,& who achieved considerable dignity in managing her own death.An intimate account of differing personal approaches to life and death.
***$\frac{1}{2}$

Y

490.   YOU AND YOUR GRIEF.Edgar M.Jackson. Harper & Row,NY.
       1962. 64pp. $ 2.50.

The advice of an experienced counsellor & pastor on coping with grief.
**

491.   YOU AND YOUR WILL:The Planning & Management of Your
       Estate. Paul P.Ashley. Mentor Books,New American
       Library,NY. 1977. 222 pp.

(Previously published by McGraw-Hill as a hardback). Revised to conform with the 1976 Tax Reform Act. Deals with wills, fiduciaries,trusts,executors,guardians,insurance & taxes. Succinctly helpful.
***

492.   YOUNG WIDOW.Jane Seskin. Ace Books,NY.1975.201pp.$1.50.

Alas,another self-therapeutic Widowbook.Loving,often over--done,often self-pitying account by a young widow of her husband's death from leukemia & how she coped with it.
*

N.B. THE WIDOWHOOD BOOK,and AN INTRODUCTION TO WIDOWHOOD
       (The Racing Pigeon Publishing Co.,London).Please note that these books are about racing pigeons,and "widowhood"is a system used in racing,involving enforced celibacy rather than actual bereavement.Also sad,but not entirely relevant to non-avian thanatology.

———o0o———

SUPPLEMENTARY LIST OF BOOKS

This list includes books very recently reviewed or notified, too late for inclusion in the main listing;and books which are definitely not recommended for reading or reference, which merit less than one star in the classification used, and were not considered to deserve even brief review.

493. THE ACCIDENT.Carol Carrick. Seabury,NY.1976.

A book for children 5-8,about how young Christopher mourns the loss of his dog who was killed by a truck.
**

494. AN ACT OF MERCY:EUTHANASIA TODAY. Richard Trubo.
      Nash Publ.Los Angeles. 1973. $ 7.95.

495. ADVENTURE IN DYING.Nancy Karo & Alvara Michelson.
      Moody,1976. $ 3.50.

496. AFTER THE FLOWERS HAVE GONE. Bea Decker.Zondervan.
      1973. $ 4.95.

497. ANN & THE SAND DOBBIES.John B.Coburn.Seabury,NY.1964.
      $ 4.95.

Danny's father tries to help him understand the death of his sister. (Ages 12+)

498. ANNIE AND THE OLD ONE.Miska Miles. Little,Brown,
      Boston. 1971.

On an Indian reservation,a girl learns a more philosophical acceptance of aging and death. (Ages 5-9)
**

499. APPOINTMENT WITH DEATH.Alvin N.Rogness & Youth
      Research Center. Thomas Nelson,NY.1972.$1.95.PB.

500. ATTITUDES ON DEATH & DYING:A CROSS CULTURAL VIEW.
      Ronald & Judy Lunceford. Hwong Press,1976.$ 8.95.

501. AWAY IS SO FAR.Toby Talbot. Scholastic Press,NY.1974.

B

502. THE BANAL & COSTLY FUNERAL.Vern L.Bullough. The
      Humanist Association,Humanist House,Yellow Springs,
      Ohio. 1960.

Evaluates mourning as a psychological need,the laws governing disposal of the dead,& high funeral costs.
***

137

503. BASIC PSYCHIATRY FOR PRIMARY CARE.Ed.Harry S.Abram.
      Little,Brown,Boston. 1976. 291pp. PB. £ 8.75.

Chapter on the Dying Patient by David Barton—surprisingly
weak.Reasonably fresh approach,but too many things are
mentioned too briefly,in too choppy a style.Levy & Clark on
the Chronically Ill,& Janowsky & Sternbach on pain,are
both good.
**½

504. BEING AND DEATH:An Outline of Integrationist
      Philosophy. Jose Ferrater Mora. University of
California Press,Berkeley. 1965.

505. BEING,MAN & DEATH:A Key to Heidegger. James W.Demske.
      University Press of Kentucky,Lexington. 1970.

506. BEGIN AGAIN.Margaret Torrie. CRUSE,London. £ 1.37.

507. BIBLIOGRAPHY OF BIOETHICS.Ed.Leroy Walters. Gale
      Research Co.,Detroit.   Vol.I, 1975. Vol.II,1976.
      Vol.III,1977.

508. THE BIRTHDAY VISITOR.Yoshiko Uchida.Scribners,NY.1975.

(For children,5-8).A Japanese family funeral.

509. BLICK NACH DRÜBEN: SELBSTERFAHRUNGEN IM STERBEN.
      Eckart Weisenhütter.(View into the Beyond:Self-
-experiences in dying). 3rd Edition. Gütersloher Verlag,
Gerd Mohn;Gütersloh,Germany. 1976.91pp. DM 5.80.

A psychiatrist at the Universities of Tübingen & Salzberg.
Following his own experiences near death,he explored those
of others .Explores death as a peak experience of
blissfulness,with"conscious collaboration";but without
telling us what"being dead"is like.Observes similar
phenomena to those Moody described later,but does not
speculate on life after death.Considers how a physician
like himself,after a near-death experience,approaches
his patients and can help them. Sensitive and highly
intelligent work.
***½

510. THE BLOOD OF THE LAMB.P. De Vries.Popular Library,NY.
      1974.

511. A BLUEBIRD WILL DO.Lolla Grace Erdman. Dodd,Mead,& Co.
      New York. 1973. $ 4.50.

512.   THE BOOK OF THE DEAD: FROM THE ANI,HUNEFER & ANHAI
       PAPYRI IN THE BRITISH MUSEUM.
       Garrett Publications,New York. 1966.

513.   BOOKS TO HELP CHILDREN COPE WITH SEPARATION & LOSS.
       Joanne E.Bernstein. Bowker,NY.1977.255pp.$ 13.95.

Designed for parents or therapists who want to help a child
deal with loss by reading a story.Part I.briefly discusses
separation & loss;Part 2 has an annotated bibliography in
3 sections: learning to face separation with regard to new
schools,new neighbourhood,going into hospital,etc.;coping
with tragic loss involving death,divorce,war,etc., and
adjustment to foster-care,adoption & step-parents.Part 3
is a bibliography on separation and loss for adult helpers.
Useful for those who believe in bibliotherapy.
***

514.   BOUNDARIES:Psychological Man in Revolution.Robert
       Jay Lifton. Simon & Schuster (Touchstone PB)1977.$2.95.

A further eloquent exploration of modern social problems in
the light of Lifton's views on the result of the breach of
our sense of immortality,the blurring boundary between
living and dead.
***

515.   THE BROKEN HEART:THE MEDICAL CONSEQUENCES OF
       LONELINESS. James J.Lynch.Basic Books,NY.1977.271pp.
       $ 10.95.

C

516.   CASE STUDIES IN MEDICAL ETHICS.Robert M.Veatch.
       Harvard University Press,New Haven.1977.424pp.£10.50.

517.   THE CAUSES OF SUICIDE.Maurice Halbwachs. Routledge &
       Kegan Paul,London. 372 pp. 1978. £ 7.75.

(Originally published in French as'Les Causes du Suicide',
Librairie Felix Alcan,Paris,1930).A significant successor
to Durckheim,studying the social causes of increasing
suicide rates up to 1927,including data on England,France,
Germany & Italy.
***

518.   THE CHILD IN HIS FAMILY.Vol.2.THE IMPACT OF DISEASE
       & DEATH. Ed.E.J.Anthony & Cyrille Koupernik. John
       Wiley & Sons,1973. 510 pp.

519.   CHILDREN IN FEAR: HOW WE TEACH THEM FEAR OF DEATH.
       Stephen Joseph. Holt,Rinehart,NY. 1974.$ 6.95.

520.   CHILDREN'S CONCEPTIONS OF AGING AND DEATH.Steve
       Fleming & Richard Lonetto. Springer,NY.1978 (in press)

521.   THE CHILD'S ATTITUDE TO DEATH.Marjorie Mitchell.
       Schocken,NY. 1966. $ 4.95.

A not very profound account of some children's attitudes
toward death in Britain in the early 1960's.

522.   CHRONIC ILLNESS IN CHILDREN:Its Impact on Child and
       Family. Georgia Travis. Stanford University Press,
       Stanford.1976. 556 pp. $ 19.50.

Written to help Social Workers deal with the psychosocial
implications of chronic illness in children,the effects on
child & family.Opening chapters outline a conceptual
framework for discussing the experience of chronic illness
in childhood,& community resources.Further chapters deal
with specific problems,outlining the medical data & psycho-
-social implications & effects,& their management.These
include asthma,chronic kidney disease,congenital heart
disease,cystic fibrosis,head injury,hemophilia,leukemia,
muscular dystrophy,& spina bifida.Generally reliable,and
comprehensive in its advice,biased toward California in its
examples & citations. It could with benefit have included
more on other varieties of cancer,& on child & early
adolescent attitudes to death.Surely useful to any Social
Worker dealing with sick children.
***

533.   CONTEMPORARY ADULTHOOD. J.Turner & D.Helms. W.B.
       Saunders,Philadelphia.1978.260pp. $ 5.95.

A suitable text for courses considering the life-span,
beyond the usual text which abandons life at adolescence.
It covers the period from late adolescence through to death.
***

534.   COPING WITH TRAGEDY:SUCCESSFULLY FACING THE PROBLEM
       OF A SERIOUSLY ILL CHILD. J.L.Schulman. Follett
       Publ.Co.,Chicago. 1976.335 pp. $ 9.55.

525.   THE CRAFT OF DYING:A Study in the Literary Tradition
       of the Ars Moriendi in England. Nancy Lee Beaty.
       Yale University Press,New Haven. 1970.

526.   CRAIG & JOAN: TWO LIVES FOR PEACE. Eliot Asinof.
       Viking Press,New York. 1971.

527.   A CRITICAL EXAMINATION OF THE BELIEF IN LIFE AFTER
       DEATH. C.J.Ducasse.C.C.Thomas,Springfield,Illinois.
       1961. 335 pp. $ 7.50.
D
528.   THE DANCE OF DEATH (Les Simulachre et Historiees Faces
       de la Mort.) Hans Holbein engravings. The Cygnet Press,
       Boston. 1974. (Also Bodley Head,London,private edition.)

529.   DAY BY DAY.Ron Shuman. The Scrimshaw Press,Oakland.
       1977. 96 pp. $ 13.95.
Very competent photojournalism,representing the pediatric
oncology unit at Children's Hospital,Stanford University.
48 black & white photographs,& a text of verbatim comments
from staff,patient meetings,& interviews.Evocative account
of life near death,for patients,families & staff. Accurate
without undue sentimentality.
****
530.   DEATH: A BIBLIOGRAPHICAL GUIDE.Albert J.Miller and
       Albert J.Acri. Scarecrow Press,Metuchen,NJ. 1977.
       420pp. $ 16.00.

Assembled by non-experts-a sort of bibliography,whose
guidance is not especially reliable or impressive.
**
531.   DEATH & BURIAL IN THE ROMAN WORLD. J.M.Toynbee.
       Cornell University Press,Ithaca,NY.1971.$ 11.50.

532.   DEATH & CONTEMPORARY MAN:THE CRISIS OF TERMINAL
       ILLNESS. Carl G.Colozzi. Wm.B.Eerdmans,Grand
       Rapids,Michigan. $ 1.45.
Written by a minister,attempting to understand those
facing death.
**
533.   DEATH & CREATIVITY:An Interdisciplinary Encounter.
       Florence Hetzler. Health Sciences Publ.Co.NY.
       1976. 351 pp. $ 8.95.
Some aspects of death & the humanities.
**
534.   DEATH & DYING: A BIBLIOGRAPHY (1950-1974) G.Howard
       Poteet. Whitston. 1976. $ 12.50.

535. DEATH AND ETERNAL LIFE.J.Hick. Harper & Row,New
      York. 1976.

536. DEATH & IMMORTALITY. Josef Pieper. Burns & Oates,
      London.(Herder & Herder,NY). 1969.

537. DEATH AND PRESENCE: The Psychology of Death & the
      After-Life. Ed. A.Godin. Lumen Vitae Studies in the
Psychology of Religion. Lumen Vitae Press,Brussels.1972.PB.
Religious implications of death & dying,with some reviews
in English of the European literature.
**

538. (Omitted.)

539. DEATH & THE MINISTRY.J.Donald Bane & A.H.Kutscher.
      Schocken,NY. 1975. $ 10.95.

540. DEATH,DYING & THE LAW. Ed.James T.McHugh. Our Sunday
      Visitor Press,Huntington,IN. 1976. 88pp.

541. DEATH:END OF THE BEGINNING? Mary Montgomery.
      Holt,Rinehart & Winston,Toronto. 1972.

542. DEATH IN LIFE: SURVIVORS OF HIROSHIMA.Robert Jay
      Lifton. Simon & Schuster (Touchstone PB)NY.
      1967,1975. $ 5.95.
Brilliant study of the hibakusha,the survivors of the Bomb.
Compelling empathy,analysis,insight,grace.An understanding
of the awful that illuminates our own existence.
****

543. A DEATH IN THE FAMILY:A GUIDE TO THE COST OF DYING IN
      NEW YORK CITY,NASSAU & SUFFOLK. Barbara Kronan. New
      York Public Interest Research Group,NY.1974.

Price ranges,information & advice for consumers,to help them
make informed purchases,with suggestions for legislators.
***

544. A DEATH IN THE SANCHEZ FAMILY. Oscar Lewis. Random
      House,NY. 1969.
In this sequel to the Children of Sanchez,the anthropologist
describes how death affects a poor Mexican family.
***

545. DEATH IN THE SECULAR CITY:A Study of the Notion of
      Life After Death in Contemporary Theology & Philosophy.
      Russell Aldwinkle. George Allen & Unwin,London.1972.

546. DEATH,SACRIFICE & TRAGEDY.Martin Foss. University of
      Nebraska Press, Lincoln,Nebraska. 1966.

547. DEATH: TEACHER'S GUIDE. Marion Nessit. Holt,Rinehart
      & Winston, Toronto.(Infinity Series).1972.

548. DIARY OF A PIGEON WATCHER.Doris Schwern.Wm Morrow,
      New York, 1976.

549. DISASTERS: Theory and Research. Ed. E.L.Quarantelli.
      Sage Publications,London. 1978. 160pp.£8.00,£3.95 PB.

550. THE DOCTOR AS JUDGE OF WHO SHALL LIVE & WHO SHALL DIE.
      Helmut Thielicke. Fortress Press,Philadelphia.1976.41pp.

551. DYING: A PSYCHOANALYTICAL STUDY With Special
      Reference to Individual Creativity & Defensive
      Organization. Tor-Björn Hagglund. Monographs of the
Psychiatric Clinic of the Helsinki University Central
Hospital. 1976. 138 pp. PB.

552. THE DYING CHILD:The Management of the Child or
      Adolescent Who is Dying. William M.Easson. C.C.Thomas,
      Springfield,Ill. 1970.112pp. $ 5.75. 1977, $ 4.75 PB.

553. DYING: FACING THE FACTS. Ed.Hannelore Wass. McGraw-
      Hill/ Hemisphere,NY,Washington. 1979.
A bright & original college text on matters relating to
death,with good review-chapters on all major aspects of the
topic.Authors include Fulton,Simpson,Davidson & Quint-
-Benoliel.Insufficient on research methodologies,but
otherwise excellent.
****
E
554. THE EDGE OF NEXT YEAR.Mary Stolz. Harper & Row,NY.1974.

555. EFFECTS OF EARLY PARENT DEATH. Ed.J.Bischwell.MSS
      Information Corp.,NY. 1973. $ 17.00.

556. THE EMERGING DEATH MYSTIQUE: THE CHALLENGE & THE
      PROMISE. Harry G.Armstron. Exposition Press,
      Hicksville,NY. 1978. 252 pp. $ 10.50.
The benefits of terminal oxygen deficiency.A routine
account of the routine stuff,with laudatory reviews from
people not involved in the field or familiar with the
literature,or qualified to judge.
*

557.   ENCYCLOPEDIA OF DEATH. J.R.Francis. Amherst Press,$4.00
An ambitious title for a mediocre product...

558.   ETHICAL ISSUES IN MODERN MEDICINE. Ed.Robert Hunt &
       John Arras. Mayfield Publ.Co.,Palo Alto.1977. 524pp.
       $ 13.95, $ 9.95 PB.

An earnest anthology.A detailed introduction by the editors
outlines ethical theory in the medical context (especially
utilitarianism,Kantian theories,religion & natural law),&
is a competent resource for any course on the subject.
Subsequent sections include exerpts from various authors,&
deal with Genetics (Brave New World,genetic engineering &
screening;Veatch,Fletcher & Ramsey);Abortion;Euthanasia
(including Shaw on dilemmas of consent in children, and
Schowalter on the adolescent patient's decision to die);
Informed Consent (Capron,Lasagna & guess who?:Veatch &
Ramsey!);Behavior Control & Psychosurgery (Skinner,Dworkin,
etc,);& Justice & Social Policy in Medicine——who lives &
dies,allocation of scarce life-saving therapies,etc.:Illich,
Kass & others. Overdependent on Veatch & Ramsey;but a most
useful,thought-provoking & varied collection.
***

559.   EUTHANASIA & THE RIGHT TO DEATH.Ed.A.B.Downing.
       Peter Owen,London. 1969. £ 3.25.

560.   THE EUTHANASIA CONTROVERSY (1812-1974)A Bibliography
       with Select Annotations. Charles W.Triche III & Diane
       Striche. Whitston, Troy,NY.1975.242pp. & 18.00.

561.   THE EVIDENCE FOR LIFE AFTER DEATH.Martin Ebon. Signet
       NY (New American Library). 1977.177pp. $ 1.50 PB.

Kitsch. Includes The Moody Phenomena,& The Pilgrimage of Dr.
Kubler-Ross. By the author of books about--Test Your ESP,
the Maharishi,Witchcraft Today,Exorcism,TM,Atlantis,Uri
Geller,Pyramid Power,etc. Gruesome "me-too" book,100%
bandwagon jumping. A sort of Teach Yourself Life After
Death in Six Easy Lessons.
minus *

562.   AN EXISTENTIAL UNDERSTANDING OF DEATH. James Park.
       Existential Press, 1975. $ 1.00.

F

563. FACING GRIEF & DEATH.William P.Tuck.Broadman,1975.$3.95.

564. THE FAMILY AND INHERITANCE.Marvin B.Sussman,et al.
      Russell Sage Foundation,NY.(Distributed Basic Books).
      1970.

What happens to a family legally on the death of a property-
-owner.Based on interviews with lawyers,will-makers and
beneficiaries.
***

565. THE FAMILY IN MOURNING: A GUIDE FOR HEALTH
      PROFESSIONALS.Ed.Charles E.Hollingsworth & Robert O.
      Pasnau. Grune & Stratton,NY. 1977. 240pp. $17.50,£12.40.

A study of one family,with congenital cardiomyopathy;then
sections on informing families of death;observations on
mourning;helping the family in mourning;& helping the
helpers;the role of liaison psychiatry. Seriously
over-ambitious.Some reasonable material on mourning in
different situations,& on pathological grief.Considers
sudden death,the death of the very elderly,violent deaths,
abortion,birth of a handicapped child,& other varieties of
loss. Also useful descriptions of some liaison programs
with obstetrics staff (dealing with the tragic birth);a
bone.marrow transplant project,& with coronary care staff.
Very superficial,many chapters are merely a page or 2 of
brief case-histories;some material unhelpful and
inaccurate. Shallow and disappointing.Too little made out
to be too much.
**

566. FIGURES OF DEAD MEN. Leonard Baskin. Preface:Archibald
      Macleish. Photo's Hyman Edelstein. University of
      Massachusetts Press,Amherst.1968.

The superb Baskin engravings of the dead.
***

567. THE FINAL MYSTERY.S.Klein. Doubleday,NY.1974.
Exploration of the meanings of death for people of different
cultures,times,religions & regions.
**

568. FOR THE LIVING.E.Jackson. Meredith Publishing Co.,
      Des Moines,IA. 1963.

569. FREUD: LIVING AND DYING.Max Schur. International
      Universities Press,NY. 1972. 601 pp. $ 20.00.

Analyzes Freud's concepts of death in relation to his own
life and fear of death.Dr.Schur was Freud's personal
doctor for eleven years before his death.
***

570. FREEDOM AND DEATH.A.Metzger. Human Context Books,
      Chaucer Publ.Co.,London. 1973. 240pp. £ 4.50.

571. FUNERAL CUSTOMS:THEIR ORIGIN & DEVELOPMENT.
      Bertram C.Puckle. Gale,Detroit.1968.$12.50.

572. THE FUNERAL ENCYCLOPEDIA.Ed.Charles Wallis.Baker.
      $ 3.95.

G
573. GLIMPSES OF THE BEYOND. J.B.Delacour. Delacorte
      Press,New York. 1974.

574. GOODBYE,GRANDPA.Ron Koch. Augsberg. 1973. $ 1.95.

575. GOOD GRIEF:A Constructive Approach to the Problems
      of Loss. G.Westberg.Fortress,Philadelphia. 1962.

576. GREEK BURIAL CUSTOMS. Donna C.Kurtz & J.Broadman.
      Cornell University Press,Ithaca,NY. 1971.

Burial customs & beliefs about death & the afterlife,based
on archeological & literary sources. Illustrated.
***

577. GRIEF & MOURNING IN CROSS-CULTURAL PERSPECTIVES.
      P.C.Rosenblatt,P.R.Walsh,D.A.Jackson. Human Relations
      Area Files,Washington,DC.1977.231pp.$9.00,$.4.50 PB.

The authors rate 78 societies on 87 variables concerning
mourning practices,& look for correlations,for example,
between the occurrance of death ceremonies & the absence of
prolonged grief;tie-breaking ceremonies & remarriage with
a former in-law,between specialists in ritual & curtailing
the expression of anger.Compares American practices quite
closely with other cultures.Somewhat oversimplified,for
such simple correlations could have a considerable number
of social or psychological causes,& this book has no means
of choosing between them.More detailed analysis of individual
cases & more sophisticated statistical technique might have
improved the degree of understanding achieved.A promising
beginning,however.
***

578. GRIEF: SELECTED READINGS. Ed. Arthur S.Carr & B.
      Schoenberg. Health Sciences Publishing Co.,NY.
      1975. $ 6.75.

579. GRIST FOR THE MILL. Ram Dass. Unity,California.1977.
Describes the author's explorations in non-drug techniques
for altered states of consciousness,including its use to
alter the quality of the dying experience.He plans a center
for the dying "where people could come to die consciously,
surrounded by other beings who (are)not freaked by death".
This may sound like an attempt by one of the fading guru's
of the 60's to join the death movement,but it warrants more
serious & critical attention.
***

580. GROVER.V.Cleaver.Lippincott,Philadelphia.1970.
Grover,after his mother's death by suicide,finds his own
way to overcome his grief. (Children,ages 8-11).

581. GROWING TIME. Sandol Warburg. Houghton Mifflin.1969.
Coping with the death of a dog.(Children,6-9).

H
582. HELPING A CHILD UNDERSTAND DEATH.L.J.Vogel.
      Fortress Press,Philadelphia. 1975.

583. HELPING CHILDREN COPE WITH LOSS:A BIBLIOTHERAPY
      APPROACH. Joanne E.Bernstein. R.R.Bowker,NY.1978.

584. HELP FOR THE BEREAVED. Curtis A.Smith. Educational
      Dev.Association.,1972. $ 1.50.

585. HEY,WHAT'S WRONG WITH THIS ONE? M.Wojciechowska,
      Harper & Row, New York. 1969.

586. HOME FROM THE WAR: Transformations of Vietnam
      Veterans.(Neither Victims Nor Executioners). Robert
      Jay Lifton. Simon & Schuster (TouchstonePB)1977.$3.95.

587. THE HOSPICE CONCEPT.R.Buckingham,J.Kron,& H.Wald.
      Health Sciences Publ.Co.NY.1977.

588. HOSPICE: CREATING NEW MODELS OF CARE FOR THE
      TERMINALLY ILL. Parker Rossman.

Written by a freelance writer whose other books are"Sexual
Experiences Between Men & Boys;Exploring the Pederast
Underground",& "Pirate Slave". Seems to be seeking to join
the mass market band-wagon.
*

589.   HOSPICE. FIRST AMERICAN HOSPICE:Three Years of Home
       Care. Robert W.Buckingham & Sylvia Lack. Hospice,
       New Haven,CT. 1978. $ 15.75.

Reviews the Hospice concept & evaluation methodology;the
history,organization,administration,training,policy and
procedure manual of the home care & volunteer program of
Hospice New Haven.The outcome of evaluation studies and
their conclusions— the sort of studies that are badly
needed.
***

590.   HOW TO FACE DEATH WITHOUT FEAR. St.Alphonse Liguori.
       Liguori Press. 1976. $ 1.00.

591.   HOW TO PREPARE FOR DEATH.Yaffa Drazin.Hawthorn.1976.
       $ 7.95.

I

592.   IDENTIFYING SUICIDE POTENTIAL. Dorothy B.Anderson &
       L.J.McClean. Behavioral Press/Human Sciences Publ.
       Corp.,NY.1971. 124 pp. $ 9.95.

593.   IF I SHOULD DIE,IF I SHOULD LIVE.Joanne Marxhausen.
       Concordia. $ 4.95.

594.   THE IMMORTALITY FACTOR.Osborn Segerberg. E.P.Dutton,
       New York. 1974.

595.   THE IMMORTALITY NEWSLETTER.26 issues,5 volumes,bound.
       The Dominion Press,San Marcos,California.$ 20.00.

596.   IMPACT OF DEATH FEAR ON AN AMERICAN FAMILY. Eric
       Bermann. Greenhaven. 1974. $ 7.95.

597.   IN A DARKNESS.James Wechsler.Norton,NY.1972. $ 5.95.

A journalist's account of his son who committed suicide.
***

598.   INDIVIDUALITY IN PAIN & SUFFERING.Asenath Petrie.
       2nd Edn. University of Chicago Press,Chicago.
       1978. 154 pp. PB.

599.   I NEVER SANG FOR MY FATHER. R.Anderson.Random House,
       New York. 1968.

J

600.   JOY BEYOND GRIEF.Colena M.Anderson. Zondervan,
       1974.

601. JUDGEMENT OF THE DEAD:LIFE AFTER DEATH IN MAJOR
RELIGIONS.Samuel G.Brandon. Scribner,NY.1969.
300pp. $ 4.95, $ 2.95 PB.

602. JULIA'S STORY: The Tragedy of an Unnecessary Death.
Fred J. Cook. Holt,Rinehart & Winston,NY.1976.
180pp. $ 7.95.

L

603. THE LAST ACT:BEING THE FUNERAL RITES OF NATIONS AND
INDIVIDUALS.William Tegg. Gale,Detroit. 1973.$ 15.00.

604. THE LAST OF THE NUBA.Leni Riefenstahl. Collins,
London. 1976. 208 pp.
Magnificent,opulent photographic account of the Nuba;Chapter
5 dealing specifically with the Death beliefs & customs of
this African tribe.
***

605. THE LAST RIGHTS:A LOOK AT FUNERALS.Ed. Francia Faust
Johannson.Maryland Center for Public Broadcasting,
Owings,Mills,Md., 1975.(Consumer Survival Kit series)
$1.00.
An assortment of articles dealing with funeral planning;
cost information,alternatives,& advice.
***

606. LEARNING TO DIE. Jon Mundy. Freedeeds Associationm
1976. $ 2.95.

607. LEARNING TO DIE,LEARNING TO LIVE.Robert Herhold.
Fortress,Philadelphia. 1976. $ 2.95.

608. LEARNING TO LIVE AS A WIDOW.M.Langner. Messmer,NY.1957.

609. LEGISLATIVE MANUAL 1977. The Society for the Right
To Die,New York. 1978. $ 2.00. PB.

Review of 1977's Right to Die legislative activity;texts of
8 new laws,with commentary;chart of the year's Bills in
47 states. Excellent summary of the current position.
***

610. LIFE AGAINST DEATH:The Psychoanalytical Meaning of
History.Norman O.Brown.Wesleyan Univ.Press,Middletown,
Conn.1959.374pp. $ 2.95 PB.Sphere Library,1968/70.
40 pence,U.K. Routledge & Kegan Paul,London,1959.
Eros,death,sublimation,anality & resurrection.A major work
of post-Freudian psychology,considering death as Freud
could not.
***

611. LIFE & DEATH IN PSYCHOANALYSIS.Jean Laplanche.
      Johns Hopkins University Press,Baltimore.

612. THE LIFE OF THE SELF:Toward a New Psychology.Robert
      Jay Lifton. Simon & Schuster (TouchstonePB)1977.$2.95.

The theme of death & the continuity of life explored with
the techniques of psychohistory;survivors & psychic numbing
as our heritage from the nuclear age;the search for an
understandable form of existence.
***

613. LIFE OR DEATH: ETHICS & OPTIONS.Edward A Shils.
      University of Washington Press,1968.

614. LIVING WITH AN EMPTY CHAIR:A GUIDE THROUGH GRIEF.
      Roberta Temes. Mandala Press,Amherst,Mass.
      1977. 80pp. $ 3.95 PB.

615. LIVING WITH DYING.Glen W.Davidson.Augsberg,
      Minneapolis. 1975. $ 2.95.

616. LOVE STORY. E.Segal. New American Library,NY.1970.

M
617. THE MAGIC MOTH.Virginia Lee. Seabury Press,NY.1972.

618. MANAGING GRIEF WISELY.Stanley Cornils. Baker
      Books. 1967. $ 8.50.

619. MAN DOES SURVIVE DEATH.D.S.Rogo.Citadel Press,
      Secaucus,NJ. 1977.

(Originally published as The Welcoming Silence,in 1973)
Some events relating to possibilities of survival.
**

620. THE MASK OF EUTHANASIA.Leah Curtin. Nurses Concerned
      For Life, Cincinnati. 1976. 72pp.

621. MOMO. Emile Ajar. Transl.R.Manheim. Collins/Harvill.
      1978. £ 4.25.

French novel which won the Prix Goncourt,& was made into a
prize-winning film.A young Arab boy is brought up by an
old Jewish woman;a study of their affection through her
senile dementia & death.Moving & surprisingly funny.
***

622. THE MORALITY OF KILLING. Marvin Kohl. Peter Owen,
      London. 1975. £ 3.25.

623. MR DEATH:FOUR STORIES.Anne Moody.Harper & Row,New
      York. 1975. $ 5.95.

624. MEANING OF IMMORTALITY IN HUMAN EXPERIENCE. William
      E.Hocking. Greenwood. 1973. $ 13.50.

625. MESSENGERS FROM THE DEAD:Literature of the Holocaust.
      Irving Halperin. Westminster Press,Philadelphia.1970.

626. THE MODERN VISION OF DEATH.Nathan A.Scott. John Knox
      Press,Atlanta. 1967.

627. THE MOMENT OF DEATH: A Symposium.Ed.Arthur Winter.
      C.C.Thomas,Springfield,Ill.1969. $ 6.00.

628. THE MORALITY OF KILLING.Marvin Kohl. Humanities Press,
      Atlantic Highlands,NJ. 1974.

629. MY FRIEND FISH. Mamie Hegwood. Holt,Rinehart & Winston,
      New York. 1975.
For children.A black 7 year-old catches a fish,decides to
keep it,& responds to its death.
**

630. MY GRANDPA DIED TODAY.Joan Fassler.Behavioral/Human
      Sciences Press,NY.1971.(pages not numbered). $ 5.95.
A boy's feelings when his grandfather dies.Somewhat didactic.
For children,4-8.
**

631. MY GRANDSON LEW. Charlotte Zolotow. Harper & Row,
      New York. 1974.
(Children,4-8).Lew isn't told of his grandfather's death,
& waits for him to return;& still mourns for him years later.
**

632. THE MYSTERY OF DEATH.Ladislaw Boros. Crossroads.1973.

N
633. NEEDS OF THE CANCER PATIENT.Ed.Joanne Parsons.Pamphlet.
      Nursing Digest,Wakefield,MA. 1976.

634. NILDA.Nicholasa Mohr. Harper & Row,NY.1973.$5.95.

635. NONNA. Jennifer Bartoli. Harvey,NY. 1975.
(Children,4-8). After their grandmother's death,children
take part in the funeral and estate decisions.
**

O
636. THE OLD DOG.Sarah Abbott. Coward,McCann & Geoghegan,
      1972.

For children,5-9. A boy's dog dies,& he feels lonely & empty.

637. ONLY A LITTLE TIME:A Memoir of My Wife. Sidney
      Werkman. Little,Brown, Boston. 1972. $ 5.95.

A psychiatrist writes about his young wife's struggle
against leukemia.
***

638. ONLY A LITTLE TIME:A MEMOIR. Sidney Werkman.
      Harper & Row, 1973. $ 2.95.

Account of the final months of the life of his son,with
a brain tumour.
***

639. ON SUICIDE.Paul Friedman. International Universities
      Press,New York. 1967. 141 pp. $ 7.50.

P
640. PAINTING IN FLORENCE & SIENNA AFTER THE BLACK DEATH.
      Millard Meiss. Harper Torchbook,NY.1964. PB.
(Originally,Princeton University Press,1951). The arts,
religion & society in the era of the Great Plague.Illus.

641. THE PARENT AND THE FATALLY ILL CHILD.M.B.Hamovitch.
      Delmar,Los Angeles. 1964.

642. PASTORAL CARE & COUNSELLING IN GRIEF & SEPARATION.
      W.Oates. Fortress Press,Philadelphia.1976.

643. THE PERSON:HIS & HER DEVELOPMENT THROUGHOUT THE LIFE
      CYCLE.Theodore Lidz. Basic Books,NY. 1976.615pp.$10.95.

Revised version of an earlier(1968)text of personality
development from a psychodynamic perspective.Heavily
dynamic rather than empirical.Three sections deal with the
theoretical background,the course of the personality across
the life-cycle,& the impact of life-stress on adjustment.
Discussion of the second half of life is far less adequate,
& a variety of recent developments & studies are omitted &
neglected.The final chapter,on death,considers the patient's
perspective & the doctor's role in caring.Omits much
important work,including Parkes & others;inadequate with
regard to bereavement & survival.A literate but out-of-date
account,even in its latest edition.
**

644. PHILOSOPHICAL ASPECTS OF THANATOLOGY. Ed.F.M.Hessler
     & J.P.Carse.Vol.I & Vol.II. MSS Information Co.,NY.
     1976. $ 13.50.

645. PHILOSOPHY OF LIFE & PHILOSOPHY OF DEATH.C.M.Flumani.
     Classical College Press,1972. $ 15.00.

646. PRACTICAL PSYCHIATRY IN MEDICINE.J.B.Imboden & J.C.
     Urbaitis. Appleton-Century-Crofts,NY.1978.304pp.£6.65.

More about general psychiatry than liaison psychiatry,so a
misleading title.Chapters on the Dying Patient & his family,
& suicidal behavior are awfully over-simplified,too brief
& inadequate,with very few references.Unusable.
*

647. THE PRICE OF DEATH: A SURVEY METHOD & CONSUMER GUIDE
     for Funerals,Cemetaries,& Grave Markers. Seattle
     Regional Office,Federal Trade Commission.U.S.Govt.
     Printing Office,Washington DC. 1975.

648. PRIMITIVE CONCEPTIONS OF DEATH & THE UNDERWORLD.
     Nicholas J.Tromp. Loyola Press. 1969. $ 11.00.

649. PROLONGEVITY.Albert Rosenfield. Alfred A.Knopf,NY.
     1976. 267 pp.

650. THE PSYCHEDELIC EXPERIENCE:A MANUAL ON THE TIBETAN
     BOOK OF THE DEAD.T.Leary,R.Letzner,R.Alpert.
     University Books,New Hyde Park,NY. 1964.

651. THE PSYCHOLOGY OF DEATH AND DYING.Richard Schultz.
     Addison-Wesley Publ.Co.,Reading,Mass.1978.
General review of death work,not especially impressive.
**

652. THE PURSUIT OF DEATH.H.Congdon.Abingdon,Nashville,1977.

Q
653. QUEST:A SEARCH FOR SELF.Sarah Cirese. Holt,Rinehart
     & Winston,NY.1977. 427 pp. $ 12.95.
A text & how-to-do-it exploration of personal growth,
including the "quests"for separateness & wholeness,intimacy,
competence,& unboundedness.Its final chapters deal with
aging & death,not especially profoundly.Handsomely produced.
**

R
654.   RACE & SUICIDE IN SOUTH AFRICA.Fatima Meer.
        Routledge,Kegan Paul,Boston.1976.304pp.$18.95.

655.   REPORT OF THE PRESIDING OFFICER ON PROPOSED TRADE
        REGULATION RULE CONCERNING FUNERAL INDUSTRY
        PRACTICES.Federal Trade Commission.Jack E.Kahn,
Presiding Officer.(16.C.F.R.Part 453;Public Record 215-46)
July 1977. 40pp. PB. FTC,Washington DC.

Intriguing reading,of the hearings,critical of current
practices in the industry.
***

656.   RESPONSIBLE STEWARDSHIP OF HUMAN LIFE:INQUIRY INTO
        MEDICAL ETHICS.II. Ed.D.G.McCarthy.Catholic Hospital
        Association,St.Louis. 1976. 138 pp.

657.   REVOLUTION IN THE BODY MIND.I.Forewarning Cancer
        Dreams & the Bioplasma Concept. Daniel E.Schneider.
        The Alexa Press, Easthampton,NY. 104pp. $ 8.95.
An unparalleled specimen of eccentricity,deliciously dotty.
A wierd set of theories & formulae involving dreams that
predict cancer,a sort of psychosomatic theory of death &
disaster,an assertion that we live for the duration of
2.796×10^9 heart beats;graphs purporting to show a
correlation between the male schizophrenic admission rate
& the growth of heart weight,& the bioplasma-paraconscious
body-mind communication-control systems,with equations for
use in urgent research on cancer,psychosis,heart disease,
stroke & homosexuality (!) A solemn work that reads
unfortunately like a complex delusional system or awkward
parody of the scientific method. Golly!
*

658.   THE ROLE OF THE COMMUNITY HOSPITAL IN THE CARE OF THE
        DYING PATIENT & THE BEREAVED.Ed.E.Gerchick. MSS
        Information Co.,NY. 1976. $ 13.50.

S
659.   SEASONALITY IN HUMAN MORTALITY:A Medico-Geographical
        Study. Masako Sakamoto-Momiyama.University of Tokyo
        Press, Tokyo. 1977. 181pp. $ 14.50.

660.   THE SHAPE OF DEATH:Life,Death & Immortality in the
        Early Fathers. Jaroslav Pelikan. Macmillan,London.1962.

661.   SISTERS. Eloise Greenfield.Crowell,NY.1974. $ 4.95.

662. THE SOCIAL MEANING OF SUICIDE. J.D.Douglas. Princeton
      University Press. 1970. $ 15.00.

663. SOCIAL STRUCTURE & ASSASSINATION BEHAVIOR:The
      Sociology of Political Murder. Ed.Doris Y.Wilkinson.
      Schenckman,Cambridge,Mass.1976. 226pp. $ 9.50.

A collection of 15 articles,ranging from ex cathedra
pronouncements by psychiatrists,journalists & historians
(who should know better) to some sobre quantitative cross-
-cultural studies of assassination.Themes include social
structure & the assassination of U.S.Presidents.Basically,
its posture is that assassination arises from social factors
rather than individual psychology. Somewhat doctrinaire.
**

664. STANDARDS FOR SUICIDE PREVENTION & CRISIS CENTERS.
      Jerome Motto,R.Brooks,C.Ross & N.H.Allen (Eds).
      Behavioral Publications/Human Sciences Press,NY.
      1974. $ 9.95.

665. STORIES FROM A SNOWY MEADOW.C.Stevens.Seabury,NY.1976.

Children's story,representing death in relatively clear
terms,using simple animal characters.
**

666. SUICIDAL BEHAVIOR.J.W.McCulloch & A.E.Phillip.
      Pergamon,NY & London.1972.123pp.$9.50,£5.50.

Very lacklustre & drab account of routine suicidology,
devoid of special features.
**

667. SUICIDAL BEHAVIORS:DIAGNOSIS & MANAGEMENT.H.L.Resnik,
      Little,Brown, Boston. 1968. $ 17.50.

668. SUICIDE & MASS SUICIDE.Joost A.M.Meerlo. E.P.Dutton,
      NY. 1968.

669. SUICIDE & MORALITY:The Theories of Plato,Acquinas &
      Kant,& Their Relevance for Suicidology. David Novak.
      Scholars Studies Press,NY. 1975. 134 pp. $ 7.50.

670. SURVIVAL & DISEMBODIED EXISTENCE.Terence Penelhum.
      Routledge & Kegan Paul,London. 1970.

T

671. A TASTE OF BLACKBERRIES.Doris Buchanan Smith.
Thomas Y.Crowell,NY. 1973. (Ages 8-11)
James dies of a bee-sting,& his best fried comes to terms
with his grief & guilt at not having been able to save him.
***

672. A TEACHING UNIT ON DEATH & DYING.(For Senior High
School & Junior College Students). Memorial Society
of Edmonton. 1975. 103pp. $ 4.00. PB.
A competent & thoughtful booklet of teaching materials on
aspects of death & funerals,with valuable advice on such
teaching,& a healthy attitude to funerals.
***

673. TEACHING YOUR CHILD TO COPE WITH CRISIS. How To Help
Your Child Deal With Death,Divorce,etc. Suzanne Ramos.
David McKay,Co.Inc.,NY. 1974. 666pp. $ 7.95.

674. TELLING A CHILD ABOUT DEATH.Edgar N.Jackson. Hawthorn
Books Inc.,NY. 1965. 94pp. $ 4.95, $ 1.95 PB.

675. THE TENTH GOOD THING ABOUT BARNEY. Judith Viorst.
Atheneum,NY. 1971. $ 4.95.

Barney the cat has died,& his owner eulogises him at the
funeral.
***

676. TEREPIA DE MUERTE (The Death Therapy).Richard Sapir
& Warren Murphy,transl.M.O.Castro. (Spanish). Fiesta
Publ.Corp.,Miami,Florida.1975. 95¢, PB.

677. THANATOLOGY COURSE OUTLINES.D.J.Cherico.MSS Informn.
Co.,NY. 1975. $ 12.50.

678. THANATOS:A MODERN SYMPOSIUM. Maurice Richardson &
& Philip Toynbee. Victor Gollancz,London.1963.

679. THANK YOU,JACKIE ROBINSON.B.Cohen.Lothrop,NY.1974.
12 year-old Sam mourns for his close friend,an old black
cook,after the experiences they have shared. (Ages 8-11).

680. THEMES IN GREEK & LATIN EPITAPHS.Richmond Lattimore.
University of Illinois Press,Urbana.1962. PB.

Explores the form,style,& diction of epitaphs,& their
expression of attitudes to death & immortality.
***

681.   THREE LEGGED RACE.Charles Crawford. Harper & Row,
        New York. 1974. $ 4.50.

682.   THROUGH DEATH TO LIFE. Mary Perkins-Ryan, Christian
        Experiences Series,Whitman Books (Pflaum Standard),
        Dayton, Ohio. 1971. PB. 75¢.

683.   THE TIME OF THEIR DYING. S.Rosenfield. Norton,NY.1977.
A journalist considers the illness & death of his parents,
only months apart.
**$\frac{1}{2}$

684.   A TIME TO LOVE...A TIME TO DIE.Prince Leopold of
        Loewenstein. Doubleday,NY. 1971. $ 6.95.

685.   A TIME TO MOURN.(Judaism & The Psychology of
        Bereavement). J.D.Spiro.Bloch Publ.Co.,NY.
        1967. $ 4.95.

686.   THE TOMB OF TUTANKHAMEN.Howard Carter. Sphere Library,
        Sphere Books. 1972 edn. 238 pp. £ 1.50 PB.

The original account of the discovery & contents of the
tomb,with contemporary photographs,& more recent colour
pictures. A stylish account of the Egyptian way of death.
***

687.   TOO YOUNG TO DIE. Donald Germann. Farnsworth Publ.Co.,
        NY. 1975. 364 pp. $ 9.95.

688.   THE TRACTATE"MOURNING"(Regulations Relating to Death,
        Burial & Mourning). Transl.with introd.& notes by
        Dov Zlotnick. Yale Judaica Series,Vol.17. Yale
        University Press,New Haven. 1966.

U
689.   UNDERSTANDING BEREAVEMENT & GRIEF.Ed. Norman Linzer.
        KTAV Publishing House,Yeshiva University Press and
        Jewish Funeral Directors of America,Inc. (Proceedings
        of the Interdisciplinary Educational Conferences of
        1974 & 1975). 1977. 253 pp. PB.

690.   UNDERSTANDING DEATH.Edgar N.Jackson. Abingdon,
        Nashville. 1957. $ 4.00.

691.   UNDERSTANDING DEATH & DYING.Ed.Sandra G.Wilcox &
        Marilyn Sutton.Alfred Publ,Sherman Oaks,Cal.1977.
        474pp. $ 12.15, $ 8.05. PB.
Reprinting over 50 articles from sociology,psychology,
medical & other literature,in chapters on definitions &

691 ctd.) meanings of death;experience of dying;grief,
mourning & social functions;death & the child;& choices &
decisions on death, with exercises,projects,questions,&
index.Includes Plato,Talcott Parsons,Dylan Thomas,Lifton,
Mary Shelley's Frankenstein,Kalish,Mansell Pattison,Kubler
Ross,Emily Dickinson,Horace,John Donne,Strauss & Glaser,
Kastenbaum,Lindemann(yet again,immortal grief!),Freud,
Plath,Nagy (so inaccurate & out-of-date that it should not
be reprinted again),Agee,Fletcher,Anne Sexton,Studs Terkel,
& others. One of the most useful texts available for
classroom use.
****
692.   UPDATING LIFE & DEATH: Essays on Ethics & Medicine.
       Ed. Donald Cutler.Beacon Press,Boston.1969.286pp.
       $ 4.50.
Includes Paul Ramsey,Joseph Fletcher,Daniel Callahan,etc.
**

V
693.   THE VALUATION OF HUMAN LIFE.Gavin H.Mooney. Macmillan,
       London. 1977. 165 pp. £ 5.95.

694.   THE VICTORIAN CELEBRATION OF DEATH. James S.Curl.
       Gale, Detroit. 1972. $ 7.00.

695.   VICTORIAN CEMETARY ART.E.V.Gillon,Jr. Dover Publ.,NY.
       1972. 173 pp. Illustrated. $ 4.00. PB.

W
696.   WHAT A MODERN CATHOLIC BELIEVES ABOUT DEATH.
       Robert Nowell. Thomas More Press,Chicago. 1972.

697.   WHAT YOU SHOULD KNOW ABOUT DEATH.Marlene Hess.
       Keats. 1974. $ 1.50.

698.   WHEN SOMEONE DIES. Edgar Jackson. Fortress. 1971.$1.50.
Jackson writes quite well on coping with grief,but in far
too many books,not sufficiently distinct in purpose,style
or content to be readily distinguishable by this reviewer.
**
699.   WHEN A PARENT DIES. Eda LeShan.Macmillan,NY.$ 6.95.

700.   WHEN DEATH TAKES A FATHER. Gladys Kooiman. Baker
       Books. 1974. $ 1.25.

701. WHEN PEOPLE DIE.Joanne E.Bernstein & Stephen Gullo.
      Dutton,New York. 1976.
Considers life,death,& loss in the instance of one woman's
death.Intended for use with Children of 5+.
**
702. WHEN VIOLET DIED.Mildred Kantrowitz. Parents Magazine
      Press,NY. 1973. 40pp. $ 4.95.
For children,4-8.The life cycle,illustrated by the death
of a bird.
**
703. WHO SHALL LIVE & WHO SHALL DIE? The Ethical
      Implications of the New Medical Technology. Dr.Adrian
      Kantrowitz,et al. Union of American Hebrew
      Congregations,New York.Pamphlet.1968.12pp. 60¢.

704. WHO SHALL LIVE? The Dilemma of Severely Handicapped
      Children,& Its Meaning for Other Moral Questions.
      L.J.Weber. Paulist Press,NY.1976. 138 pp.

705. WHY DID HE DIE? Audrey Harris. Lerner. 1965.
A book for children 5-9,about a child dealing with the
death of a friend's grandfather.
**
706. WIDOWHOOD IN AN AMERICAN CITY.Helena Z.Lopata.
      Schenckman Publ.Co.Inc.,Cambridge,Mass. 1972.
      $ 9.95, $ 6.95 PB.

Y
707. YOU & YOUR GRIEF.Edgar N.Jackson.Channel Press,
      1961. $ 2.50.

708. YOU LIVE AFTER DEATH.Harold Sherman. Fawcett/Gold
      Medal.NY. 1949/1956/1972. 175pp. $ 1.50. PB.

"Will show you how to use your own logic to gain an
understanding of the afterlife---you can attain·a belief
in immortality beyond contradiction or dispute.And you
can begin today to prepare yourself for survival beyond
the grave".
Makes Coue and Norman Vincent Peale look like pessimists.
*

————oOo————

SUBJECT INDEX

Within each category,the books are arranged in order of
rating stars,roughly in order of quality,from the best
to the worst. (Note: O includes books not rated!)

1   BIBLIOGRAPHIES
     *****- This book itself-41,145.
     ****-17,242,337.
     **½-246.
     **-39,184,418,530.
     *-6,40,456.
     0-507,534.

2 DEATH
2.1   GENERAL BOOKS ON DEATH
     *****-138,152,181,213,332,352.
     ****½-116.
     ****-103,112,164,167,186,386,476,553.
     ***-21,101,104,122,149,153,157,158,163,183,206,236,
         252,330,375,382,637,638,691.
     **½-83,380.
     **-108,130,141,143,144,185,224,315,379,399,480,532,
         643,651,653,701.
     *-20,211,556.
     0-495,499,501,510,511,540,541,546,548,554,557,568,
         570,574,593,599,602,606,607,615,616,617,623,626,
         627,632,634,649,652,659,661,676,678,687,690,697.

2.2   DEATH & PHILOSOPHY
     *****-152,332.
     ****-106,118,126,336,457,483.
     ***-28,45,74,127,205,277,347.
     **½-270.
     **-117,170.
     0-504,505,545,562,644,645,669,670.

2.3   DEATH & HISTORY
     ****-346,381,439,469,483.
     ***½-148,412.
     ***-46,47,125,150,179,193,229,254,266,284,368,382,
         640,680.
     **½-171.
     **-140,155.
     *-140,155.
     0-512,525,531,660,694,695.

3. DYING

3.1 ATTITUDES TO DEATH,PSYCHOLOGY OF DEATH

*****-138,213,352,363,364,393.
****-115,164,249,309,336,346,396,397,447,542,553.
***½-54,322,344.
***-13,24,111,120,163,166,264,306,317,347,390,392,
    401,415,420,447,455,514,523,610,612.
**-119,170,208,215,643.
*-128,210,282,316.
0-500,515,551,562,596,611.

3.2 SOCIOLOGY OF DEATH

*****-138,213,372.
****½-116,209.
****-27,96,336,462,469,483,553.
***½-148.
**½-270.
**-16,140,468.
*-80,310,657.

3.3 PERSONAL ACCOUNTS

*****-231,473.
****½-335.
****-159,199,259,314.
***-15,194,223,269,275,313,343,429,445,569.
**½-268,325,683.
**-169,197,208,230,237,240,292,357.
*-7,482.
0-684.

3.4 DEATH & CHILDREN

*****-213,248.
****-72,176,288,479,529.
***½-255.
***-59,70,87,198,360.
**-69.
*-71,192,247.
0-513,518,519,520,521,524,552,580,582,641,673.

3.5 DEATH & THE OLD

***-8,91,350,385.
**-94.
*-257,310,318.

3.6   MISCELLANEOUS,Including Self-Help,on Dying

       *****-457.
       ****-82.
       ***½-412.
       ***-21,47,77,421.
       **½-433.
       **-2,26,84,100,464.
       *-348,377.
       0-590,591.

4.   DEATH EDUCATION

4.1   GENERAL

       ****-177,553.
       ***½-113,161,187.
       ***-79,333.
       **-217.
       0-547,677.

4.2   CHILDREN,JUNIOR SCHOOL

       *****-248,450,451.
       ****-103,288.
       ***-129,228,326,671,675.
       **½-51,453.
       **-1,2,18,293,298,493,498,508,581,629,630,631,635,
          636,665,702.
       *-430,485.
       0-497,583,673,674,679,681,705.

4.3   HIGH SCHOOL,COLLEGE

       ****-177,386,553.
       ***½-113,161.
       ***-8,672.

4.4   UNIVERSITY
       None.

4.5   CLINICAL,COUNSELLING TRAINING (Including Medical
      & Nursing

       ***½-187.
       **-452.
       *-361.

4.6   TEXTBOOKS & TEACHING MATERIALS (See also separate
      index of teaching materials)

       *****-231.

5. TERMINAL CARE & COUNSELLING

5.1 GENERAL

*****- 320,352,413.
****-73,-82,202,207,396,398.
***½-187,405.
***-57,59,85,89,90,166,183,195,256,300,376,395,403,
    406,589.
**½-61,188,190,598.
**-95,100,272,329,399.
*-60,63,367,454,588.
0-513,587,633,658.

5.2 MEDICAL

*****-363,364.
****-30,81,196,213,241,328,397,398.
***½-54.
***-58,111,263,338,378,391,394,455.
**½-341,503.
**-119.
*-646.

5.3 NURSING

****-53,213,358.
***½-245,255.
***-102,360.
**½-61,190.
**-185,189,359.

5.4 PSYCHOLOGICAL,SOCIAL

***-356,522,579.
0-611.

5.5 RELIGIOUS

***½-56.
***-373,579.
**-374.
0-642.

6. LOSS,GRIEF & BEREAVEMENT

6.1 GENERAL

*****-124,154,213,320.
****-146,542.
***½-203.

6.1 ctd :
    ***-24,90,137,191,317,420,425,471,577.
    **½-433.
    **-10,18,235,273,565.
    *-109,233,282,321,404.
    0-518,555,563,575,578,585,586,600,642,685,689,
      699,700.

6.2   PERSONAL ACCOUNTS,WIDOWHOOD

    *****-234.
    ****-29,48,134.
    ***½-324,400,487.
    ***-3,165,362.
    **-11,273,463,608.
    *½-220.
    *-492.
    0-496,506,706.

6.3   PROFESSIONAL & CLINICAL ASPECTS,THERAPY

    ****-34,72,219.
    ***½-35.
    ***-355,471.
    **½-341.
    *-192.

6.4   COUNSELLING,CONSOLATION,SELF HELP

    ****-29,213.
    ***½-324,446,472.
    ***-64,165,236,239,243,267,304,311,312,326,334,
      373,471.
    **½-52,325.
    **-11,33,50,88,156,221,232,303,307,369,427,448,
      490,698.
    *-180,244,262,316.
    0-584,614,618,699,707.

6.5   WILLS,PROBATE,LAW

    ****-260.
    ***-261,491,564.
    **½-52.
    **-448.
    *-121,488.

9.2   CLINICAL MANAGEMENT,COUNSELLING & PREVENTION

  ****-98,213,327,440,443,444.
  ***½-467.
  ***-75,238,384,437,470.
  **-204,452,666.
  *-434.
  0-592,664,667.

9.3   SUICIDE & ART,PHILOSOPHY,LITERARY ACCOUNTS

  *****-31,414.
  ***½-36.
  ***-38,436,441,458.
  **-435.

9.4   PERSONAL ACCOUNTS

  *****-31.
  ***½-442.
  ***-597.
  **½-428.
  **-10,417.
  0-526.

10.   MEDICAL ETHICS RELEVANT TO THANATOLOGY

  *****-66,201.
  ****½-209.
  ****-96,142,413.
  ***½-342.
  ***-42,43,465,558.
  **-44,173,265,305.
  *-172,383.
  0-507,516,550,613,622,628,656,692,693,703,704.

————o0o————

AUTHOR INDEX

(By principal author or editor)

Abbott-636
Abrahamsson-368
Abram-503
Abrams-356
Adams-26
Adler-481
Agee-154
Ajar-621
Alden-76
Aldwinkle-545
Allentuck-91
Alsop-429
Alther-287
Alvarez-414
Amulree-365
Anderson,CM-600,DB-592,
        R-599
Andrus-486
Anon.-337,512,595
Anthony,E-518, S-176
Aries-483
Aring-330
Armstrong-556
Arvio-92
Ashbrook-406
Ashley-491
Asinof-526
Asquith-156
Austin-208

Bacon-252
Bane-539
Bartoli-635
Barton-182
Ball-103
Barnard-353
Barth-407
Baskin-566
Bataille-120
Bayly-475
Beaty-525
de Beauvoir-473

Beck-384
Becker-170
Beckman-7
Behnke-174
Bendann-415, E-590
Bender-386
Bermann-415, E-590
Bernstein-246,JE-701,513,583
Bettelheim-449
Bichat-382
Bischwell-555
Boase-155
Boros-632
Bowers-95
Bowlby-24,420
Bowman-12
Brand-200,276
Brandon-601
Brim-186
Brodie-201
Brody-318
Brown-610
Browne-266
Browning-189
Buckingham-587,589
Budge-193
Bullough-502
Burton-59

Caine-304,487
Calhoun-100
Callenbach-311
Campbell-342
Camus-347
Caplan-446
Carr-235,466,578
Carrick-493
Carrington-158
Carter-686
Cartwright-300
Castles-185
Caughill-190

—————o0o—————

JOURNALS

OMEGA: THE JOURNAL OF DEATH AND DYING. Edited :Dr Robert
   Kastenbaum. Baywood Publishing Company,43 Central
   Drive,Farmingdale,NY 11735.
$35 per volume(4 issues,quarterly)+ $2.00 post,overseas.
per volume. Back issues- $ 40 per volume.
This has established itself as the major and most
prestigious journal in the field,of high standards,with
good research and key opinions.

DEATH EDUCATION: Pedagogy,Counseling,Care. Edited:Hannelore
   Wass.   Hemisphere Publishing Corp.,1025 Vermont
   Aveune NW,Washington DC 20005. Quarterly.
Libraries & institutions:$42 per annum;individuals:$22 p.a.
A most promising new journal,with good quality material.

ESSENCE: Journal of Aging,Dying & Death. Edited:Richard
   Lonetto & Stephen Fleming,Dept.of Psychology,
   Atkinson College,York University,4700 Keele St.,
   Downsview,Ontario M3J 2RJ, Canada.   Quarterly.
$ 12.00 p.a.($5 for students).+$4 postage outside
Canda & U.S.A.
The third of the highly reputable thanatology journals.

DEATH NEWS REPORT .180 S.Broad St.,Prescott,Wisconsin,
   54021. $14 p.a. Monthly journal dealing with topics
relating to death.Not recommended.Failed to provide any
review copies,or even to reply to correspondence.
FORUM FOR DEATH EDUCATION & COUNSELLING NEWSLETTER.
Forum Membership-$ 10 p.a. P.O.Box 1226,Arlington,VA 22210.

SUICIDE & LIFE THREATENING BEHAVIOR.Quarterly.$15 p.a.
       (individuals) 11431 Kingsland St,Los Angeles,CA 90066.
LIFE EXTENSION MAGAZINE. 663 W.Barry,Chicago,Ill.60657.
       $ 9 p.a. (for those who prefer to avoid death).
St Francis Burial Society Newsletter, 3421 Center St.,
   Washington DC 20010. $12 p.a. Quarterly.
THE BIOETHICS DIGEST.P.O.Box 6318,5632 Connecticut Ave.,NW,
   Washington DC 20015. $ 60 p.a.,12 issues. Provides,
very expensively,a series of summaries abstracted from some
of the world literature on bioethics.They claim to screen
over 3,000 articles,books,etc.each month,selecting 200 for
abstract.Includes some material on death & dying,as well as
other ethical issues,experimentation,abortion,etc.Also
promises"bioethical opinions written by noted experts". !

From the Foundation of Thanatology.
Warning. Over the course of years,numerous readers have
experienced problems with Foundation of Thanatology
journals,which have often appeared & criculated irregularly
with changes of title,frequency & format.It has not always
been easy to establish or maintain a regular subscription.
Here is a recent listing provided by the Foundation.

ARCHIVES OF THE FOUNDATION OF THANATOLOGY.Quarterly
(formerly Tri-annual) Vol.VII,1978.$30 per volume,single
issues $ 7.Canada-$34 p.a.,Foreign-$34 p.a.
Back issues- $ 7.50 per issue,$ 30 per volume.
Formerly published by Alan R.Liss Co.NY,now published by
Foundation Book & Periodical Division,P.O.Box 1191,
Brooklyn,NY 11202.

ADVANCES IN THANATOLOGY. (Formerly The Journal of Thanatology)
Cloth-back Annual.Due 1978.Price-$15 per issue,Canada $ 16,
Foreign-$ 18. Back Issues-$ 7.50 per issue,$ 30 per volume
(+ $ 2 foreign).Published by MSS Inf.Corp.(formerly Alan
R.Liss Co.,NY)
THANATOLOGY ABSTRACTS. (Formerly Funeral Services Abstracts!)
Cloth,Annual.Due 1978.$15 per number,Canada $ 17,Foreign
$ 19. Published MSS Information Corp.
THANATOLOGY NEWS. Quarterly (irregular(newsletter,Vol.III,
1978.sent to members of the Foundation.
The Thanatology Librarian (begun by Highly Specialized
Promotions,Brooklyn.
The Thanatology Book Review Journal,planned for 1978
has been cancelled.

ETHICS. Ed. Warner A.Wick.The University of Chicago Press,
1103o Langley Avenue,Chicago,Illinois 60628.
Quarterly: $ 14 p.a. institutions,$ 10.50 individuals,
        $ 8.40 students.

The JOURNAL OF MEDICINE & PHILOSOPHY (Society for Health
        & Human Values).University of Chicago Press,5801
        Ellis Avenue,Chicago,Illinois 60637. $ 15 p.a.
        Quarterly. Vol.3,No.1,March 1978,on the Nature of
        Death.

————oOo————

FILMS

1. <u>ABYSS</u>. 17 min. Color.
     by Gilbert Dassonville.A mountain-climber's struggle to
reach high ground after falling 130 feet.Considers man's
tenacious will for survival & life,even against major odds.
Rental-$25, Purchase-$275
Phoenix Films,New York.

2. <u>ACCIDENT</u>.16½ min. Color. 1974
     The survivor of a plane crash talks about how it
affected his attitudes toward life & death,having been so
nearly killed.Effects in life of the threat of death.Now,
life is"now",& he feels more fully aware of it.
Rental-$22, EMC-$17
Doubleday Media,California, & E.M.C.— No.9184

3. <u>AFTER OUR BABY DIED</u>. 21 min. Color. 1975.
     (Sudden Infant Death Syndrome).Looks at the death of a
baby through the eyes of the bereaved family.Those they
meet—Emergency Room staff,doctors,nurses,police— are
sympathetic,but could do more to help.Considers why,where,
& how more could have been said,& said differently,to aid
them. Pity it wasn't still more positive in its approach.
1976 American Film Festival Blue Ribbon Winner in Mental
Health. Dr Marie Valdes-Dapena & Dr B.Beckwith;& Togg Films
Inc.,for Dept H.E.W.,Bureau of Community Health Services,MD.
Free Loan: Modern Talking Picture Service,NY.

4. <u>AFTER THE FIRST</u>. 14 min. Color.
Sportsman father gives his son of 12 a hunting trip on his
birthday.Boy is aware of appreciating nature,enthusiastically
learns to handle a shotgun.As he kills a living thing for
the first time,there is growth in distance between father
& son."After the first time,it gets easier".Opens discussion
on many issues. Blue Ribbon Award,American Film Festival.
Rental $ 17
Association Films,Texas

5. <u>AGUA SALADA</u>.12 min. B & W.
In Brazil,an old fisherman leaves shore in a small boat,his
20 year old son helping him push his nets into the water.
Later,he pulls them in,tossing fish into the boat.Suddenly,
pulls the body of his son from the net.No narration,no
dialogue,but the shocking immediacy of sudden death.
Rental-$25
Viewfinders Films,Illinois.

6. <u>ALL THE WAY HOME</u>.103 min. B & W.
Based on James Agee story.Problems of aging,maintaining
religious convictions,dealing with death,& family
relationships.The effects of death on a young boy of 6.
Rental-$40,$55
Films Incorporated

7. <u>A MAN.</u> 21 min. B & W.
Produced & directed by Len Grossman & Michael Chait. A
moving film about Mike,young man in a men's consciousness
raising group,experiencing the death of his father.
Originally on portable videotape equipment,so video image
& sound not always of high quality.Good for focussing
on such issues as:Why do men hold back feelings? How do
they come to learn to do so? How dies society encourage it?
Why do men fear touching & giving support to one another
even in time of crisis?
Rental-$30, purchase-$245
Polymorph Films,Mass.

8. <u>THE AMERICAN WAY OF DEATH</u>.40 min. B & W.
Documentary about American funeral customs.

Obtainable for rental from:Denis Boyd,Public Relations
Officer,Memorial Society Association of Canada,2525 West
Mall, University of British Columbia, BC, U6T 1W9

9. <u>ANGER AFTER DEATH</u>.28 min. Color.
Improbable & amateurish,muddled & confusing.Depicts a World
War I soldier briefly returning to life,the chemist who
manufactured weapons,the scientist who developed the Gas.
Unusable.   Rental- $ 17
Canadian National Film Board,& Contemporary/McGraw-Hill.

10. <u>ANNA & POPPY</u>.15 min. Color. 1976
A young girl's first experience of death,on the loss of her
grandfather.Looks back on her fond memories of "Poppy",
asking:Why did he die? Why did he leave me now? Is there a
heaven? Reconciled by the recall of his love.
Rental $ 15.95. Sale-$ 196
Association Films.

11. <u>ANNUAL FESTIVAL OF THE DEAD</u>.14 min. Color.
Silent film showing the Dogon people of Mali in a
celebration of the achievements of their dead warriors.
Rental $ 19.
New York University Film Library, also EMC

12. AT 99. 24 min. Color. 1975
Louise Tandy Murch portrayed at 99 years.Her birthday party,
her daily chores,& yoga.She discusses being old,alone but
not necessarily lonely,& death.
Rental $ 24
EMC, No. 9313.

13. AU FOU.10 min. Color. 1968
Clever animation by Yoji Kuri,showing brief,macabre,
episodes of black humour illustrating the many forms and the
absurdity of death.
Rental-$16
EMC,No.8299.

14. AVRIL.20 min. Color. 1976
Intended to help General Practitioners improve their
understanding of the continuing care of patients with
terminal illness.A woman of 50 is interviewed about her
attitudes towards how she & her family cope with her
approaching death.
Dorset Area Health Authority,Dept.of Teaching Media,
University of Southampton, & Merck,Sharp & Dohme Ltd.

15. BALLAD WITHOUT END. 12 min. Color. 1973
The reactions of a young soldier who killed an unarmed
member of the enemy forces,& then decides that war is
barbaric.He rejects war,violence & killing,& decides that
life & survival are more important than"courage",Civil War.
Rental-$ 20
Phoenix Films,NY.

16. BASHERT.
Washburn Films,NY.

17. BETWEEN THE CUP AND THE LIP. 11 min. Color.
Animated film on death,funerals & funeral processions,
grieving & bereavement.An endless procession of figures,
interspersed with the snuffing out of a candle,representing
expiration.
Rental-$15, Purchase-$ 150.
Mass Media Associates,Baltimore & St.Louis.

18. BIG BOYS DON'T CRY.9 min. Color.
No narration or dialogue.A boy kills a bird while playing
cowboy.Inserts of death scenes in war in contrast .
Rental- $ 10.
Perspective Films.

19. <u>BIG SHAVE</u>.6 min.Color. 1968.
A young man wakes in the morning,goes into the bathroom,
begins to shave--and shaves himself to death.Black humour.
Rental-$ 12
EMC- No. 7676

20. <u>BIRTH & DEATH</u>.2 parts,total 119 min. B & W.1971
The 2 parts contrast a young couple having their first
baby,including a sequence in the delivery room ;while
Part II,Death,focusses on a terminal cancer patient,his
family,staff & other patients.
Together-- Rental $ 75, Purchase- $ 600.
Birth- 76 minute version-rental $ 45,sale $ 350
    shorter edited version,40 mins,rental $ 35,sale $ 275.
Death (43 min.) rental-$ 35, purchase- $ 275.
Filmakers Library,NY.

21. <u>BOARDED WINDOW</u>.18 min. Color.
An elderly hunter is buried by his rustic cabin which has
only one window,which has been boarded over for years.When
he was young,his wife died,& he lovingly prepared her body
& dug the grave. Somewhat macabre.
University of Michigan AV Center, & EMC.

22. <u>BRIAN'S SONG</u>. 75 min. Color. 1975.
The story of the death of Brian Piccolo,26 year-old player
for the Chicago Bears.The effects on himself,his wife,& his
best friend.Features James Caan & Billy Dee Williams,&
won 16 major awards. Stresses brotherhood,compassion.
Rental-$ 150, Purchase-$ 1195
Learning Corporation of America,NY & Univ.of Michigan
AV Centre,& Kent State University.

23. <u>BUT JACK WAS A GOOD DRIVER</u>. 15 min.Color. 1974.
Dramatized conversation between 2 teenagers after the
funeral of a friend,killed in an automobile accident.They
realize his death was not accidental & that they had
ignored his"cries for help".Opens discussion of
adolescent suicide.
Rental-$ 17
EMC-No.9195,CRM Educational Films,California.

24. <u>CASE OF SUICIDE</u>.30 min. B & W. 1968
Study of 17 year-old wife & mother who killed herself,
considers causes,interviews those close to her,& discusses
how she might have been helped.
Rental-$19.
EMC,No.7885 Also sold by Time/Life Media, $ 275.

25. <u>CATTLE;WAITING;& RENASCENT; ACT OF SEEING WITH ONE'S</u>
    <u>OWN EYE</u>--Stan Brakhage; DEUS EX--Stan Brakhage.
Grove Press Film Division,New York.

26. <u>CHICKAMAUGA</u>. 33 min. B&W. 1967.
Ambrose Bierce Civil War short story.A deaf boy's encounter
with war & death,not understanding the magnitude & finality
of death,uncertain what is wrong with his dead family.He
plays soldier among the dead & dying on a battlefield,then
returns to find his home burned & family killed.Won
several awards.
Rental-$20.50 (EMC $18),purchase-$ 225.
Contemporary/McGraw Hill Films; EMC No. 8540.

27. <u>A CHILD'S EYES.</u> 9 min. Color.
Simple but stirring collection of children's reactions to
the assassination of President Kennedy;their drawings and
comments (5 & 6 year-olds).
Rental-$12.50, Sale-$ 135.
McGraw-Hill/Contemporary Films.

28. <u>CHIPPER</u>.27 min. Color or B & W.
A parable.A young man,Chipper,meets the angel of death
disguised as a waiter in a restaurant,who helps him
struggle through the "stages of dying",towards acceptance.
Too rigid by far in its understanding of stages,so it can
be misleading. Also a religious tract.
Rental-$19.00, Association Films.
Rental $ 9.95 B&W,&18.95 color,Sale $160 B&W,$ 325 color,
    Paulist Productions.

29. <u>CIPHER IN THE SNOW</u>. 24 min. Color. 1974
A little boy is rejected & ignored by family,teachers,and
school-mates,until one day he drops dead in the snow.Opens
discussion on the individual needs of children.Won several
awards.
Rental-$20.
EMC,No.9197. Also,University of Iowa.

30. <u>CONFRONTATIONS OF DEATH</u>.35 min. Color.
Made during a seminar at which participants attempted to
discuss their own feelings about death;listening to music,
showing slides,writing their own eulogies.(Narcissistic?)
Rental-$22.
Oregon Division of Continuing Education Film Library,
    also University of Iowa.

31. COPING. 22 min. Color. 1974.
A young boy with terminal leukemia,has adjusted well to his
coming death,with his parents.Shows how family support can
help the individual to cope.
Rental- $ 16. EMC,No. 9191

32. CRUNCH,CRUNCH. 9 min. Color.
Animation. Life/death cycle;the evolution of life & society
with the preying of one life form on another for survival;
life producing death,to maintain life.
Rental- $ 15. Pyramid Films.

33. CYCLE. 5 min. Color. 1971.
Animation in freehand style.Cycle of life,humanity situated
between primal dust and infinite universe.No narration or
dialogue. Won awards.
Rental;$ 13. EMC- No. 9881.

34. THE DAY GRANDPA DIED.11½min. Color. 1970.
A 9 year-old boy's reactions to the death & funeral of his
Grandfather.Jewish context,upper middle-class.Parent-child
interactions in response to the loss,and how ritual helps.
Rental-$12.00 (EMC $ 15), Purchase-$ 150.
BFA Educational Media, & EMC,No. 9190.

35. A DAY IN THE DEATH OF DONNIE B.18 min. B & W .1970.
A typical day in the life,& death,of a young.poor,Black
heroin addict.Harlem slums,comments from mother,neighbours
& police,who all expect his death.He hustles money for his
next "fix". Folksong lyrics accompany it. Award-winner.
Rental-$13,EMC,No.7790. National Institute of Mental
Health, Rental $ 7.50, Sale $ 32.50.

36. DAY OF THE DEAD. 15 min. Color.
Festival for the Day of the Dead,with a party,plays,food
& flowers. A different cultural approach.
Rental-$ 7.00. Univ.of Southern California & Pyramid Films.

37. THE DAY MANOLETE WAS KILLED. 19 min. 1957.
Examines ideas of death & courage.A bullfighter loses his
life while displaying or proving his'manhood'&'fearlessness'
August 1947 when Manolete the legendary came out of
retirement to meet the challenge of the young Luis
Dominguin.He is seen preparing for the fight,talking of his
fear,but goes out."The crowd kept demanding more of him,&
more was his life.So he gave it to them".Award-winner.
Rental-$16.50,Films Inc.;$ 15,EMC,No.7205.

38. THE DEAD BIRD. 13 min. Color.
4 children find a dead bird,& bury it.
Bureau of AV Instruction,PO Box 2½93,Madison,Wisc.53701.

39. DEAD BIRDS. 83 min. Color. 1963.
Detailed study of the Dani,who live in the mountains of
Western New Guinea.Their values are based on an elaborate
system of inter-tribal warfare & revenge,like our
Department. When a warrior is killed,the victors celebrate
& the victims plan revenge.The wars will never end,for they
are necessary to satisfy the ghosts of the dead.
Rental-$40. Contemporary/McGraw-Hill; EMC,No.6606.

40. DEAD MAN. 3 min.
By Robert E.Neale & Richard Black.No sound.The camera moves
slowly around the body of an old man lying in a morgue.
Stark,though the point of it all is unclear.Only to be used
by an experienced & skilled teacher.
Rental: Foundation of Thanatology,New York.

41. THE DEAD RESTORED. 29 min. Color.
Dramatization of a daughter's death in a car accident,her
parents finding comfort in Biblical promises of life
beyond the grave.May be useful for Bible study groups.
Dawn Films, free loan.

42. DEAR LITTLE LIGHTBIRD. 19 min. Color.
Made by a poet & film-maker,about the short life of his son
Skippy,a "blue baby".Very simple,like a home-movie,& more
affecting for this.The baby dies. By Leland Auslander.
Rental-$ 17, Viewfinders.
Leland Auslander Films--Rental-$15,Sale-$ 235.

43. DEATH. 23 min. B & W. 1966.
Sir John Gielgud recites Shakespeare's comments on death
from various of his plays.
Rental-$ 7.50. University of Colorado Film Library.

44. DEATH.(see BIRTH & DEATH). 40 min.B&W.1968.
Documentary,originally for NET.Witnesses the suffering,
dying & death of Ambro Pearsall-follows him to the morgue
& the funeral director.Filmed at Calvary Hospital,Bronx.
When he asks for attention,nurse says"Youre not the only
patient in the hospital,you know.." Direct,& suitably
annoying.
Rental $ 35,Sale $275.Filmmakers Library,EMC,Univ.Iowa
& University of Michigan.

45. DEATH & SUNRISE. 10 min. Color. 1962.
Animation;stylized cartoon of classic Western gunfight
between the sheriff and the bad guys.
Rental-$ 14. EMC,No.7974.

46. DEATH BE NOT PROUD.99 min. Color. 1976.
Based on John Gunther's account of his son of 16's
experiences with a brain tumour.Includes processes of
dying,anticipatory grief,quality of life,family
relationships,& the needs of the dying.Robby Benson as
Johnny was nominated for an Emmy,& the original TV movie
was well reviewed.
Rental-$90, Long-term lease-$ 1150.
Learning Corporation of America,NY;Mass Media; Budget Films.

47. DEATH ITSELF MUST DIE. 29 min. Color.
A young girl,after her parents' deaths,finds comfort,with
her aunt,in Biblical promises of resurrection & the
destruction of death. For Bible study groups.
Dawn Films, free loan.

48. DEATH NOTIFICATION.23 min. Color.
Training film for police officers,usable by others,about
how not to notify death to people,& how it can be better
done.Some dramatized episodes & didactic material.Useful
discussion guide available with film.
Rental-$50, Sale-$ 365. Harper & Row Media Films,NY.

49. DEATH OF A PEASANT.10 min. Color. 1972.
Dramatized portrayal of true story of a Yugoslav peasant
who chooses death on his own initiative rather than
execution by the Nazis.No narration or dialogue;closely
edited & tense.Opens discussion on martyrdom,cheating
death,etc.
Rental-$15,Sale-$150. EMC,No.8722;& Mass Media;Univ.Maryland.

50. THE DEATH OF PRESIDENT KENNEDY.22 min. B&W. 1964.

Screen News Digest exerpt;reviews life of JFK,the trip back
to Washington after the assassination,& the lying-in-state.
Can be used to evoke publically shared mourning experiences.

51. DEATH OF THE WISHED-FOR CHILD. 28 min. Color. 1977.
Produced Bill Goveia-Script Glen Davidson. Bereaved parents
(especially the mother)whose child dies soon after birth,
tell their story.Not very imaginative in its presentation,
& rather sententious in its commentary;but considerable in
impact.Interviews with Linda & her husband.Shows how

51. ctd.) destructive inappropriate even if well-intended
interventions can be;the problems of caregivers,often
unaware of their own difficulties;Linda's need to see & hold
her dead baby was ignored;she was not allowed to attend the
funeral. Useful with health sciences professionals and
students,& with bereaved parents.
Glen W.Davidson,P.O.Box 3926,Springfield,Illinois 62708.

52. DEATH,PART V. 26 min. B & W.
Role-play scenes depicting meanings of life & death.Needs
follow-up discussion.
Rental-$ 12.50. Association Films,Inc.

53. DEATH TAKES A HOLIDAY.
Universal 16,New York.

54. DECISIONS: LIFE OR DEATH.3o min. B & W.
Religious & medical professionals discuss the ethics of
heart transplants & other developments of medical
technology.Fr.Charles Curran & Michael de Bakey.
Rental-$17.50,Sale-$145.
Association Films, & Macmillan Films.

55. DEPRESSION/SUICIDE.24 min. Color. 1976.
"YOU CAN TURN THE BAD FEELINGS INTO GOOD ONES". Considers
leading causes of death among teenagers.Young people who've
attempted suicide describe their experiences & how they
got themselves out of their depression.
Rental-$ 25. EMC,No.9614.

56. DIGNITY OF DEATH. 30 min. Color.
St Christopher's Hospice & pain control.
Rental/Sale: ABC News,New York.

57. DO I REALLY WANT TO DIE? 31 min. Color. 1976.
English subtitles. Produced & Directed by Fons Gransveld.
People who contemplated & attempted suicide speak frankly
about their behavior and feelings,& what led to their
suicide attempt.Questions many common misconceptions about
suicide,& how such crises might be helped.
Rental-$ 40, Purchase-$385.
Polymorph Films, Boston.

58. DYING. 97 min. Color.
Very powerful,moving documentary,with 4 sequences.Mark's
widow describes a party they held in his room shortly
before he died;SALLY,despite an obvious brain tumour,shows

58. ctd.) little fear;HARRIET & BILL squabble & she
expresses great bitterness;& Rev.BRYANT,a Black minister,
faces his imminent death with courage & dignity;it concludes
with his funeral,& the farewell from his wife & parishioners.
A very tender & powerful film-one of the finest available.
Rental-$100 as 16 mm film. Sale-$ 565 as VC.
WGBH-TV,Boston.

59. THE DYING PATIENT.60 min. B&W.
Interviews with patients,& a psychiatrist discussing the
dynamics of the interview.
Rental-$50,Sale-$250. Office of Medical Education,
University of California, Irvine, California 92664.

60. THE DYING PATIENT. 68 min. Color.
The clinical approach to the dying patinet.
Rental-$25. Medical Education Resources Program,Indiana
University School of Medicine.

61. ECHOES. 11 min. Color.
In the family cemetary,11 year-old Ellen finds the gravestone
of 11 year-old Mary,who died in 1883.Thinks about her;
searching the ancestral house,finds her picture & doll.
Places the doll & a fresh flower on the grave;realizing life
is continuous,she following her ancestors,& due to be
followed in turn by others. Discussion Guide available.
Sale-$150. Guidance Associates.

62. EMILY,THE STORY OF A MOUSE. 5 min. Color.
An attempt to convey a concept of death to primary school
children.Mice are born,become mature,have children,& die,
in less than a year.When she dies,Emily returns to the soil
& nourishes plants & her own children & grandchildren.
Rental-$15. Viewfinders.

63. EMOTIONAL REACTIONS TO CANCER IN CLINICAL PRACTICE.
    26 min. Color.
Conversations between patients & doctors about the nature of
the illness,treatment,pain,social adjustment,& psychological
problems.
Rent-free. American Cancer Society, Cleveland,Ohio.

64. END AND THE BEGINNING. 27 min. B & W. 1956.
By James Agee. Depiction of Lincoln's death,carefully
documented,& the progress of his funeral train across the
country,accompanied by Whitman's"When Lilacs Last..."
Rental- $ 14. EMC,No. 5709.

65. THE END OF ONE. 7 min. Color. 1976.
Seagulls scavenge for food from a huge garbage dump,soaring
& swooping.A lone bird limps frailly along a polluted
stretch of beach,stumbling & dying.The others compete in
raucous uncaring unconcern. Allegorical.Award-winner.
Rental-$ 15. Learning Corporation of America.

66. ETERNALLY YOURS. 12 min. Color.
Visually evocative study of death as impersonal,but
universal experience,and cremation.
Creative Film Society,California.

67. EVERYBODY RIDES THE CAROUSEL.72 min. Color.
Animation.The 8 stages of life,based on Erik Erikson (yawn)
available in 3 24-minute parts.I.Newborn to childhood, II-
School to Young Adulthood, III.Grown-ups to Old Age & Death.
Rental-each part $ 25,all 3 $ 60. Purchase:$350 each part,
      $ 900 all three.
Pyramid Films,California.

68. THE EXCUSE. 16 min. Color. 1975.
About American poet Ruth Stone,who reads her poetry & talks
about her feelings as a widowed mother with 3 daughters.
Reminisces about her dead husband Walter,also a poet,
who inexplicably committed suicide in 1959.
Rental-$ 18, Sale-$ 210. EMC,No.9176.

69. FACING DEATH. 20 min. Color.
A panel of doctors discuss the psychological problems of
informing the patient & family of a terminal illness.
Free Loan, National Medical Audiovisual Center Annex.

70. THE FALL OF THE HOUSE OF USHER. 30 min. Color.
From Poe's tale;melancholy,gloomy,tale of crypts & death.
Rental $ 29. EMC.

71. THE FAMILY OF MAN. 45 min. Color. 1968.
8 part series (originally for TV):Birth,Children,Teenagers,
Weddings,Married Life,Old Age (2 parts),& Death. Looks at
the life-cycle in cross-cultural terms. Death,looks at
death & burial in Northern India,Britain,Botswana,New
Guinea & Hong Kong. Rental-set of 8-$200,Old Age or Death-
-$50. Purchase-set of 8- $ 2100, Old Age or Death-$ 500,or
$ 350,as VC. Death,rental from EMC,$30.
Time-Life Multimedia, NJ. & EMC.

72. THE FATHER. 30 min. Color. 1972.
Adaptation of Chekov's story of the old man so alienated
by his miserable life that he is unable to share his grief
over his son's death.Burgess Meredith as the old man,a
horse-carriage driver in New York,in this version.
Rental- $ 17, EMC,No.9196.

73. FEMOMENIL.
Mass Media,2116 N.Charles St.,Baltimore,Maryland 21218.

74. THE FINAL PROUD DAYS OF ELSIE WURSTER.30 min. B&W.
A film which follows Elsie,retired public health nurse,
through her final months of life in a nursing home.
Rental-$ 13. Penn State University,AV Services.

75. THE FOLLOWING SEA. 11 min. B & W.
Virgin Islands.Sam the fisherman is dead & his son Charles
attends the funeral with his family,thinking about how the
old man's wisdom rolls on like the sea,if we look for it.
Rental-$ 10, Sale-$90. Contemporary/McGraw-Hill.

76. FRIGHTENED CHILD. 19 min. B & W. 1967
Relatives have soured an 11 year-old's mind against her
father,& have made her feel responsible for her mother's
death.She is frightened & depressed.Staying in a foster
home,she accepts the fact that folk do care for her,and
that her father cares too.
Rental- $13,   EMC,No. 4674.

77. FUTURE UNKNOWN. 15 min. B&W.
Shows the emotional problems of a young woman hospitalized
for a recurrent malignancy.She & her husband suspect but
can't discuss it;staff avoid her.A nurse helps her express
her feelings,& gives her support. Discussion guide with film.
Rental- $ 10. University of Pittsburgh School of Nursing.

78. GALE IS DEAD. 51 min. Color.
Teenegae death from drugs.Fine British TV documentary;
interviews with Gale before her death,with friends and
others who tried to help.
Rental. Sale-$ 275. Time-Life Films,New York.

79. THE GARDEN PARTY.24 min. Color. 1973.
Based on Katherine Mansfield short story,changed from England
after World War I,to New England after World War II.A vain,
aristocratic family deals with death with a mixture of sorrow,
condascension,fear,guilt,& detachment.Elaborate plans for a

79. ctd.) garden party are under way when news comes that
a neighbour has been killed in an accident.The teenage
daughter wants to cancel the party,but mother refuses.
Instead,the girl is sent to the neighbour's house with a
basket of food.She sees the widow & unwillingly is taken up
to see the dead man,her first meeting with death.
Rental-$ 25,Purchase $ 325,ACI Media,NY.Rent-$12,University
of Illinois; Rent-$ 9.25 University of Arizona Bureau of
AV Services. Also Univ of Southern California Film
Distribution Center.

80. THE GIFT OF LIFE.19 min. Color.   1972.

A poetic expression of life,birth to death,in the Christian
perspective,with scriptural quotations.
Rental-$ 20. Pyramid Films.

81. GIFT OF LIFE/RIGHT TO DIE. 15 min. B&W. 1968.

NET. Considers medical ethical problems,where one person
must die,& another receives an organ transplant.Laymen and
clinical personnel discuss euthanasia for malformed infants
& people suffering from incurable disease. Explains the
concept of Brain Death.
Rental-$ 12,$7,$ 4.40.   EMC,No.7320,& Indiana University
Audio-Visual Center;& Visual Aids Service,Division of
University Extension,University of Illinois,Champaign,IL.
61822.

82. THE GRANDFATHER. 16 min. B&W. 1968.
Portrait of a 93 year-old man,the oldest inhabitant of his
village in Friesland (Netherlands).He reminisces about what
he has learned in life,about war,old age,& death.
Rental-$ 13. EMC, No. 8914.

83. THE GREAT AMERICAN FUNERAL. 54 min. B&W.
The famous CBS documentary on funerals.Funeral practice in
Western society in the last 50 years;the industry in
detail,its costs,benefits,& alternatives.
Rental-$ 12.50 (plus $ 1.95 handling)
Mass Media Associates, St Louis.

84. THE GREAT PLAN (What Death Means).20 min. Color.
A grandfather helps Tik & Susan cope with the impending
death of their grandmother.
Rental-$ 12.50. BFC Films, NY.

85. GREAT TREE HAS FALLEN.22 min. Color. 1973.
The eight-day funeral of the King of the Ashanti in Ghana;
its traditional customs,dances & music.
Rental-$20. EMC, No. 9633.

86. GRIEF. 50 min. Color.
A collection of responses to death,as bereaved people discuss
their feelings of anger,disbelief,sadness and fear.
Concord Films,England.

87. GRIEF THERAPY. 19 min. Color. 1976.
CBS '60 Minutes' item about Donald Ramsey's work (Clinical
Psychologist in Amsterdam) on a particular type of grief
therapy. He treats a woman whose grief at the death of her
12 year-old daughter has left her suicidal 2 years later.
Condensded view of intense week-long re-grief therapy.
Rental-EMC-$19,U.Mich.$ 10.75. Purchase-$ 275.
Carousel Films,NY for purchase. EMC No.9634. & University
of Michigan Audiovisual Education Center.

88. THE HIGHEST BIDDER. 28 min. B&W.
Modern allegory of death.At the weekly bridge game,an
enigmatic stranger arrives instead of Abe,their regular
fourth player.A phone call informs them that Abe is dead,
and they recognize the stranger as Death.
Rental- $ 9.95.   Association Films.

89. HOSPICE. 30 min. Color.
A film by Arnold Behr. Student's comment:"A very nice
hospital,but it's not clear that people die there". Often
poor sound quality.Sometimes inaccurate (e.g.their ward-
rounds are not very different from what many others of us
do).Splendid patients--one should see more of them.The
staff seems rather too perfect,the comments & scenes often
too "marvellous",too coy. It's as if everyone is taking
euphoriant medication.Self-congratulatory,prim,prissy.
And a bit too long.
Rental- £ 10 per day. St Christopher's Hospice,London.

90. HOSPITAL. 84 min. B & W.
Graphic cinema-verite documentary by Frederick Wiseman,who
made Titicut Follies and Primate.A day in an urban hospital,
with lives,diseases and deaths.The drugged,the unconscious,
the stabbed,the shot,the lost.Shows great sympathy for all
the people trying to cope with it.Opens many issues relating
to terminal care in the hospital.
Rental- $100, Sale-$ 750. Zipporah Films, Boston.

91. <u>HOW COULD I NOT BE AMONG YOU?</u> 30 min. Color. 1970.
Prize-winning portrayal of Ted Rosenthal,30 year-old poet
who learns he has leukemia.Interviews and free verse,black
& white & color film & stills. A song of dying & incomplete
life,crying"live while you can".Emotionally intense,ending
abruptly with the sound of a slide projector and close-up
shots of the poet alternating with a blank screen.In fact
the end of the story is very different from the impression
given.He didn't die in 1970 at 31 as it seems.He went into
remission after making the film,and lived to late 1972 at
the age of 34,divorcing his wife and remarrying weeks before
his death in hospital. A moving cinematic and poetic death
which is <u>not</u> a documentary.Powerfully moving and of great
value in <u>teaching</u>. By Thomas Reichman.American Film
Festival Blue Ribbon Winner 1972.
Rental $ 41/$ 35; purchase-$ 410/$390. EMC rental-$25.
EMC No.8527,Also Univ.Minnesota,Indiana Univ.,Univ.Wisconsin
-La Crosse; SUNY Media Library,Buffalo,NY ($ 14 rental);
Benchmark Films, & Viewfinders,Evanston, Illinois.

92. <u>HOW DEATH CAME TO EARTH</u>. 14 min. Color.
Colorful film of animated Indian paintings,showing the Asian
legend about the problems of a world without death,and
how death arrived. Charming.
Canadian National Film Board. 106C-071-951

93. <u>HOW MANY LIFETIMES?</u> 28 min.
Basic concepts of theosophy,considering the patterns and
purposes of life.
Rental-$ 20, sale-$ 300.
The Theosophical Society in America.

94. <u>I HEARD THE OWL CALL MY NAME</u>. 78 min. Color. 1974.
Film made for TV;adaptation of novel by Margaret Craven. A
bishop decides to send a terminally ill young priest
(unaware of his prognosis)to a small Indian village to learn
more about the meaning of life and death;& explores Indian
approaches to death & dying. Tom Courtenay & Dean Jagger.
Rental- $ 110 (EMC $ 65) Long term lease-$ 1150.
Learning Corporation of America,NY. EMC No. 1103.

95. <u>IKIRU</u>. 140 min. B&W.
Excellent Japanese film,English subtitles.The existential &
emotional crisis of a middle-aged widower,bureaucrat,who
discovers he has cancer,but achieves personal growth in his
last months.   Macmillan Films,Mt Vernon,NY.

96. I NEVER SANG FOR MY FATHER. 92 min. Color.
Feature film,dealing with the approaching death of a
father,& how a family deals with it.
Macmillan Audio Brandon, Mt Vernon,NY.

97. I NEVER SAW ANOTHER BUTTERFLY. 15 min. Color.
A Czech film of children's drawings made in the
concentration camps of Europe in the 1940's,showing both
happiness and death.
Rental- $ 12.50, Sale-$ 200.
Macmillan Films.

98. IN MY MEMORY. 15 min. Color. 1973.
A young girl's concerns about the death of her grandmother.
(Aimed at 8-10 year-old children).
Rental $ 3.50, Sale $ 150.
University of Wisconsin-La Cross; & Agency for Instructional
Relevision, Bloomington,IN.

99. AN INVESTMENT IN SIGHT. 19 min. Color.
An Eye-Bank Film.Story of a boy with impaired vision who
receives a corneal transplant and his vision improves.
Rental-$ 6.60. Media Library,AVC,Iowa.

100. JOSEPH SCHULTZ. 13 min. Color.
Re-enacting a true episode,when a German soldier refused to
serve on a firing squad and was,therefore,killed by his
fellow soldiers.Raises the issue of man's willingness to
die in order to preserve his values and moral principles.
Rental-$ 18.50. Purchase-$ 185.
Wombat Producations,NY. & Univ.Michigan, & EMC.

101. A JOURNEY. 12 min. Color.
Brief,powerful,symbolic representation of death & dying
as universal and inescapable.
Rental-$ 16.50, Purchase-$ 165.
Wombat Productions,NY.

102. JOURNEY'S END. 28 min. Color. 1974.
Dramatized,documentary-style,presentation of the difficulties
resulting for a family when a man,desiring to ignore death,
fails to make any plans for his funeral or Will.Film guide.
Rental-$ 22 (EMC),or $ 25.00 for 3 days,purchase-$295.
EMC No. 9192,Also Univ.Southern California.

103. JOY OF LOVE. 9 min. Color.
Wordless depiction of courtship,marriage,old age & death.
The old widower lives on with memories of his wife as young.
Rental-$ 4.95. Univ.of Michigan AV Center.

104. JUST A LITTLE TIME. 21 min. Color.
A terminally ill woman & her nurse(specialist in Oncology),
discuss the problems & rewards in their relationship.
American Journal of Nursing Film Library.

105. JUST LATHER,THAT'S ALL. 21 min. Color. 1976.
Based on a short story by Columbian writer Hernando Tellez.
Award winning study in suspense,awaiting death.A Latin
American army captain strolls into a barber shop for a
shave,lies back in the chair,& chats about his activities
traching down & killing revolutionaries.The barber quietly
& methodically prepares his razor. Then you realize that
he is a revolutionary....
Rental-$ 25. Learning Corporation of America.

106. A LAST & LASTING GIFT. 26 min. Color.
About the idea of bequeathing your body for medical &
scientific education & research;reviews the uses of donated
body tissues & organs.Includes an interview with a recipient
of a donated body part,who can now see again.Recommends
memorial services.
Rental-$ 25 / $ 20.
San Diego Human Resource Center,P.O.Box 5322,San Diego,CA
92105; Inland Empire Human Resourse Center,2 West Olive
Avenue, Redlands,California 93373.

107. LAST LEAF. 20 min. B&W. 1952.
Segment from Hollywood feature film "O.Henry's Full House",
about an unappreciated old painter who sacrifices his life
to keep a sick young woman alive.Introduced by John Steinbeck.
Rental-$ 12. EMC No. 8920.

108. LEO BEVERMAN. 13 min. Color.
A severely disabled man's courageous struggle to live; the
will to live.
Rental- $ 38.
Centron Educational Films,Kansas.

109. LES MISTONS. 18 min. B&W. 1958.
Truffaut's first film,about the brief period of growing-up
of some small-town pre-teen boys,as they become aware of
sex & death.   Rental-$ 20. Pyramid Films.

110. <u>LIFE IN A TIN</u>.
By Bruno Bozetto.An animated film about life & death.
Films Incorporated,NY.

111. <u>LIFE ON DEATH ROW</u>.9 min. B&W 1968.
Death Row,in San Quentin Prison.Sketches of the prisoners,
film of the views from their cells,their thoughts &
feelings.Introspection,forced to confront themselves,faced
with the constant awareness of impending execution.
Rental- $ 11. EMC- No. 7332.

112. <u>THE LIFE THAT'S LEFT</u>. 29 min. Color.film or VC.
Excellent.Nothing superfluous.Direct,clear,honest,
brilliantly well-organized & tightly edited.A powerful
series of interviews showing a range of experiences of
grief,including Harry who now wants to die too,and the later
remark:"I don't <u>want</u> my life to be the same---I don't <u>want</u>
to get over it!"
Rental-£ 6.30 (film) £ 3.90 (VCR)
Purchase-£ 180 film,£100 VCR--Philips or Sony U-matic.
CTVC,Watford,England.

113. <u>LIVING AND DEATH</u>. 29 min. B&W 1971.
Considers the nature of fear in relation to living,loving &
death.Krishnamurti lectures that fear of the future is
because we haven't cleared our minds of the past.If we
totally assimilate & understand each experience as it
happens,he assures us that we can overcome fear.
EMC-No. 8350,Rental-$ 15.
Rental-$ 9.50,Purchase $ 165. Also Field Service Division,
Indiana University AV Center,Bloomington,Indiana 47401.

114. <u>LIVING (VIVRE)</u>. 8 min. B&W.
Carefully selected newsreel excerpts of faces showing the
shocking impressions war leaves on its witnesses.No
dialogue,but impressive music.
Rental- $ 10. Contemporary/McGraw-Hill.

115. <u>THE LONG VALLEY:A STUDY OF BEREAVEMENT</u>. 56 min.Color.
BBC Television documentary (Project No.66256/7130).Produced
Martin Freeth;advisors Colin Murray Parkes & Michael Simpson.
December 1976. Thorough study of bereavement,with detailed
interviews with the bereaved,excerpts from C.S.Lewis,Parkes,
Pincus,etc.Very moving,but with good intellectual content,
too. BBC Enterprizes,Kensington House,Richmond Way,
London W14 OAX,England. <u>WARNING:</u> Though"Enterprizes" is
supposed to market BBC programmes for TV & educational uses,

115 ctd.) it usually seems extraordinarily unenterprizing,
and has dragged its heels about making this & other
outstanding documentaries available for sale or rental to
teachers.Keep nagging them persistently,as the material is
very well worth getting.

116/117. THE LOTTERY. 18 min. Color. 1969.
Based on Shirley Jackson's short story,chilling,symbolic,in
which the "winner" of an annual lottery is stoned to death.
Raises issues about violence,traditions & rituals.
Additional Film: The Lottery-Commentary. EMC No.7841,
Color, 10 min. provides commentary by James Durbin.
Rental-$ 20, EMC No.7814. Rental-$ 13.50,Sale-$ 265.
Encyclopedia Britannica Educational Corp.,Chicago.

118. THE LOVED ONE. 116 min. B&W.
Brilliant satire on American funeral practices,of great
value in teaching.
Rental-$ 75. Films Inc.

119. LOVE TO KILL. 14 min. Color. 1976.
Edited exerpt from Columbia feature film Bless the Beasts
and the Children (Stanley Kramer).About attitudes to
hunting & killing for pleasure.Six young boys are repulsed
by killing for sport,take action,but themselves become
victims of the violence in society.Provokes controversy.
Rental-$ 25. Learning Corporation of America.

120. MAGIC & CATHOLICISM. 34 min. Color.
A fatal accident during the festival of Santiago in Bolivia
leads to a combination of Catholic responses,burning candles
to the Saint,with ancestral religious response,with magical
rites and sacrifices.
Rental-$ 25. EMC.

121. MAGICAL DEATH. 28 min. Color. 1974.
Ethnographic study of voodoo death,spiritual manipulation
and coercion by the shamans of the Yanomama Indians in
Southern Venezuela. Award winner.
Rental-$ 13. EMC-No. 9285.

122. THE MAGIC MOTH. 22 min. Color.
From Virginia Lee's book.The death of a child & how family
members react;grieving,fears & uncertainties.One of her gifts
is a cocoon from which a moth emerges when she dies.
Discussion guide included.
Rental-$ 35, Sale-$ 350. Centron Educational Films,& Iniv.
Wisconsin--La Crosse.

123. <u>MAN APART: THE MURDERER</u>. 35 min. B&W.
Interviews with murderers,& families & friends of both
murderers and victims.Murderer & victim often know
each other.
Sale only- $ 275. Time/Life Multimedia.

124. <u>THE MARK WATERS STORY</u>.26 min. Color. 1969.
True story of a Honolulu newsman dying of lung cancer who
writes his own obituary.Acted & directed by Richard Boone.
Rental-$ 14,EMC No.9212.Aso VC rental/sale,Public
Television Library,475 L'Enfant Plaza SW,Washington DC 20024.

125. <u>THE MARVELS OF CREATION</u>. 29 min. Color.
A 9 year-old girl,delighting in nature & science, discovers
death.Her parents ask a Bible student to explain why death
exists,& how it fits God's design.For Bible Study groups.
Free Loan. Dawn Films.

126. <u>THE MASQUE OF THE RED DEATH</u>. 10 min.
Animation of paintings.Poe short story,dealing with man's
perceptions of death,& his fear & denial of dying.
Rental-$ 15,purchase-$ 160. McGraw-Hill Films,NY.
Also Rental-$ 5.50,University of Michigan AV Center.

127. <u>MATINEE</u>. Perspective Films,Chicago.

128. <u>A MATTER OF TIME</u>. Indiana University AV Center.

129. <u>MEDICINE,MORALITY & THE LAW: EUTHANASIA</u>. 30 min.B&W.
3 case studies,presented to an interdisciplinary panel which
discusses the legal & moral aspects of them.
Rental- $ 7. Sale- $ 90. Univ.of Michigan TV Center.

130. <u>THE MERCY KILLERS</u>. 30 min. B&W.
Discussion of euthanasia by physicians,clergymen,& four
terminally ill patients.Poor sound quality.
Rental-$ 25,Purchase-$ 250. Time/Life Multimedia,NY.
or Time/Life Films. Rental $ 11, Univ.of Illinois,Visual
Aids Department.

131. <u>THE MOCKINGBIRD</u>. 39 min. B&W 1963.
Ambrose Bierce short story,Civil War.A private in the Union
Army on night guard sees an indistinct moving figure and
fires.Next day he searches for his victim & finds the body
of his twin brother in Confederate uniform.No dialogue.Awards.
Rental- $ 19. EMC, No. 8612.

132. THE MORTAL BODY. 12 min. B&W.
Non-verbal,but visually powerful view of the life-cycle,
birth to death,& the transience of human existence.
Yugoslav Film.
Rental- $ 18,Purchase-$ 100. Filmmakers Library,NY.

133. MOURNING FOR MANGATOPI. 56 min. Color.
From the Australian Institute of Aboriginal Studies,
documentary of a mortuary Pukamani ceremony of the Tiwi
tribe of Melville Island,for Mangatopi,the tribal leader.
Rental- $ 32. EMC.

134. THE MYSTERY THAT HEALS.3o min. Color.
Exploration of Jung's concept of continuation of the psyche
after death; observes Jung in his old age.
Rental- $ 30, Sale-$ 300. (EMC rental-$ 22)
Time-Life Films,NY.

135. MY TURTLE DIED TODAY. 5 min. Color.
Animated film for children.
Rental: $ 9. Bailey Film Assoc,Santa Monica.CA.

136. NAMING OF PARTS. 5 min. B&W. 1972.
Based on the superb poem by Henry Reid.Young military
trainee receiving instruction on the use of an M-14 rifle
as instrument of war & death,while his thoughts reflect on
the value of life & the beauty of nature.May be interpreted
optimistically or pessimistically
Rental-$ 11. EMC,No. 8481.

137. NEVER GIVE UP. 28 min. Color. 1974.
The photographer Imogen Cunningham at 94,at home & walking
around San Francisco,considering her life,friends,thoughts
about death;intercut with her photographs.Positive aging
rather than mere giving up.
Rental- $ 26, EMC No. 9359.

138. NIGHT AND FOG. 31 min. B&W. 1955.
Alain Resnais documentary.Life & death in the Nazi
concentration camps;shocking & moving.Death,war, & survival.
Delicate counterpoint of sound & images,still & motion
pictures,narration & music,living & dead.French,English
subtotles. Won many important awards.
Rental-$ 3o,Sale-$ 350. (EMC rental-$ 22).
Contemporary Films/McGraw-Hill,NY & EMC No.8482.

139. NIGHT OF THE ASSASSINS. 30 min. B&W.
A chronicle of the day Lincoln was shot.
Rental- $ 12.50. Assoc.Films (EW-423).

140. NOVEMBER. 10 min. Color. 1972.
Visually beautiful depiction of late Autumn moods & scenes
with recurring images of death,natural and violent;and
images of resurgent Spring.
Rental- $ 14. EMC- No. 8276.

141. AN OCCURRENCE AT OWL CREEK BRIDGE. 27 min. B&W.1962.
Ambrose Bierce's short story of a man's feelings,perceptions,
thoughts & relaizations as he is hanged,in the split second
between life & death;or maybe not. Won several awards.
Rental-$ 20,(EMC $ 17),Sale-$ 250.
Contemporary/McGraw-Hill; & EMC No. 7091.

142. OLD,BLACK AND ALIVE! 28 min. Color. 1975.
Seven elderly Black people discuss their insights on
aging,& how their religious faith minimizes the fear of death.
Rental-$ 25. EMC No. 9361.

143. THE OLD WOMAN.2 min. Color. 1973.
Animation,no narration. Cheerful look at a sprightly old
woman who refuses to obey death when he comes to call .
Rental- $ 2.65. ACI Films,Inc.,& Univ.of Michigan AV Center.

144. OMEGA. 13 min. Color. 1970.
Deals with a man's death from this life,& re-birth into a
more surreal dimension;pictorial representation of death
& re-birth,in music and pictures.
Rental-$ 20, Sale-$ 175. Pyramid Films, California.

145. ONE IN THREE-HUNDRED FIFTY:SuddenInfant Death.30min.B&W.
Stresses mainly the need to discover the cause of SID
through research,though also reflecting how tactless others
can compound the suffering of parents whose infant suddenly
dies of unknown cause.
Rental: National Foundation for SID,1501 Broadway,NY 10036.

146. THE PARTING. 16 min. Color.
The death rituals in a Yugoslav Montenegro mountain village.
A middle-aged man has died,is washed,dressed in his uniform,
laid out.Some mourners are professional,paid to grieve.
Rental- $ 22, Sale-$ 220.
Wombat Productions Inc. & Viewfinders.

147. PASSING QUIETLY THROUGH.26 min. B&W.
Award-winning film,exploring the relationship between a
dying old man & his nurse.Rare in that it also considers
geriatric sex.
Rental-$ 35, Sale-$ 200. Grove Press Evergreen Films;
also Films,Inc.

148. PEEGE. 28 min. Color. 1974.
A young man home for Christmas accompanies his family to
visit his dying grandmother in a nursing home.At first,it
is very awkward,but once the rest of the family leaves,he
stays and succeeds in communicating his love for her.
Award winning.
Rental- $ 20. EMC,No. 9179. & Phoenix Films,Princeton,NJ.

149. PLANTING THINGS I WONT SEE FLOWER. 26 min. Color.
A family struggling to cope with the impending death of
the mother.
Rental-$ 20, Sale-$ 225. United Methodist Film Office.

150. POINT OF NO RETURN. 24 min. B&W. 1965.
Argues that each man has the obligation to prevent suicide,
& calls for more suicide prevention programs.A case
hostory of acted out & discussed by a panel of psychiatrists.
Rental-$ 7.50, Sale- $ 135. International Film Bureau.

151. THE PRICE OF LIFE. 13 min. Color.
Three vignettes illustrating the problems of the sacredness
of human life versus human dilemmas:fighting a"necessary &
just"war,can you kill enemy combatants?;retarded persons
become an insufferable burden; your wife is determined to
have an abortion. Poses questions for discussion.
Rental- $ 15.95. Association Films.

152. PRIMITIVE PEOPLE:AUSTRALIAN ABORIGINES. PART III:
     THE CORROBOREE. 17 min. B&W.
A funeral corroboree is planned by the old man;the dead are
wrapped in paper bark,placed on a high platform,& an
elaborate ritual is held to placate the spirit.
Rental- $4. Kent State University AV Service.

153. PROBLEM: TO THINK OF DYING. 59 min. Color.
Interviews with Lynn (Widow) Caine & Orville (Make Today
Count) Kelly on their experiences & how their philosophy
of life has been revised.
Rental- $ 20.75, Sale-$ 550. Indiana University AV Center.

154. <u>PSYCHOSOCIAL ASPECTS OF DEATH</u>.39 min. B&W. 1971.
Intended for training health care professionals in dealing
with terminally ill patients.Dramatized story of a leukemic
patient,his wife,& the nursing student for whom it is a
first experience of death.His wife is pregnant & wants him
to see the baby.He dies unexpectedly,& the nurse has to
learn to cope.
Rental $ 11.25 / $ 9.50. Sale-$200. Indiana Univ.AV Center.

155. <u>RABBIT</u>. 15 min. Color.
A nine year'old boy has the problem of what to do when the
Easter gift of a baby rabbit has become huge by the end of
Summer.He leaves it in the woods to fend for itself,& the
next day finds it dead.
Rental-$ 19,Sale-$190. Viewfinders, & Eccentric Circle.

156. <u>THE RED KITE</u>. 17 min. Color.
A man buys his daughter a kite.On the bus they meet a
drunken priest who starts talking as they pass a cemetary.
Rental- $ 22.50. Viewfinders.

157. <u>RETREAT.</u> 11 min. Color. 1971.
A Vietnam veteran goes for a walk in the woods to retreat
from the nightmare of war,but finds that every sound he
hears triggers a memory of the horror.He struggles to
disengage from the memories,to survive.
Rental- $ 6.50. University of Illinois.

-58. <u>RIGHT HERE,RIGHT NOW</u>. 15 min. B&W
A janitor in an apartment house is killed;his neighbours
share their memories of him & how he influenced their lives.
Rental- $ 15. Franciscan Communications Center.

159. <u>THE RIGHTS OF AGE</u>. 28 min. B&W.
Looks at the kinds of social services needed by the aged,
focussing on the problems of one lonely widow.
Rental-$ 12.50, Sale- $ 185.
International Film Bureau,Chicago.

160. <u>THE RIGHT TO DIE</u>. 56 min. Color. 1974.
Originally an ABC documentary,giving a well-balanced
discussion of issues.Examines actual cases in which life is
being prolonged by machines or a suffering patient wants
to die.Issues of euthanasia explored.Includes a doctor's
interview discussing with a young boy his impending death
from cystic fibrosis.   Univ. Michigan.
Rental-$55(EMC$37)Sale-$600. Macmillan Films,EMC.No.9193.

161. THE RIGHT TO LIVE: WHO DECIDES? 17 min. Color/B&W.1976.
Edited exerpt from Columbia feature film"Abandon Ship" with
Tyrone Power.Poses questions about the morality of making
life & death decisions about others.A ship has sunk,one
officer survives,with more passangers & crew members than
the one lifeboat is equipped to carry.Somewhat dated &
corny.Handily,the survivors include old & young,strong &
sickly,one black & one pet dog. Nonetheless,it raises such
questions as the legitimacy of authority,relationships
between the value of life & social utility,etc.Provocative.
Rental-$ 25. Learning Corp.of America,also R.O.A's Films,
Univ. of Arizona Bureau of AV Services (rental $ 7.25).

162. ROBLIN'S MILLS. 9 min. Color. 1976.
Based on Al Purdy poem.An old man shares his memories with
a young boy as they wander through an old village and
graveyard,& pay respects to the dead who have shaped their
world.
Rental- $ 15. Learning Corporation of America.

163. SALLY: 1893-1974. 60 min. Color.
A unique funeral service,life centred,as a tribute to Sally
McGinnis.At the casket are the things she loved most,her
hats & golf-clubs.Eulogies,poems,songs,& a tea party!
Rental- $ 25, Sale-$ 425.
Univ.of Oregon,Divn.of Continuing Education Film Library.

164. SAMSAVA: THE WHEEL OF LIFE AND DEATH. 10 min. Color.
Short Indian film on the cycle from birth to funeral.
Canadian National Film Board, 106C-0172-014.

165. THE SEVENTH SEAL. B&W
Ingmar Bergman's famous allegory of Death.
Janus Films,NY.

166. SILENCES. 12 min. Color. 1972.
Prize-winning Yugoslav film about the ambiguities & dilemmas
of war.A peasant helps a German soldier wounded by partisans.
Then discovers that in the meantime,the Germans have
destroyed his village & massacred his family.In rage,he
murders the soldier he has saved.
Rental- $ 16.   EMC,No.9264.

167. SOON THERE WILL BE NO MORE ME. 10 min. Color. 1972.
A young mother's fear of dying,especially how it will affect
her children.Legacy to her baby daughter,compiled from her
husband's still photographs & her writings.Song by Dory

167 ctd.) Previn. Lyn Helton,the original of "Sunshine".
Rental- $ 15,(EMC $14) Purchase-$ 130.
Churchill Films,L.A.,EMC No.9185,Univ.Wisconsin-La Crosse,
University of Illinois.

168. SPECIAL KIND OF CARE. 13 min. Color.
The impact of terminal disease on the whole family,as a
father has to tell his children that mother is dying.
Rental-$ 20. American Journal of Nursing Film Library.
c/o Association Films.

169. SPIRIT POSSESSION OF ALEJANDRO MAMANI.27 min.Color.1975.
Portrait of an old Bolivian man of property & status,but not
content as he nears death.His confrontation with old age &
death is anguished & he believes he is possessed by evil
spirits.1975 Blue Ribbon Award,American Film Festival.
English subtitles.
Rental-$ 21 EMC, $ 36.50 Filmmakers.
EMC No. 9310, & Filmmakers Library.

170. STAR SPANGLED BANNER. 5 min. Color. 1970.
Slow motion study of a soldier's death in battle,scenes as
news of his death reaches his family;set to the Anthem.
Rental- $ 10. Pyramid Films.

171. STILLBIRTH. 12 min. Color. (or VCR). 1976.
Bel Mooney,a journalist,talks about her experience of
stillbirth."Then the nurse came & told me:'You had your
baby.It was a little boy & he isn't alive..." The reactions
of Bel & the staff.The depth & variety of her emotions were
startling & moving;guilt,anger,frustration,a numbing sense
of failure,& an unexpectedly deep grief.
Contact: Ros Peedle,CTVC,Hillside,Merry Hill Road,Bushey,
   Watford,WD2 1DR,England.

172. THE SUICIDAL PATIENT. 60 min. B&W.
University of California,10962 Le Conte Ave,Los Angeles,
California 90024.

173. SUICIDE:BUT JACK WAS A GOOD DRIVER. 15 min. Color.
After the funeral of a friend killed in an auto accident,
2 teenagers realize his death was probably a suicide,& they
hadn't listened to his attempts to get help. (Also under B).
Rental- $ 17. EMC.

174. <u>SUICIDE CLINIC: A CRY FOR HELP</u>.38 min. B&W 1969.
Examines the problems of a suicide clinic,discusses the
psychological needs & problems of suicide attempters,the
need to identify suicidal persons & provide help.
Rental-$ 15,$12.50,$7.75. Sale- $ 165. Indiana University
AV Center,Bloomington,IN; Association Films, EMC No.8364.

175. <u>SUICIDE: IT DOESN'T HAVE TO HAPPEN</u>.20 min. Color.1976.
Using real case histories,shows how a sympathetic high
school teacher persuades a suicidal student to join a "rap
group"at a local suicide prevention center.There the
student learns about typical symptoms,how help is available,
& hears others tell how they dealth with their problems.
Rental-$ 21. EMC No. 9491

176. <u>SUICIDE PREVENTION & CRISIS INTERVENTION.</u> 12 films
Directed by Allen J.Enelow. Deal with identifying,managing
& evaluating potentially suicidal people;covering interview
techniques,didactic material,& knowledge tests.
<u>Case History A-The Only Way.</u> A 30 year-old housewife,after
a hysterectomy,attempts suicide.Interview film 1-$ 145,
Content film-2 - $ 145.
<u>Case History B-20 Years & Out.</u> A 55 year-old machinist grows
depressed,irritable & accident-prone. Interview film-3- $145.
Content Film 4- $ 145.
<u>Case History C-Test No. 1.</u> An alcoholic salesman feeling
hopeless. Test Interview Film-5 -$125.Test content film 6-
-$ 125.
<u>Case History D-Impulse.</u> A young waitress,"born loser",
attempts suicide.Interview Film-7:$145,Content film-8:$145.
<u>Case History E-Adolescent Crisis.</u>College co-ed,history of
bad relations with parents & rape when younger. Interview
film-9:$145; Content Film-10 : $145.
<u>Case History F.Test No.2.</u> Twice divorced mother,financially
insecure,& her affair has ended. Test Interview Film-11:
$ 125; Test Content Film-12- $ 125.
Complete set,purchase- $ 1,325. Rental- $ 25 each.
Response sheets for each film:150 sets-$6 ;Response Sheets
& content check-lists for each:150 sets--$ 9.
Charles Press Publishers,Inc.

177. <u>SUICIDE PREVENTION IN THE HOSPITAL.</u> 30 min.B&W.
How hospital staff can help to prevent suicide.
Sale- $ 52. National Audiovisual Center,General Services
Administration.

178. <u>TERMINAL PATIENTS:THEIR ATTITUDES AND YOURS</u>.Color.
Reviews the attitudes of professional staff to caring for
the terminally ill,& the experiences of two patients.
Rental: $ 7.50. Abbott Laboratories,Professional Relations.

179. <u>THINGS IN THEIR SEASON</u>. 79 min. Color.
A woman's encounter with terminal illness,& what she learnt.
Peg,played by Patricia Neal,is about to die of leukemia,&
her husband Carl deals with the truth of his love for his
family.Impending tragedy is a catalyst for happiness that
might otherwise never ave been realized.
Rental-$75,Long term lease-$750. Learning Corp.of America,
Also Mass Media.

180. <u>THOSE WHO MOURN</u>.5 min. Color. 1973.
A woman's struggle to understand & accept the sudden and
accidental death of her husband.Grief,mourning,violence &
war,with an affirmative & hopeful end.Religious tone,but
not heavily stressed. Teaching guide available.
Rental-$10,sale-$ 70. ($ 10 & $ 80,Association Films)
Franciscan Communications Center,Los Angeles. Telekinetics.

181. <u>THOUGH I WALK THROUGH THE VALLEY</u>. 30 min. Color.1972.
Documentary of the last 6 months in the life of a devout
Christian middle-aged College professor with cancer.Explores
his feelings & those of his family.Strong religious emphasis
Some awfully pious attitudes & fundamentalist preaching
which spoils it for some.
Rental-$ 25 (EMC $ 23) Purchase-$ 325.
Pyramid Films;EMC No.9182;Gospel Films;Church Films Service;
and Mass Media.

182. <u>THRESHOLD</u>. 25 min. Color. 1970.
An experience of the threshold between life & death helps
a young man realize & understand love.Symbolic approach.
John Carradine as Death.
Rental- $ 25. Pyramid Films.

183. <u>TO A VERY OLD WOMAN</u>. 10 min. Color. 1976.
Based on poem by Irving Layton. Frail but serene old woman
plays solitaire,feeds birds,plays with a child.Greets death
as a natural completion of her life.
Rental- $ 15.
Learning Corporation of America.

184. TO BE AWARE OF DEATH.15 min. Color. 1974.
Issues relating to funerals,wakes,communication with the
dead,life after death,facing the death of a loved one,or
one's own death.A montage of comments by young people.
Rental-$ 20, Sale-$200. Billy Budd Films,NY.
Also University of Minnesota AV Library Service(Rental-$8)

185. TO DIE TODAY. 50 min. B&W. 1971.
Elizabeth Kubler-Ross discusses death & dying & how she
deals with the terminally ill patient,expounds her theory
of the 5 stages.Includes an interview with a patient who
has recently learned he has Hodgkins Disease (who doesnt
really show any of the 5 stages,but is valuably ambiguous).
Over-sentimental at times,often visually dull,& too long.
Rental-$ 35,Sale-$ 275. Filmmakers Library,NY. & U.Michigan.

186. TOMORROW AGAIN. 16 min. B&W. 1971.
Loneliness in old age.No dialogue or narration.Grace lives
in a "retirement"hotel.She fantasizes her illness & possible
death,which could gain her the attention she craves.
Rental- $ 15. Pyramid Films.

187. TWO DAUGHTERS. 22 min. Color. 1976.
Based on August Strindberg story.After the death of her
young daughter,a woman returns to the apartment where they
had lived together.She is flooded with memories of the
daughter's life,illness & death;& of her own strained
relationship with her own mother.She wanders aimlessly
through Stockholm,deep in her emotions & memories.Later,
sitting on a bench in a busy square,noisy drunks interrupt
her.Annoyed,she then realizes she is surrounded by life
& vitality.Now her memories are more positive.Swedish with
English subtitles.   Rent- $ 21. EMC No. 9430.

188. UNTIL I DIE. 30 min. Color. 1970.
Concise representation of the work of Kubler-Ross,her theory
of stages,an interview with a patient(much more ambivalent
than he is presented).Visually effective.Sound quality
variable & sometimes poor.
Rental-$ 18,EMC No.9189;Rent-$25,AJN Film Library,c/o
Assoc.Sterling Films,600 Grand Ave.,Ridgefield,NY o7657.
Also University of Wisconsin, & University of Iowa.

189. <u>THE UPTURNED FACE</u>. 10 min. Color.
Stephen Crane's short story about the death of a young
soldier in the Spanish-American War,& his comrade's
reactions to it,& to the dead body,the lifeless upturned
face.Study Guide available.
Rental-$15,Sale-$150. Pyramid Films,California.

190. <u>VIOLENCE:JUST FOR FUN</u>. 14 min. Color. 1976.
Edited extract from Columbia feature film"Barabbas",dealing
with the gladiators & the arena.Why do people find
excitement & entertainment in the spectacle of violence and
death?   Rental-$25. Learning Corp.of America.

191. <u>A WALK UP THE HILL</u>. 30 min. Color.
A doctor,after a paralyzing stroke,asks that no life-
-preserving measures be undertaken for him.The question is
left open to allow for audience discussion.
Rental-$ 25. Church Films,Spokane.

192. <u>THE WAR GAME</u>. 49 min. B&W.
A documentary style portrayal of the results of a nuclear
war,as if being reported as it occurred.(English TV original)
Rental- $ 75. Contemporary/McGraw-Hill,NY.

193. <u>WARRENDALE</u>. 105 min. B&W.
Young people with emotional disturbances,& how they respond
when someone close to them has died.The similarities and
differences between'normal' and emotionally disturbed
responses to grieving.
Rental-$100, Sale-$ 750. Grove Press Film Divn.NY.

194. <u>WHAT CAN I SAY?</u>   31 min. B&W
How a nurse can handle the questions of the dying patient,
and cope with her own anxiety.
Rental-$ 15, American Journal of Nursing/Association Films.

195. <u>WHAT MAN SHALL LIVE AND NOT SEE DEATH?</u> 57 min. Color.
1971 film documentary,exploring a terminally ill patient's
feelings & worries about her approaching death.Includes
St Christopher's Hospice & the Kubler-Ross 5.
Rental-$ 42 (FI),$36(EMC),$18.75 (UI),Sale-$ 575 (FI).
Films Incorporated,EMC No.9186,Univ.Iowa;Also NBC,Kent State
Univ.,Mich.State Univ.,Univ.Illinois,Arizona,& Minnesota.
NBC Educational Enterprizes,NY: Rental-$26,Sale-$530.

196. <u>WHEN A MAN DIES.</u> 29 min. Color.
The Hereafter;the soul,heaven & hell.Very orthodox
bible study.
Free Loan: Dawn Films.

197. <u>WHEN PARENTS GROW OLD.</u> 14 min. Color. 1976.
Edited exerpt from Columbia feature film"I Never Sang for
My Father",with Gene Hackman & Melvyn Douglas.Resp onsibility
to aging parents.A young man on the verge of marriage is
faced with a suddenly widowed father whose health is failing,
& must decide where his responsibilities lie.
Rental-$ 25. Learning Corp.of America.Also ROA's Films,Wisc.

198. <u>WHEN YOU SEE ARCTURUS.</u> 27 min. Color.
Rich architect is so bored with life,he decides to kill
himself.Visits the Thanatos Society which helps people
make "the final passage".Then the senseless murder of his
son convinces him that life is serious,& he throws away
the suicide potion.   Rental-$19, Association Films.

199. <u>WHERE IS DEAD?</u> 20 min. Color. 1975.
The death of a young boy & its impact on his 6 year-old
sister--feelings of separation,confusion,fear & guilt,and
grief.Her family helps her achieve understanding.
Rental-$20 (EMC) Purchase-$ 255 (E.B.) EMC-No.9573.
Encyclopedia Britannica Educational Corporation,Chicago.

200. <u>WHO CARES?</u> 20 min. Color.
A short,sharp,emotive film about the effects of cancer on
patient & family,& the NSCR(Charity)'s work in creating
special Hospice-type units attached to regular general
hospitals,Macmillan units,to care for terminal patients.
National Society for Cancer Relief,London.

201. <u>WHO DO YOU KILL?</u> 51 min. B&W. 1967.
Story of young Black couple in Harlem whose child is bitten
by a rat & loses a great deal of blood on the way to hospital
mainly because white cab drivers will not stop for them.When
the child dies,the mother is shattered,father puts aside his
rage & grief to help her.   Rental-$ 19. EMC-7191.

202. <u>WHOSE LIFE IS IT,ANYWAY?</u> 53 min. Color. 1975.
Film of TV play--a young paraplegic man wants to be allowed
to die.Portrays arguments & struggle between doctors and
patient.Beautifully articulated review of major issues.
By Brian Clark (Granada TV International).
Rental-$40(EMC)$24(U.Mich.) $60 (Ecc.C) Sale-$650 (Ec.C).

202 ctd.) Eccentric Circle Cinema Workshop,EMC No.9224,
and University of Michigan AV Educational Center.

203. WHO SHOULD SURVIVE? 26 min. Color. 1972.
Explores issues of euthanasia,specifically the example of a
mangoloid infant who is allowed to die.A panel of experts
discuss legal,scientific & ethical points of view.Dramatic
reconstruction of the actual case incident.Best to use the
first half,posing the problem,& avoid the rather dull
discussion,& do it yourself. Produced by the Joseph P.
Kennedy Foundation. Rental-$ 23,Purchase-$ 150.
EMC;Media Center,University Extension,University of
California,Berkeley,Cal.94720. Also,Patricia Furman,209 E
Broad Street,Falls Church,Va 22046.

204. WHY DID GLORIA DIE? 27 min. Color. 1972.
The problems of Native Americans who leave the reservation
to settle in urban areas.Tragic life of 27 year-old Chippewa
woman who died of hepatitis in Minneapolis.The contributors
to her death are shared by other urban American Indians.
Rental-- $ 23. EMC No. 8901.

205. WIDOWS. 43 min. B&W 1972.
Bu Edward A.Mason.Interviews several widows,discussing their
responses to their husband's deaths,& how they came to terms
with loss.Frank,clear & emotive.Made in cooperation with the
Widow-to-Widow program.Widows of various ages,races and
economic situations.
Rental $25 (EMC $ 19) Purchase $ 240. Mental Health Training
Film Program,Harvard Medical School,33 Fenwood Road,Boston,
Mass. 02115. EMC No. 8624.

206. WILL DRAFTING. 40 min. B&W.
An attorney demonstrates the drafting of wills,interviewing
2 clients with diverse estates and needs.
Rental-$ 23,Sale-$ 310.
EMC,Berkeley.

207. THE WILL TO DIE. (Part I) 28 min. Color.
The potential suicide,his signals of needing help and
understanding.Interviews Ed Shneidman,Norman Farberow,
Manuel Pardo & Joseph Hirsch.
Rental- $ 20, Sale-$ 150.
Assoc.Films. (BSP-101).

208. THE WILL TO DIE. (Part II) 28 min. Color.
Interview with a middle-aged woman who has attempted
suicide & remains at risk.
Rental- $ 20, Sale-$ 150.   Association Films.

209. WORKING WITH DEATH SERIES. Color. (or VC)
4 units for training professionals & counselling---
Death & the Doctor-20 min; The Dying Patient-19 min; The
Family-15 min.(+user's guide);Living With Dying-15 min.
(for the terminal patient,with User's Guide).
Rental available. Purchase- Videocassettes or Super 8mm
film--$ 750; 16 mm film-- $ 800.
Professional Research Association,Los Angeles,California.

210. YOU SEE,I'VE HAD A LIFE. 30 min. B&W. 1972.
A 13 year-old boy with leukemia,his & his family's feelings
& responses,as he lives a normal life for as long as
possible.Candid,sometimes humorous. Special Academy Award.
Ben Levin.
Rental-$ 29 (EMC $ 19), Purchase- $ 290.
Ben Levin,600 Lorraine Ave.,Oreland,Pa.19075.
EMC No.9005; Univ.Illinois,Univ.Iowa.

211. THE YOUNG MAN AND DEATH. 16 min. Color.
Choreographed drama of encounter with death.Ballet by
Rudolf Nureyev & Zizi Jeanmaire.She,as Death,pursues & is
pursued by the young man,till he grovels at her feet.Then,
turning her back on him,she fastens a rope to a beam,leaving
him to hang himself.
Rental- $ 20, Sale- $ 200.   Macmillan Films Inc.

212. YOUTH,MATURITY,OLD AGE,DEATH. 8 min. Color. 1975.
Marcel Marceau,in symbolic mime,on the cycle of human life.
Rental- $ 14. EMC No. 9511.

————oOo————

FILM DISTRIBUTORS AND LIBRARIES

ABC News, 7 W 66th Street,New York, NY 10023.
ACI Films,Inc.,35 West 45th Street,New York, NY 10036.
Agency for Instructional TV,Box A,Bloomington,IN 47401.
American Journal of Nursing Film Library,c/o Associated
    Sterling Films,600 Grand Avenue,Ridgefield,NJ 07657.
American Cancer Society,Williamson Building,215 Euclid Ave.,
    Cleveland,Ohio.
Association Films,8615 Directors Row,Dallas,Texas 75247
    and 600 Grand Avenue,Ridgefield,NJ o7657.
Bailey Film Assoc.,2211 Michigan Avenue,P.O.Box 1795,Santa
    Monica,California 90404.
BBC TV,"Enterprizes",Kensington House,Richmond Way,
    London W14 0AX, England.
Benchmark Films Inc.,145 Scarborough Rd.,Briarcliff Manor,
    NY 10510
BFC Films,475 Riverside Drive,New York,NY 10027.
Billy Budd Films Inc.,235 East 57th St.,New York,NY 10022.
Brigham Young University,Educational Media Services,
    290 Herald R.Clark Building,Provo,Utah 84602.
Budget Films,81 Santa Monica Blvd.,Los Angeles,CA 91029
Bureau of AV Instruction,P.O.Box 2093,Madison,Wisc.53701.
Centron Educational Films,1621 West Ninth Street,
    Lawrence,Kansas 66044.
Church Films,2923 North Monroe St.,Spokane,Washington 99205.
Churchill Films,662 North Robertson Blvd,Los Angeles,CA 90069.
Concord Films,Nacton,nr Ipswich,Suffolk,England.
Contemporary/McGraw-Hill Films,Princeton Rd.,Hightstown,
    NJ 08520; & 828 Custer Ave.,Evanston,Illinois 60202.
    & 1221 Avenue of the Americas,New York,NY 10020.
Creative Film Society,7237 Canby Ave.,Roseda,Cal.91335.
CRM Educational Films,1104 Camino del Mar,Del Mar,CA 92014.
CTVC,Hillside,Merry Hill Rd.,Bushey,Watford WD21DR,England.
    Phone 01- 950-4426.
Doubleday Media,P.O.Box 11607,Santa Ana,California 92705.
The Eccentric Circle,P.O.Box 1481,Evanston,Illinois 60204.
The Eccentric Circle Cinema Workshop,P.O.Box 4085,416
    Fourth St.,Greenwich, CT 06830.
EMC,Extension Media Center,University of California,
    Berkeley,California 94720 / 90015.
Encyclopedia Britannica Educational Corporation,425 North
    Michigan Avenue,Chicago,Illinois 60611.

Films Inc.,1144 Wilmette Avenue,Wilmette,Illinois 60091;
    & 440 Park Ave.,South,New York, NY 10016.
    & 35-01 Queens Blvd,Long Island City,NY 11101
    (212) 937-1110.
    & 5626 Hollywood Blvd.,Hollywood,California 90068.
Filmmakers Library Inc.,290 West End Ave.,New York,NY 10023,
    (212)877-4486;& 743 Alexander Rd.,Princeton,NJ 08540.
Foundation of Thanatology,67 Park Avenue,Room 11-B,
    New York, NY 10016.
Franciscan Communications Center,1229 South Santee Street,
    Los Angeles,California 90015.
Gospel Films,P.O.Box 455,Muskegan,Minn.49443.
Grove Press Film Division,53 E.11th St.,New York,NY 10003,
    (212)677-2400;& 96 W.Houston St,New York,NY 10014.
Harper & Row Media Films,10 E.53rd St.,New York, NY 10022.
Inland Empire Human Resource Center,2 West Olive Avenue,
    Redlands,California 93373.
International Film Bureau,332 South Michigan Avenue,
    Chicago,Illinois 60611.
Janus Films,745 5th Avenue,New York, NY 10022.
Learning Corporation of America,1350 Avenue of the Americas,
    New York, NY 10019.
MacMillan Films,Inc.,34 MacQuestern Parkway South,Mt.
    Vernon, NY 10550. (Also,MacMillan Audio Brandon).
Mass Media Associates,1720 Chouteau Avenue,St.Louis,
    Mo. 63103.
Mass Media, 2116 N.Charles St.,Baltimore,MD 21218,
    (301) 727-3270.
McGraw-Hill Films,1211 Avenue of the Americas,NY 10020.
Modern Talking Picture Service,2323 New Hyde Park Rd.,
    New Hyde Park,NY 1104o.
National Foundation for SID,1501 Broadway,New York,NY 10036.
NBC Educational Enterprizes,30 Rockefeller Plaza,New York,
    NY 10020.
New Line Cinema,121 University Place,New York,NY 10003
    (212) 674-7460.
Office of Medical Education,University of California,
    Irvine,California 92664.
Oregon Division of Continuing Medical Education Film
    Film Library,P.O.Box 1491,Portland,Oregon 97201.
Perspective Films,369 W.Erie St.,Chicago,Illinois 60610,
    (312) 332-7676.
Phoenix Films,470 Park Avenue South,New York,NY 10016;
    & 743 Alexander Rd.,Princeton,NJ 08540.
Polymorph Films,331 Newbury Street,Boston,Massachusetts
    02115; (617) 262-5960.

The Public Television Library,475 L'Enfant Plaze SW,
    Washington DC. 20024.
Pyramid Films,Box 1048,Santa Monica,California 90406.
ROA's Films,1696 North Astor St,Milwaukee,Wisc.53202.
Telekinetics,1229 South Santee St.,Los Angeles,CA 90015.
Time/Life Media,43 W.16th St.,New York, NY 10011; and
    100 Eisenhower Drive,Paramus,NJ 07652.
Time/Life Multimedia,1271 Avenue of the Americas,NY 10020.
Universal 16, 445 Park Avenue,New York, NY 10036.
UCLA,10962 Le Conte Avenue,Los Angeles,California 90024.
University of Colorado Film Library,Bureau of Educational
    Media,University of Colorado,Boulder,COL 80302.
University of Illinois Visual Aids Service,Division of
    University Extension,1325 South Oak St.,Champaign,
    Illinois 61820.
University of Indiana,Field Service Division,AV Center,
    Bloomington,Indiana 47401.
University of Iowa,Media Library,AV Center,C-5 East Hall,
    Iowa City, IA 52242.
University of Michigan AV Educational Center,416 Fourth
    Street, Ann Arbor,MI 48109.
University of Southern California,Division of Cinema,
    Film Distribution Section,University Park,
    Los Angeles,California 90007.
Viewfinders Films,P.O.Box 1665,Evanston,Illinois 60204.
Washburn Films,9 E.32nd St.,New York,NY 10016.
    (212) 686-6622.
WGBH-TV,125 Western Avenue,Boston,Mass.02134.
Wombat Productions,77 Tarrytown Rd,White Plains,NY 10607.
Zipporah Films,54 Lewis Wharf,Boston,Mass.02110.

———oOo———

AUDIO-VISUAL MATERIALS

A. AUDIOTAPES AND AUDIOCASSETTES

1. **AGING & DYING:A POSITIVE VIEW.**5 Cassettes,30 min each.
Interviews with various people about their opinions on
these subjects. Sale-$ 15.
Aging & Dying Tapes,No.1111,New Dimensions Foundation,
  59 Montgomery St.,San Francisco,California 94111.

2. **THE AMERICAN FUNERAL.** 28 min. Audiocassette.
Discussion of whether funeral practices serve a useful
purpose,why people often pay more than they can afford,&
why it should need more funeral directors to bury
proportionately less people today than in 1900.A mortician,
a sociologist,& a minister participate.
Sale- $ 12.95. Center for Cassette Studies.

3. **COPING WITH DEATH & DYING.** 5 x 30 min.
A review by Elizabeth Kubler-Ross of her experiences in
terminal care;including the 5 stages,the "three languages"
used by the terminally ill in conveying their awareness of
finiteness.One deals with children,& thefinal tape contains
a discussion between Dr Ross & an Emergency Room nurse on
sudden unexpected death.
Sale-$ 38 USA,$ 40 Canada,U.S.Currency.
Ross Medical Associates,1825 Sylvan Court,Flossmoor,
Illinois 60422. (312) 798-2559.

4. **DEATH & DYING.** Kubler-Ross presents her views on
death,denial & the 5 stages.
Sale-$ 9.95. Trainex Audio Anthology.

5. **DEATH & DYING.** 2 Audiocassettes.
American Health Congress programs discussing personal,
ethical & policy issues concerning treatment of the dying,
problems of prolonging life (or death),rights of dying
patients, and the role of hope.
Sale- $ 20. Teach 'Em Inc.

6. **DEATH AND LIFE.** 60 min. Audiotape or cassette.
Interviews with individuals about their thoughts about
death & life.
Sale,only for non-broadcast use: Canadian Broadcasting
Corporation (CBC) Learning Systems,Box 500,Station A,
Toronto,Ontario,Canada. $ 15.95. Also Center for Cassette
Studies.

7.   DEATH,GRIEF & BEREAVEMENT.   Audiocassettes developed
by the Center for Death Education & Research,University of
Minnesota,consisting of interviews,lectures & discussions.
Accompanying literature for each tape includes biographical
sketch of the speakers,synposis,questions & bibliography.
DGB-1.Dialogue on Death.59 mins.Robert Fulton,R.Slater,etc.
DGB-2.Stages of Dying. 32 min. Dr Elizabeth Kubler-Ross.
DGB-3. Death & the Family,from the Caring Professions Point
    of View. 30 min.
DGB-4.Social Reconstruction After Death. 21 min.
DGB-5.The Meaning of Death in American Society.29 min.
    Dr Herman Feifel.
DGB-6.Today's Funeral Director. 25 min.
DGB-7. A Psychosocial Aspect of Terminal Care:Anticipatory
    Grief. Dr Robert Fulton. 32 min.
DGB-8.Death & the Self. 28 min.
DGB-9.Facing Death with the Patient:An On-going Contract.
    31 min.
DGB-10.Religious Faith & Death:Implications in work with
    the Dying Patient & Family.32 min.Carl Nighswonger.
DGB-11.The Role of the School in Death Education. 27 min.
    Dr Daniel Leviton.
DGB-12.Bereavement & the Process of Mourning.54 min.Irion.
DGB-13.The Widow in America:A Study of the Older Woman.
    42 min. Dr Helena Lopata.
DGB-14.Talking to Children about Death. 57 min.
DGB-15.Crib Death:Sudden Infant Death Syndrome.A
    Documentary. 59 min.
DGB-16.Death & the Child. 45 min. Dr Edgar Jackson.
DGB-17.Conversation with a Dying Friend. 50 min.
DGB-18.Adolescent Suicide-A Documentary.Norman Farberow.
    54 min,
DGB-19.Conversation with Lynn Caine,Widow. 28 min.
DGB-20. The Widow-to-Widow Program.35 min.Silverman.
DGB-21.Help & Self-Help. 49 min.
DGB-22. Journey to St Christopher's:A Hospice for the
    Dying. 29 min.
DGB-23. Dr Cicely Saunders..A Medical Pioneer. 40 min.
DGB-24.St Christopher's Hospice:A Living Experience.39 min.
Cassettes-$ 15 each.Complete series-$ 360. A 12-cassette
storage-binder included with orders of 6 or more tapes,two
with orders of 13 or more. Otherwise $ 7.00 each.
Packages- Issues in Clinical Care for Psychiatrists,
    Psychologists & Counsellors:Numbers:2,7,9,10,16,20,21,
    23,24. $ 135.

Pastoral Counselling- 2,3,10,20,21,22. - $ 90.
Death & the Child- 3,11,14,15,16,& 18. -$ 90.
The Widow- 12,13,19,20,21. -$ 75.
The Role of the Funeral Director- 1,6,12. & 45.
The Dying Experience- 2,5,10,17,23,24. -$ 90.
Psychosocial Aspects of Death- 1,4,5,7,8,12. -$90.
Dying with Dignity- 6,17,22,23,24. -$ 75.
The Charles Press Publishers,Inc., & Center for Death
Education, University of Minnesota.

8.   DEATH:ITS PSYCHOLOGY.60 min. Audiotape or cassette.
A terminally ill woman talks with her husband about her
feelings & acceptance of her fate.Overemphasis on the KR5.
Center for Cassette Studies-$ 16.95. Also CBC,Toronto.

9.   DEATH,THE ENEMY.
Interview with Ed Shneidman,on death,dying & suicide.The
usual wet interviewer seemingly inevitable with
Psychology Today tapes;Shneidman on his usual good form.
$ 6.95.
Psychology Today Reader Service,1 Park Avenue,New York,
NY 10016. Also Landsford Publ.Co., $ 12.95.

10.   DO PERSONS HAVE THE MORAL RIGHT TO COMMIT SUICIDE?
      60 min. A psychiatric nurse practitioner discusses
the moral issues of suicide. Sale-$ 9.95. PSF Prod.Corp.

11.   DRAMA OF DEATH: COUNSELING THE DYING & THEIR FAMILIES.
      2 Audiocassettes or 1 LP record.
Suggestions on how to help the dying patient & family,in a
hard-cover case with study guides.
Sale-$ 12.95, Creative Resources,Box 1970,Waco,Texas.

12.   EVERYDAY HEROICS OF LIVING & DYING.Cassette.
Interview with Ernest Becker,on fear of death,creativity,&
his own approaching death.Not particularly interesting,though
it has been consistently over-valued by some critics.
$ 6.95,/$ 12.95. Psychology Today Reader Service,1 Park Ave.,
New York, NY 10016 ; or Landsford Publ.

13.   INTERVIEWING & CRISIS INTERVENTION TECHNIQUES.Produced
by Allen J. Enelow.6 Audiocassettes about interview and
intervention techniques,suitable for various professionals
& paraprofessionals or volunteers. Simulated dialogues.
Includes:-MaryJo,17:19 min.Example of low suicide intention;
Jack Dugan,18 min. High suicide intentionality. Package of
6 audiotapes + 30 response sheets (5 per tape) $ 60.
Instructor's guide. Charles Press Publishers,Inc.

14.   JUST A LITTLE TIME.   Audiocassette + study guide.
A nursing conference to develop a plan of care for a
terminal patient.Related to the AJN film of the same title.
American Journal of Nursing,Ed.Services Division.

15.   LIFE AFTER LIFE. Audiocassette.
Raymond Moody discusses his interminable views on terminal
experiences. Is there audiotape after death? Nothing new
nothing special.   Sale-$ 9.50. Human Development Associa :es,
Inc., 1660 Union National Plaze,Little Rock,Arkansas 72201.

16.   LIFE CYCLE: THE DEATH. 30 min. Audiotape.
Dr Vivian Rakoff,not much known as an expert on the subject,
discusses various aspects of attitudes towards death at
different ages & philosophies.Not recommended.
Sale,for non-broadcast use only:$ 7. CBC,Toronto.

17.   MERCY KILLING. 30 min. Audiotape.
Panel discussion,on technical & moral aspects of euthanasia,
Sale,non-broadcast use only:$ 7. CBC,Toronto.

18.   MINISTERING TO THE TERMINALLY ILL.1975. J.Bayly,G.L.
Addington,Bal Mount,& M.O.Vincent. David C Cooke Publ.Co.
3 Audiocassettes. Taped seminars,discussing orthodox modern
views of death & bereavement--the death-denying society,the
five stages,grief & suffering,& the death of children,
stressing especially the Christian approach to these
problems.Booklet with summaries & questions for study.

19.   ON DEATH,GRIEF & BEREAVEMENT. 17 tapes,as listed
above,$ 15 each,: Center for Death Education & Research,
1167 Social Science Building,University of Minnesota,
Minneapolis,Minnesota 55455.

20.   THE RIGHT TO LIFE. 27 min. Cassette.
Discussion of euthanasia & abortion from a religious point
of view. $ 6.95. Thomas More Associates,180 North Wabash,
Chicago,Illinois 60601.

21.   UNTIL I DIE. 30 min. Cassette.
Audio version of the Kubler-Ross film reviewed above.
Sale-$ 9.50.American Journal of Nursing,Ed.Services Divn.

22.   WHAT IS DEATH? 30 min. Dr John Theobald discusses
death.Very religiously oriented.
Sale-$ 14.95. Center for Cassette Studies.

23. <u>WRITING A WILL</u>. Part I- 25 min, Part II-27 min.
Experts discuss timing & need for a will,& ways to plan a
valid,legal will.
Sale-$ 12.95 each part. Center for Cassette Studies.

24. <u>YOU HAVE SIX MONTHS TO LIVE</u>.   26 min.
What happens to people who have a short time to live,what
new dimensions to life they may gain.
Sale- $ 12.95. Center for Cassette Studies.

————oOo————

Record: <u>PEACE BIRD</u>.   Deanna Edwards.
A professional singer & volunteer music therapist with the
terminally ill & elderly.Simple & affectionate songs,
including: Peace bird,Teach me to die(And I'll teach you to
live);Catch a Little Sunshine;Folks Don't Kiss Old People
Any More;and the Right to Live. Unpretentious but
professional. A little saccharine for some tastes.
Telekinetics,1229 South Santee St.,Los Angeles,
California 90015. Compatable Stereo. Cat.No. 9151. $ 5.95.

————oOo————

B.   <u>VIDEOTAPES AND VIDEOCASSETTES</u>

1.   <u>ATTEMPTED SUICIDE:WHAT CONSTITUTES APPROPRIATE MEDICAL
     CARE ?</u>   B&W. 3/4" Videocassette. 60 min.
Panel discussion on the basis of a case history,by an
interdisciplinary group--philosophy,psychiatry,medicine
& emergency room staff.
Sale:$68. Dr Bernard Towers,Dept.of Pediatrics,School of
     Medicine,UCLA,Los Angeles, California 90024.

2.   <u>CHILDREN'S CONCEPTIONS OF DEATH</u>. 28 min. Color.
3/4 " VC (U-Matic) Review of the developmental acquisition
of concepts of death,emphasizing 3 general stages.Outdated.
Loan,Sale-$ 150. Univ.of Wisconsin,Milwaukee,Sch.of Nursing.

3.   <u>CONFRONTING DEATH</u>. 58 min. VC.
Interviews several authorities,including Kubler-Ross,on
personal & social aspects of death.Very heavy religious
emphasis. rental: $ 9.95.
Thomas More Associates,180 North Wabash,Chicago,Ill.60601.

4.   CONSCIOUS DYING. 30 min.
Interview with Ram Dass on his ideas about working with
the dying. I'm not sure why.
Rental: $ 35 for 5 days,Sale:$150.
Interface,63 Chapel St.,Newton,Mass.02158.

5.   CRIB DEATH--OR SUDDEN INFANT DEATH SYNDROME.
3/4 " VC U-matic. B&W   47 min.
A physician,Dr Barbara Brunner,talks about SIDS.
Rental-$30,Sale:$95.   Georgia Regional Medical TV Network,
A.W.Calhoun Medical Library,Emory University.

6.   DEALING WITH THE TERMINALLY ILL PATIENT.16 min.B&W.3/4".
Only available to NCME subscribers.Kubler-Ross discusses her
5 stages & other experiences. Network for Continuing
Medical Education.

7.   DEATH & DYING. Four 3/4" VC(Also 8mm or 16mm film).
Death & the Doctor (28 min),The Dying Patient(19 min),
The Family (15 min).Public education program-Living with
Dying (18 min). 3 for professionals-& 750,1 public-$350.
Professional Research,Inc.

8.   DEATH OF A SIBLING. 19 min. Color.
2 doctors discuss the attendant problems.But too remote;
better to have spent the time talking to the siblings.
Rental,subscribers only, NCME,15 Columbus Circle,NY 10023.

9.   AN EQUAL KNOCK ON EVERY DOOR. 30 min. color.
Program on arranging details of the funeral,& coping with
grief.Practical & theoretical aspects covered.
WKYC-TV,Public Affairs Dept.

10.   GUIDELINE FOR CONSENT:The Uniform Anatomical Gift Act.
Videocassette,3/4".B&W,15 min.
Discussion of medico-legal aspects of transplantation.
NCME Subscribers only.

11.   IMPLICATIONS OF NURSING THE DYING PATIENT.55 min.Color.
Discussion of the nurses role in terminal care.
Rental:Milwaukee Regional Medical Instructional TV System,
Inc.,500 West National Ave.,Milwaukee,Wis.53193.

12.   I WANT TO DIE. 19 min. Color.
Guidelines for evaluating & managing suicidal & depressed
patients,discussed by psychiatrists.
NCME Subscribers only.

13. <u>IRREVERSIBLE COMA</u>. B&W. 16 min.
Discussion of the definition of death.
NCME Subscribers only.

14. <u>LEARNING TO LIVE WITH DYING</u>. Color. 39 min.
Medical students,doctors & a minister discuss the
management of terminally ill patients & their families.
Rental-$25. NCME Subscribers only.

15. <u>LEAVES FROM A DIARY.</u> 21 min.
Thoughts & experiences of a new cancer patient.Script by a
Registered Nurse who has recently discovered she has cancer,
& considers her anguish on realizing her disease is probably
fatal. In matter-of-fact but affecting prose,she describes
in diary form her experiences in hospital.
CCTV by Swedish County Councils (in Swedish).
Landstingsförbundet(Federation of Swedish County Councils),
ITV-Gruppen,Box 6606,111 34 STOCKHOLM,Sweden.Tel:08/236560.

16. <u>LEUKEMIA IN ADULTS 2.</u> 12 min.
Reviews different leukemia types,treatments & complications.
Emphasizes the patient's need for information,exemplified
in scenes between patient & staff. (in Swedish).
Landstingsförbundet,Stockholm.

17. <u>THE LINGERING HEART</u>. 30 min. Color.
Foster Shaw,a young husband & father,dying of leukemia,
helps other terminal patients.
WKNC-TV Public Affairs Dept.

18. <u>MANAGEMENT OF THE TERMINALLY ILL: THE FAMILY.</u>16min.B&W.
Elizabeth Kubler-Ross.
NCME Subscribers only.

19. <u>THE MARK WATERS STORY</u>. 26 min. Color. 1969. 3/4" VC.
Acted & directed by Richard Boone,the story of a man dying
of lung cancer,who writes his own obituary.
Rental/Sale: Public Television Library,475 L'Enfant Plaza
West,SW, Washington DC 20024.

20. <u>MUST WE REDEFINE DEATH?</u> B&W 60 min. 3/4 " VC.
Long & not especially interesting panel discussion.
Sale: $ 68. Dr Bernard Towers,School of Medicine,UCLA.

21. THE PATIENT'S RIGHT TO DIE. 60 min. B&W. VT or VC.
Lecture,in Christian Theological terms,on moral-ethical
dilemmas,on preservation of life,active & passive euthanasia.
Available in several video formats,without charge,on
borrower's own raw stock tape. Walter Reed Army Medical
Center, Videotape Library.

22. PICKING UP THE PIECES: ONE WIDOW SPEAKS. 29 min. Color.
Interview with Lynn Caine,author & professional widow.
Reviews her book. (WHED TV) Rental- $68.
Public Television Library,Washington.

23. PLEASE LET ME DIE. Color. 30 min. VT or VC.
Interview with a 27 year-old man who was blinded & severely
maimed in an explosion & fire 10 months earlier.Alert,
intelligent,articulate,he argues a compelling case for being
allowed to die.Life-sustaining treatments are extremely
painful.Hard to watch,& its distribution is restricted to
professional audiences in medicine,law,psychology,sociology,
or similar fields.Extreme impact,leading to inevitable
debate on the right to refuse treatment,& the value of life.
Rental-$ 25 (applicable to sale price). Sale-$ 100.
Library of Clinical Psychiatric Syndromes;Dr.Robert B.White,
Department of Psychiatry,University of Texas Medical Branch,
Galveston,Texas 77550.

24. THE ROTHE TAPE. 30 min. Color. 3/4" VC.
Discussion of death with Marcus Rothe,22 year-old college
student,who talks of his hopes & hopelessness.He has already
survived surgery for a leg tumour,lung tumour,& amputation
of one leg.He is preparing for exams——& dies the following
month.Valuable discussion of the dimensions of meaning and
purpose in life.
Rental- $ 10. Dept.of Pastoral Care,Shands Teaching Hospital.

25. SINCE THE AMERICAN WAY OF DEATH. 59 min. Color. VC.
Fast paced documentary investigating the funeral industry;
training of funeral directors,funerals in Chicago's black
ghetto,a Jewish group looking for simple funerals;the high
cost of cremations in some areas. CWTTW-TV.
Rental-$ 95. Public Television Library,Video Program Service.

26. STOPPING TREATMENT WITH OR WITHOUT CONSENT.62 min.B&W.
Dr Joseph Fletcher,minister,discusses 8 levels of initiative
on ethics of euthanasia.30 min lecture then medical discussion.
Rental:$30. Georgia Regional Medical TV Network,Emory Univ.

27. <u>SUICIDE— PRACTICAL DIAGNOSTIC CLUES.</u> 13 min.B&W.
Identifying the potential suicide.
NCME Subscribers only.

28. <u>TEACHING DEATH: AS A PROCESS OF AWARENESS & COPING.</u>
B&W. 3 lesson series discussing techniques of teaching others
how to care for the dying. Rental/long-term lease-$20 each.
Nebraska TV Council for Nursing Education,1800 N.33rd,
Lincoln,Nebraska 68503.

29. <u>TERMINAL ILLNESS.</u> (Leinbach-Eisdorfer Series). 6 VC,B&W.
Interviews with 39 year-old Gary Leinbach,Prof.of Medicine
at the University of Washington who was a terminal patient,
discussing his illness & his reactions to it. Interviews
with the patient (25 min),role of the physician (41 min),
Pain management (37 min),Religion & the Clergy (35 min),
the Grieving Process Part I (25 min) Part II (45 min).
Rental- $ 25 each or $150 for the series.
University of Washington Press,AV Division.

30. <u>THE THREAT OF SUICIDE.</u> 27 min. Color. 3/4" VC.
Assessing suicide risk & managing the patient. NCME.

31. <u>TO THINK OF DYING.</u> 58 min. 3/4" VC
Conversations about death between Orville Kelly (Make
Today Count) and Lynn (Widow) Caine. (KTCA-TV.
Rental- $ 95. Public Television Library,Video Program Service.

32. <u>WHO SPEAKS FOR THE BABY?</u> 20 min. Color. 3/4" VC.
A mongoloid baby needs life-saving surgery for heart & gut
problems,but the parents don't wish to consent to surgery.
Pediatrician seeks court order to operate.Is this his duty?
Should the child live or die? Discussion. NCME.

33. <u>WORKING WITH DEATH SERIES.</u> 4 units in color.VC or
Super 8mm or 16mm film. See under film reviews.
Rental or purchase: $75) Super 8, $ 800 16 mm.
Professional Research Associates,Los Angeles,California.

————oOo————

27. SUICIDE — PRACTICAL DIAGNOSTIC CLUES, 13 min. b&w.
    Identifying the potential suicide.
    NCME Subscribers only.

28. TEACHING DEATH... A PROCESS OF AWARENESS & COPING.
    b&w. 3 lesson series discussing techniques of teaching others
    how to care for the dying. Rental/Purchase. Each lesson $20 each.
    Nebraska... Central for Nursing Education. 200 N. 33rd.
    Lincoln, Nebraska 68503.

29. TERMINAL ILLNESS (Leinbach-Eisdorfer Series), 6 VC,b&w
    Interviews with 33 year-old Gary Leinbach, Prof. of Medicine
    at the University of Washington who was a terminal patient,
    discussing his illness & his reactions to it. Interviews
    with the patient (76 min) role of the physician (41 min),
    Pain management (37 min) Religion & the Clergy (33 min),
    the Grieving Process Part I (25 min) Part II (45 min).
    Rental $5 P. each or $110 for the series.
    University of Washington Press, AV Division.

30. THE THREAT OF SUICIDE, 27 min. Color, b&w. VC
    Assertive suicide... & managing the patient. NCME.

31. THE DILEMMA OF DYING, 58 min. 3/4". VC
    Four patients about death between D-vitterkally (Make
    Today Count) and Kevin (J-down) Corner. (KTCA-TV.
    Rental $49. Public Television Library Video-Program Service

32. CHILD OPERATION - OR THE BABY? 20 min. Color 3/4" VC
    A unmarried baby needs life-saving surgery for several gut
    problems, but the parents don't wish to consent to surgery.
    Pediatrician seeks court order to operate. Is this his duty?
    Should the child live or die? Discussion. NCME.

33. WORKING WITH DEATH SERIES: 4 units in color VC or
    Super 8mm or 16mm film. See under film reviews
    Rental or purchase: VC/Super 8, $ 800 16 mm.
    Professional Research Associates,Los Angeles,California.

———000———

TEACHING MATERIALS,KITS,etc.

1.   CANCER: FOCUSSING ON FEELINGS. Series S-105. Filmstrips (FS) + cassettes or records (AC or LP). + Instructors Manual, with presentation guidelines,questions,objectives,script narrations,topics for discussion,study questions & bibliographies. + Selected Readings (a selection of articles) i.Viewpoint:the Nurse. a.a nurse who takes her feelings home,b.a nurse working with a patient whose spouse refuses to tell him about his terminal illness,c.a nurse who becomes totally emotionally involved with a terminal patient. 19 min. ii. Viewpoint: The Nurse. a. A student nurse with negative reactions to a cancer patient;b.dealing with a patient who longers on;c.caring for a teenager with leukemia.16 min. iii. Viewpoint:the Patient. a-young boy with leukemia,vaguely aware of what is happening,b-an older woman prepares for death;c-a laryngectomy patient's feelings about surgery & rehabilitation. 22 min. iv. Viewpoint:the Patient. a-a salesman who learns he has cancer of the larynx;b-a patient facing amputation;c-adjusting after radical face & neck surgery. 27 min. Complete set (AC or LP) $ 285. Individual programs-$70. Additional Instructors manual-$4,Readings-$5. Concept Media.

2.   CARE FOR THE DYING & BEREAVED: HOW CAN WE HELP? 3 filmstrips,+ AC or LP. Part I-Walk in the World for Me;intended to help health care professionals explore the impact of terminal illness on patients & families; Part II:The Critically Ill Patient & Grief,deals with Grief,mourning & recovery. Sale- $ 79.50.   Guidance Associates.

3.   CARE OF THE DYING PATIENT. Filmstrip + AC or LP) Discusses the physical,emotional & spiritual needs of the dying patient as well as what to do after death,in preparing the body,etc. Sale-$70 with LP,$75 with AC.Trainex Corp.

4.   CARE OF THE DYING PATIENT. 2 Filmstrips + LP or AC. Deals with the nurse-patient relationship,signs of impending death,& after-care. Sale- $ 48. Training Aide Educational Systems.

5.   CARE OF THE TERMINALLY ILL. Filmstrip + LP or AC. Case study of a terminally ill patient,rigidly stressing the 5 stages.Considers the reactions of patient,family & staff. Sale-$55 with AC,$30 with LP.Career Aids,Inc.

6.   CHANG-CHING DIES A HEROIC DEATH.   From "The Red
Detachment of Women",a modern Revolutionary ballet.
Book with script,photographs,& recording,available from:
Guozi Shudian,China Publications Centre,P.O.Box 399,Peking.

7.   CHILDREN IN CRISIS: DEATH. 5 filmstrips + 3 AC or 1 LP.
Script by Richard Obershaw. Death as a reality of life,
expressing grief,ages of understanding,explaining death to
children,& the importance of funerals.5 audio script
booklets,& discussion guide. Real people are shown,not
animals or cartoons,interracial cast,clear & with repetition.
Broad but shallow.List of resources not good.Preview.
Sale:$ 58 with AC,$ 53 with LP. Parents Magazine Films.
Dept.F, 53 Vanderbilt Ave.,New York,NY 10017.

8.   COPING WITH FATAL ILLNESS. Filmstrip or slides.
Illustrations of the needs & feelings of terminal patients,
& how we can communicate with them.
Sale-- $ 28 as FS, $ 33 as SL. Educational Perspectives Ass.

9.   CROSS-CULTURAL ASPECTS OF DEATH. FS or SL + AC.
How different societies deal with dying & death as reflected
in their rites & ceremonies.Looks at similarities   and
differences. Sale-- $ 28 as FS, $ 33 as SL.
Educational Perspectives Associates.

10.   DEATH AS A MORAL & ETHICAL ISSUE. FS or SL + AC.
Suicide & euthanasia,understanding & coping with them;
relatively objective & open-ended.
Sale- $ 28 as FS,$33 as SL. Educational Perspectives Assoc.

11.   DEATH AS A PRACTICAL MATTER. FS or SL + AC.
Economic effects on the survivors,after a death.Insurance,
wills,legal matters,funerals.Practical consumer interests.
Sale-$28 as FS,$33 as SL. Educational Perspectives Assoc.

12.   DEATH & DYING: CLOSING THE CIRCLE. 1976.5 FS+AC or LP.
The Meaning of Death:Attitudes & modern technology,
immortality & confronting our emotions.
A Time to Mourn:A Time to Choose:-rites & rituals of death,
their origins & purposes,the needs they meet.
Walk in the World for Me-Doris Lund,author or Eric,discusses
her son's struggle with leukemia.
Dealing with the Critically Ill Patient,& Dealing with Loss

12 ctd.) & Grief. Robert Jay Lifton,Consultant.
$ 99.50 for the set. Guidance Associates,757 Third Avenue,
New York, NY 10017.

13. DEATH & THE CREATIVE IMAGINATION. FS or SL + AC.
Views of death from artists,poets,authors & musicians.
Not terribly creative or imaginative.
Sale-$28 as FS,$33 as SL,Educational Perspectives Assoc.

14. DEATH: A PART OF LIFE.George G.Otero.Teaching Unit.
Useful unit,including activities,exercises,role-play
situations,suggestions for using resources.Death rites &
customs,in cross-cultural perspective,too.
Center for Teaching International Relations,Graduate School
of International Studies,University of Denver, Denver,
Colorado 80210. $ 4.

15. DEATH,GRIEF & MOURNING. FS or SL + AC.
Grief,funerals,healthy & unhealthy mourning.
Sale-$ 28 as FS,$ 22 as SL. Educational Perspectives Assoc.

16. DEATH: THE LAST TABOO. Unit on Thanatology.
E.Rudolph. TIME Education Program,Rockefeller Center, New
York, NY 10020.   Not bad.A historical survey of death
through the ages & different religions,with some teaching
suggestions,questions & activities.(An unfortunate example
is illustrated of the cheap & nasty classroom gimmick of
getting a student to lie in a coffin:the sign of a desperate
teacher).Inserts are spirit-master (printing,not other-world!)
pages for duplication,of a questionnaire on attitudes to
death,the Living Will,two TIME Essays,fragments of student
poetry on death,a section of Tolstoy's Ivan Illych,& a
bibliography (some old & unobtainable references,& the weak
book by Hendin).

17. DEVELOPMENTAL CONCEPT OF DEATH. FS or SL + AC.
Discusses the evolution of concepts of death from early
childhood on,& the influences on such concepts.
Sale-$28 as FS,$33 as SL. Educational Perspectives Ass.

18. EARLY AMERICAN CEMETARIES. FS + AC.
Illustrations of old graveyards,including a free copy of
the book "The Last Word",reviewed above.
Sale-$22. Educational Perspectives Associates.

19. THE FUNERAL IN AMERICAN CULTURE. FS or SL + AC.
Traces the historical roots of funeral practices from
Colonial times,then considers modern practices & funeral
directors.Also considers alternative practices.
Sale-$28 as FS,$33 as SL. Educational Perspectives Assoc.

20. GRAMP: A MAN AGES & DIES. FS + AC or LP.
Based on the great book,reviewed above.
Sale-$ 25,Human Relations Media Center;also Sunburst
Communications.

21. THE INDIVIDUAL,SOCIETY & DEATH.(Student Anthology).
193 pp. PB. $ 2.50. Highly elementary choice of material,
often amateurishly written.Heavy emphasis on funerals,from
the National Funeral Director's Association point of view.
Not a shred of critical thinking mars the unnatural
tranquillity of the material.

22. LIFE & DEATH STUDIES: A Starter Set. Bantam Books,NY.
$ 25. Teacher's Guide:Death Out of the Closet,Stanford &
Perry,reviewed above. 1 copy each of-Plath's Bell Jar,
Blinn's Brian's Song,Voltaire's Candide,Agee's Death in
the Family,Levit's Ellen,Rubin's Emergency Room Diary,
Wolitzer's Ending,Thmas' Biology Watcher,Lifton & Olson ,
Lord's Night to Remember,Solzhenitsyn's Ivan Denisovitch,
Crane's Red Badge of Courage,Leck's Reincarnation, and
Caine's Widow.

23. LIFE & DEATH STUDIES: A CURRICULUM PROGRAM.
Bantam Books, New York. $ 61.00
Teacher's guide-see above.6 copies of Agee & Levit,3
copies of Plath,Blinn,Rubin,Wolitzer,Lewis' Grief Observed,
Lifton & Olson,Crane & Caine.

24. LITERATURE OF THE SUPERNATURAL:WORLDS BEYOND REASON.
160 SL in 2 carousels,+ 2 AC or 2 LP,Teacher's Guide.
Considers works of literature dealing with supernatural
beings,satanic figures,gods & angels.
$ 109.50. The Center for the Humanities,2 Holland Avenue,
White Plains, NY 10603.

25. LIVING WITH DYING. Bantam Books,New York. A series of
11 x 14" photographs of aspects of death for use in teaching.
Set of 24 pictures: $ 20.

26. LIVING WITH DYING. 2 FS + LP or AC.
Concepts of death,attempts to deny it,individual experiences,
& the inevitable 5 stages. Naive.
Sale-$50 per set. Sunburst Communications,Pound Ridge,
NY 10576; Also Human Relations Media Center.

27. LOSS & GRIEF. S-121. FS + LP or AC,Instructor's Manual.
a-loss:Discussion of components of loss,positive & negative.
25 min. b-The Grief Process-emotional,physiological and
behavioral components,& maladaptive grief states- 29 min.
c- When Someone is Grieving-how to break bad news,how to
recognize grief,how to respond. 33 min. Dramatized
episodes:— d. The Child Who Left Us:Amy.Anticipatory grief
in a father whose 5 year-old daughter is dying of leukemia,
contrasted with the mother's response. Portrait of Peter:
Family with a 4 year-old boy with Down's syndrome,loss of
the idealized child through birth of the defective child.
26 min. e-A Sense of Place:John & Gwen.Loss of community
on moving home,New England to California;The Child Who Was
Let Go:Carol."Anniversary reaction" of mother who gave child
for adoption 15 years earlier;The Empty Nest:Ruth-a woman
who was family nurturer faces loss of her now obsolete role.
- 29 min. f. A Marriage Ending:Frank & Jenny. The multiple
losses experienced by a couple before,during & after
separation & divorce;effects on children,family & friends,
20 min.; g-My Son's in Trouble:James.Maturational and
situational loss,a delinquent teenage boy is in prison,the
effects on him & his mother; If I Take Care of Myself:
Harvey. Recurring cycles of loss & grief of a man with
multiple sclerosis,its effects on him & his family: 29 min.
Sale: Complete set (AC or LP) $ 455. Individual programs:
$ 70. Additional Instructor's Manual-$ 7.
Concept Media.

28. MAN'S ATTITUDES TOWARD DEATH. FS or SL + AC.
Contemporary attitudes to death,in historical and
psychological perspective. Sale-$ 26 as FS, $ 33 as SL.
Educational Perspectives Associates.

29. PERSPECTIVES ON DEATH. Multimedia kits. David Berg &
George G.Dougherty. 1972. (P.O.Box 213,De Kalb,Illinois
60115). 30 student anthologies,30 student activity books,
a teacher's resource book,2 sound FS + AC,& 2 other AC.
$ 150.AV package alone-$ 55.

29 ctd.)   Student Anthology reviewed above,as The
Individual,Society & Death.
Student Activity Book. $ 1.50 PB. 54 pp. Very elementary &
simple.Brief Death Attitude/Information Inventory,room for
notes on guest speakers & on the tape presentations,some
very trite quotations,pro-Funeral Director bias.
A"Funeral Home Data Sheet"to record "data" gained from
visiting the Director.Lists the equipment needed for
embalming,preparation for viewing & disposal.A "Cemetary
Data Collection Record"to record epitaphs,the oldest &
youngest dead you can find,the most recent grave,& a survey
of ages at death,and "list the ecological benefits of the
cemetary"; a vocabulary of death ("patricide,insecticide...
...inurnment");a Deathword Puzzle! (20 across.Too great a
dosage,may cause death (abbr.);39 across.May the Lord Have
      on Your Soul; 43 across.American Medical Association
(abbr.); 5 down.Place where bodies are buried.). Likely to
be of very little use except to those trying to duplicate
the authors' course;most teachers should be able to be less
macabre & more personally useful.
Teacher's Resource Book. PB.69 pp. $ 2.00. Some guidance on
how to run the authors' course,including How to Contact
Guest Speakers (with suggested invitations & questions).A
very simple,barely adequate Daily Lesson Guide for the 30
day course,answers to the deadly Deathword Puzzle,& a final
examination with some very trivial questions.Maybe the most
widely marketed course,but not a particularly good one.
None of the material would be useable above a grade-school
(primary-school) level,if that.

30. PERSPECTIVES ON DEATH. 2 FS + LP or AC. Part I.Towards
Acceptance-attitudes to death,religious beliefs,philosophy,
science & arts in this context. Part II-The Right to Die--
medical,legal & moral questions. Sale- $ 50.
Human Relations Media Center; Sunburst Communications.

31. PERSPECTIVES ON DYING. S-107. FS + AC or LP.
1.American Attitudes toward Death & Dying.Interaction with
the dying person;denial & cultural factors:urbanization,
advances in medical science,& secularization. 17 min.
2. Psychological Reactions of the Dying Person. The response
to a fatal illness;coping mechanisms of denial,regression,
and intellectualization. 30 min.
3.Hazards & Challenges in Providing Care.Unexpected death,
and prolonged dying needing symptom control. 28 min.

31. ctd.) 4. Guidelines for Interacting with the Dying Person.How to meet basic psychological needs:personal dignity,security,some hope,self-expression;listening.22min. 5.Viewpoint:the Dying Patient. 31 min. 6. Viewpoint:The Nurse. 26 min. Personal discussion with patients and nurses,open-ended format.
Plus: Instructor's Manual & Role-Playing Cards,+ Personal Questionnaire (pack of 20),provocative questions to arouse personal awareness,+ Supplementary text:Confrontations of Death (see separate review). Sale: Complete set(AC or LP) -$ 398.Individual programs-$ 70. Extra Manual & Cards-$ 6; Extra Confrontations-$ 8.Extra Questionnaires (5 packs of 20 each)-$7.   Concept Media.

32. THE POETRY OF DEATH.FS + AC.
None contemporary.Reflects death in poetry of writers like: Poe,Masters,Shakespeare,Whitman,Rosetti,Tennyson,Arnold, Donne,Stevenson,Herrick,Landor & Bryant. Dull readings, badly and stagily read;some guitar accompaniment. Unimaginative,Flat,elocution-style emotionless readings. 2 cassette versions,one with an audible & intrusive tone to warn you to change the pictures,one with an inaudible advance tone.Filmstrips have some good,evocative color pictures. 60 on each.
Spectrum Educational Media,308 Linden Lane,Mattoon,Illinois 61938, or 105 Beverly,Morton,Illinois 61550.

33. REDESIGNING MAN: SCIENCE & HUMAN VALUES. 6 FS+AC or LP.
Recent advances in biomedical sciences & future projections. 2 relevant to death: Part III,Transplants & Implants,& Part VI,Search for Immortality: Cryonics,& whether death is needed to give meaning to life.
Sales: $ 135 for the series. Harper & Row Media, also Human Relations Media Center.

34. RELIGIOUS VIEWPOINTS ON DEATH. FS or SL + AC.
Jewish,Protestant, & Catholic views on dying,death & the afterlife,post-death rites & ceremonies.
Sale: $ 28 as FS, $33 as SL. Educational Perspectives Assoc.

35. THE RIGHT TO DIE. FS + AC.
Moral,legal & practical implications of extending life by technology,with cases & discussion-guide.
Sale- $ 24. Career Aids,Inc.

36.   SANDCASTLE. FS + AC or LP. 1971.
On death in the family;intended for children ages 10-12,
discussion between a father & his 2 children after the
death of the mother.
Image Publications,Miles-Samuelson Inc.,15 E.26th St.,
New York,NY 10010.

37.SCIENCE & SOCIETY: BIOMEDICAL ENGINEERING. 2 FS+LP or AC.
Life-support machines,transplants,genetic surgery;social
effects of intervention,definitions of death & making
choices. Sale- $44 as LP,$ 50 as AC. Schloat Productions.

38.   SUICIDES: CAUSES & PREVENTION. 2 FS + AC or LP.
I.Causes:psychological,philosophical,sociological theories;
     Durkheim,Freud & Menninger.
II.Prevention: typical warning signs,ways to handle the
suicidal person,misconceptions,& functions of a suicide
prevention center. Sale: $ 50. Human Relations Media Center.

39.   A TEACHING UNIT ON DEATH & DYING. For Senior H.S. & Jr.
College Students. 1975. Memorial Society of Edmonton,5326
Ada Boulevard,Edmonton,Alberta T5W 4N7. $ 4.50.

40.   THAT UNDISCOVERED COUNTRY.Wayne De Mouth & Robert
Hullihan. The Perfection Form Company,Logan,Iowa. 1975
66pp PB. An uninspiring collection of pieces for classroom
use,some rather ordinary essays,& a generally awful
collection of verse. I know it's far easier & cheaper to
stick to very old,out-of-copyright material,but much of it
is unusable.Among the weedy verse: The Cremation of Sam
McGhee,Browning's Prospice & Evelyn Hope,Henley's Invictus
("I am the master of my fate,I am the captain of my soul"
Ughh) William Cullen Bryant's awful Thanatopsis.They're
ghastly stuff to inflict on kids. Better are Emily
Dickinson's "Because I could not stop for death",The Bustle
in a House, & I Heard a Fly Buzz. Some questions & class
activities suggested. Not recommended.

41.   UNDERSTANDING DEATH. 5 FS + AC.
4 programs for children:Life & Death;Exploring the Cemetary;
Facts about Funerals; & A Taste of Blackberries.One program
for parents & teachers.
Sale- $ 81 for the series.Educational Perspectives Assoc.

42.   WITH HIS PLAY CLOTHES ON.47min.FS.Bill Goveia.AC.
Order of the Golden Rule Service Corp.,P.O.Box 3586,Spring-
-field,Ill.62708.The impact of bereavement,loss of child.

————oOo————

EUROPEAN LITERATURE

A. FRENCH

1. James Agee. Une Mort dans la Famille.Flammarion,1975.
2. Alvarez,A. Le Dieu Sauvage:Essai sur le Suicide.
   Mercure,1972.
3. Annales. Economies Societies Civilisation.(Armand Colin)
   Jan.-Fev.1976.(issue of quarterly journal) 237 pp.
Including Guidieri on Melanesian rituals,Schmitt on suicide
in the middle ages,Chaunu on dying in Paris (16th,17th &
18th centuries),Chartier on 'Arts de Mourir,1450-1600',
Roche on'La Memoire de la Mort,Ars Moriendi,& Vovelle on
methodological problems in estimating attitudes to death.
4. Anthony EJ & Koupernik C. L'Enfant Dans La Famille.
   Masson & Cie,Paris.1974 (120 Blvd.Saint Germain,VIe).
5. Aries,Phillippe. Essais sur l'histoire de la mort en
   Occident du Moyen Age à nos Jours. Seuil,Paris.1975.
6.Baechler,Jean. Les Suicides. Calman-Levy (3 rue Auber,
   Paris 9e. (A very thorough political study of suicide).
7. Baudrillard. L'echange Symbolique et la Mort. Essai de
   Sociologie. Editions Seuil,1975.
8. Barrière,I et Lalon,E. Le Dossier Confidentiel de
   l'Euthanasia. Coll.Points.,Seuil,Paris.1975.
9. de Beauvoir,S. Un mort très douce. Gallimard,1964.
10. Berger,Maurice et Francoise Hortala. Mourir à l'Hôpital:
    Infirmières d'aujourdhui. Le Centurion,219pp,1974.
11. Blanchot,Maurice.L'Arret de Mort.Gallimard,Paris,1948.
12. Brehaut,Jacques. Thanatos:Le malade el la médecin devant
    la mort. Editions Robert Laffont,6 Place Saint-Sulpice,
    75279 Paris. PB. 349 pp. 1976.
13. Castets,Bruno.La Loi,L'Enfant et la Mort. Essai de
    psychopathologie de l'enfant. Editions Fleurus,31 rue
    de Flaurus,Paris,6e. 1971. PB. 243 pp.
14. Castets,Bruno.La Mort de l'autre. Essai sur
    l'aggressivite de l'enfant at de l'adolescent.
    Bibliotheque de Psychologie Clinique.Eduart Privat,
    14 rue des Arts,Toulouse. 1974. 250pp.
15. Charlot,Monica. Vivre Avec la Mort. Editions Alain
    Moreau,3 bis quai aux fleurs,Paris 4.1976.320pp.PB.
16. Chauchard,Paul. Le Combat de la Vie et de la Mort.
    Editions Saint-Paul,6 rue Casette,7500 6 Paris.1976.173p.
17. Esprit:La Mort a Vivre.(Issue 3,Mar.1976).pp 409-644.
    This issue of the journal includes original articles
    and a short French Bibliography.

18. Fabre-Luce,Alfred.La Mort a Changé.Gallimard,1966.324pp.
19. Godin,A(ed).Mort et Presence.Etude de psychologie.
    Editions de Lumen Vitae,Bruxelles (186 rue Washington,
    1050 Bruxelles. 1974. 338 pp.
20. Heuse,Georges Guide de la Mort. Masson,Paris. 1975.
21. Jankélévitch,Vladimir. La Mort. Flammarion,26 rue
    Racine,Paris 6. 426 pp. 1966.
22, Jolivet,Régis. Le Problème de la Mort chez M.Heidegger
    et J-P Sartre. Abbaye Saint Wandrille:Editions de
    Fontenelle,1950.
23. Kubler-Ross,E. Les Derniers Instants de la Vie. Editions
    Labor et Fides,Geneve (140 Blvd St Germaine,Paris).
    280 pp. 1975.
24. Laplanche,Jean.Vie et Mort en Psychoanalyse.Flammarion,
    Paris. 1976.
25. Mehl,Roger. Le Vieillissement at la Mort. Presses
    Universitaires de France,Paris. 1962.
26. Menahem,Ruth. La Mort Apprivoisee. Editions
    Universitaires,16 rue Maget,75006 Paris,1973,170pp.PB.
27. Meynard,L. Le Suicide.Presses Universitaires de France,
    108 Blvd.St.Germain,Paris. 123pp. 1970.
28. Morin,Edgar. L'Homme et la Mort dans l'Histoire.
    Editions du Seuil,27 rue Jacob,Paris 6.352 pp. PB
    1970. (1st edition,Editions Correa,Paris,1951).
29. Moron,Pierre. Le Suicide. Presses Universitaires de
    France. 125 pp. 1975.
30. Portail,Jean. Savoir Mourir. Editions IOS,106 rue de
    Bas, Paris 7. 1974.
31.Quidu,Marguerite. Le Suicide. Etude Clinque/Perspectives
    Preventives.Les Editions Sociales Francaises,17 rue
    Viete,Paris 17.
32. Raimbault,Emile. La delivrance. Editions Mercure de
    France. 257 pp. PB. 1976.
33. Raimbault,G. L'Enfant et la Mort. Privat,Toulouse.1975.
34. Schur, Max. La Mort dans la vie de Freud. Gallimard.1975.
35. Serge-Leclaire. On tue en enfant.Un essai sur le
    narcissisme primaire et la pulsion de mort. Seuil,1975.
36. Sabatier,Robert. Dictionnaire de la Mort. Editions Albin
    Michel,22 rue Huyghens,Paris. 540 pp. 1967.
37. Sarda,Francois. Le Droit de Vivre et le Droit de Mourir.
    Editions Seuil. 225 pp. 1975.
38. Shestov,Leon. Les Révélations de la Mort. Dostoyevsky-
    -Tolstoy. 1923.
39. Spithakis,Roger.La Vérité et le Cancer.Ed.Resma.Paris,
    166pp. 1973.

40. Sporken,Paul. Le Droit de Mourir. Le nouveaux problemes de la vie. Desclee de Brouwer. 1974. 174 pp.
41. Thibault,Odette. Maitrise de la Mort. Jean-Pierre Delarge. Editions Universitaires. 1975.
42. Thomas,Louis-Vincent. Anthropologie de la Mort. Payot, 106 Blvd.St.Germain. 535 pp. 1975.
43. Toulat,Jean. Faut-Il Tuer par Amour? L'Euthanasie en Question. Editions Pygmalion,198 Blvd St.Germain. Paris. 250 pp. 1976.
44. Voivenel,Paul. Le Médecin devant la douleur et devant la mort. Librairie des Champs-Elysees,Paris.1934.
45. Vovelle,Gaby. Vison de la Mort et de l'au-dela' en Province d'après les autels des âmes du purgatoire, XVe-XXe siècles. A.Colin. 1970.
46. Vovelle,Gaby. Mourir autrefois:attitudes collectives devant la mort aux XVIIe et XVIIIe Siècles. Gallimard,Julliard,coll.Archives. 1974. 251 pp.
47. Vuillemin,Jules. Essai sur la Signification de la Mort. Presses Universitaires de France,Paris. 1948.
48. Ziegler,Jean. Les Vivants et la Mort. Essai de sociologie. Seuil,Paris. 1975.

B. SCANDINAVIAN

1. Åkesson,Elvor. Nür barnen frågar om Lidande och dod. Verbum,Stockholm. 1971 PB. 51 pp.
2. Alandh,Tom. Dödentalar man ju inte om.Sveriges Radios Forlag. 1975. 144pp PB.
3. Anderson,Poul. Levandedöd. Bokförlaget Tusch,Malmo. 1973. 77 pp. PB.
4. Anon. Tala om döden. Verbum,Stockholm. 1967. 159 pp.
5. Autton,Norman. Själavärd i dödens närhet. Verbum, Stockholm.1968. 141 pp. PB.
6. Becker,Ernest. Dödensproblem. Lindqvist,Stockholm. 1975. 357 pp. PB. (Denial of Death).
7. Blomquist,Clarence. Medicinsk Etik. Natur och Kultur, Stockholm.1971. 386 pp. (incl.abortion,euthanasia, and suicide).
8. Bjerg,Svend. Doden. Berlingske Forlag,Kobenhavn.1975. Competent review of meanings of death:natural, unnatural,social & political.
9. Ekner,Reidar. Efter Flera Tusen Rad. Författarförlaget. 1974. 71 pp. PB.
10. Elwing,Ann-Marie. Sjuksköterskan- med människa inför döden. Svensk Sjukskoterskeforenings förlag,Stockholm. 1972. 76pp. PB.

11. Fabricius,Johannes. Dødsoplevelsens Psykologi. Rhodos,
    Copenhagen. 1972. 125 pp. PB.
12. Fabricius,Johannes & Rene Ferney. For Egen Hånd—
    Selvmordet Gennem Tiderne. Rosenkilde og Bagger,
    Denmark. 1978. PB. pages unnumbered. A strange strip
    cartoon about suicide,its history & methods. Why?
13. Fair,Charles. Det Døende Selv. Atlantis Bøgerne.
    Thaning & Appel. 1964. PB. (orig.The Dying Self)
14. Feigenberg,Loma. Terminalvård.En metod för psykologisk
    vård av döende cancerpatienter. Liberläromedel,
    Lund. 1977. 231pp.
15. Feigenberg,Loma. Om döden. HR. 1976.84pp.
16. Fehrman,Carl. Diktaren och Döden. Bonniers,Stockholm.
    1952. 434 pp. PB.
17. Frederiksson,Dorrit. Leunard Dog Ung. Verbum,
    Stockholm. 1973. 112 pp. PB.
18. Furberg,Mats. Tankar om Döden. Aldusserien. Aldus/
    Bonniers, Stockholm. 1970. 129 pp.
19. Hagerfors,Anna Maria. När vi ska Dö. Forum.1975.86pp.
20. Hinton,John. Att Dö. Bokförlaget PAN/Norstedt,
    Stockholm. 1969. 204 pp.
21. Jenhoff,Annie. Dags. Askild & Kärnekall,Uppsala.
    1976. 107 pp.
22. Johannssen,Birgitta & Carsson,Gun-Britt. Barns tankar
    om Döden. Natur och Kultur,1976. 73 pp. PB.
23. Keleman,Stanley. Den Daglige Død. Forlaget Fremad,
    København. 1976. 128pp. PB.
24. Koch,Bent & Rald,N.J. Den Sidste Fjende - En Bog om
    Døden. Kristeligt Dagblads Forlag,København,1969.205pp.
25. Kubler-Ross,E. In för Döden. Frågor och svar. Bonniers,
    Stockholm. 1975. 174 pp. PB.
26. Kubler-Ross,E. Forfattern besvarer spørgsmål om døden
    og den Døende. GB. 1975. 156pp.
27. Lavik,Nils Johan & Ramvi Ivar (eds) Liv of Død.
    Nomi Forlag,Stavanger. 1970. 188 pp.
28. Lepp,Ignace. Människan inför dödens mysterium.
    Håkon Ohlssons,Lund. 1974. 170pp.
29. Leunbach,B & Bellunder,Sten Didrik. Mor,var är de döda?
    Bonniers,Stockholm. 1964. 44 pp. illus.
30. Malmquist,Ole.(ed) Døden:medicinsk,juridisk,praktisk.
    Nyt Nordisk Forlag,Arnold Busck.1973.178pp.
31. Melin,Margareta & Söderberg,Per. Johanna och Leif.
    Berlingske Bocktryckeriet,Lund.1972. 32pp. PB.

32. Michelsen,Ole & Thorgaard,Jørgen. Om Livet og Døden.
    Lundhardt & Ringhof,København.1974. 154 pp. PB.
33. Ninka (Anne Wolden-Raethinge). Den Vanskelige Død.
    Gyldendal,København.1974. 138pp. PB.
34. Parkes,Colin Murray. Når den nårmaster Dör:studier i
    vuxnas sorg.Wahlström & Widstrand,Stockholm.1976.
    257 pp. PB.
35. Sjoquist,Eric. Livet efter detta (en intervjuserie).
    Gumnessons,Falkoping. 1966. 95 pp. PB.
36. Sollerman,Erik. Livets kamp och dödens drama.
    Bokförlaget Libris,Örebro. 1971. 230 pp.
37. Stensnäs,Inge. Att Möta Döden.(En introduktion för
    Vårdspersonel). Natur och Kultur,Stockholm.1974.61pp.
38. Strandberg,B. Barmhjertighedsdrab og Laegegerning.
    Gyldendal,København. 1965. 132 pp. PB.

C. GERMAN

1. Ansohn,Eugen.Die Wahrheit om Krankenbett.Anton Pustet,
   KG, Munchen,1965.
2. Boden,H.J. Literatur und Selbstmord.Cesare Pavese--
   Klaus Mann--Ernest Hemingway. Stuttgart,1965.
3. Bowers,M.et al. Wiekönnen wir Sterbenden Beistehen.
   (transl) Kaiser-Grünewald. 173 pp.
4. Briesemeister,Dietrich.(ed) Bilder des Todes. Verlag
   Walter Uhl,Unterscheidheim.1970.
Magnificently,sumptuously illustrated with superb engravings
from the early Dance of Death to the 19th Century.Minimal
text,so very accessible to anyone.
5. Fuchs,Werner. Todesbilder in der Modernen Gesellschaft.
   Suhrkamp Verlag,Frankfurt/Main.1969. 228 pp.
6. Hahn,Alois. Einstellungen Zum Tod und Ihre Sociale
   Bedingtheid.(Eine Sociologische Untersuchung).
   Ferdinand Euke Verlag,Stuttgart.1968.162 pp.
7. Jüngel,Eberhard. Tod. Kreuz-verlag.Stuttgart.1971.175pp.
8. Korschelt,E. Lebens dauer Altern und Tod. 3rd ed. Jena:
   Verlag von Gusta v.Fischer.1924.
9. Metzger,Arnold. Freiheit und Tod.Max Niemeyer Verlag,
   Tubingen. 1953.
10. Pieper,J. Tod und Unsterblichkeit.Munchen.1968.
11. Ringel,E. Der Selbstmord.Abschluss einer Krankhaften
    psychischen Entwicklung. Wien-Disseldorf. 1953.
12. Rost,Hans. Bibliographie des Selbstmords.Literar Institut
    von Haas & Grabherr,Augsberg.Abteilung Buchverlag.1927.

13. Schaefer,Hans,Manfred Pflanz & Hans Strortzler.
    Was ist der Tod? 11 Beiträge und eine Diskussion.
    Piperverlag,Munchen. 1969. 192 pp. PB.
14. Stumpfe,Klaus Dietrich. Der Psychogene Tod. Hippokrates
    Verlag,Stuttgart. 1973.100pp.PB.
15. Thielicke,Helmut. Tod und Leben:Studien zur Christlichen
    Anthropologie. J.C.B.Mohr.Tubingen. 1946.
16. Thomas,K. Handbuch der Selbstmord verhusting.Stuttgart.
    1964.
17. Zwingmann,Ch. Selbstvernichtung. Frankfurt am Main,1965.

D. DUTCH

1. Rapport Euthanasie en de bejaarde mens. Uitgave van de
    stichting landelijk orgaan v.d.geref.gezindte voor de
    bejaardenzorg. Utrecht,1968.
2. Euthanasie: zin en begrenzing van het medisch handelen.
    Pastorele handreiking.Boekencentrum,'s-Gravenhage.
    1972. Nederlandse Hervormde Kerk.
3. Ansohn,Eugen.Spreken en zwigen aan het ziekbed. Dekker
    & Van de Vegt,Nijmegen-Utrecht.1968.143pp.PB.
(excellent account of truth & hope in medicine).
4. de Beauvoir,S. Een zachte dood. Hilversum.1966.
5. van den Berg,J.H. Medische macht en medische ethiek.
    Callenbach,Nijkerk.1969.49pp.PB.illus.
(argues the need for a new medical ethics,arising from the
new problems,with examples,of euthanasia,hemicorporectomy,etc)
6. Berger,W.J. Leven bijstaan van stervenden. Openbare les.
    Nijmegen-Utrecht. 1968.
7. Bowers,M.et al. De Pastor aan het Sterfbed (transl).
    Nijmegen-Utrecht. 1969.
8. H.A.H.van Till-d'Aulnis de Bourouill. Medisch-juridisch
    aspecten van het einde van het menselijk leven.
    Kluwer, Deventer. 1970. 161 pp. PB.
9. Braaksma,Dick,P.de Bruijn,& G.Salemink.Omgaan met de
    Dood. Uitgave MFAS,Amsterdam. 1969.
10. Buskes,J.J. Waarheid en leugen aan het ziekbed.
    Amsterdam,1964.(Truth & lying at the sick-bed).
11. Downing,A.B. et al. Euthanasie,het recht om te
    sterven.(transl). Spectrum,Utrecht. 1969.
12. Eade,Carp. De Dubbelganger. Utrecht. 1964.
13. Frijling-Schrender,E.C.M. De Psychiater en de Dood.
    Hoofdstukken uit de hedendaagse psychoänalyse.Arnhem.
    1968.

14. de Geus,C.A. Huisarts en Kankerpatient.Nijmegen.1970.
15. Hofstede,Peter. Tot onze diepe droefheid.Documentaire
    over de dood.een Anthos-boek.Baarn.1970.
16. Kubler-Ross,E. Lessen voor Levenden.Gesprekken met
    Stervenden. Ambo,Bilthoven.1970.(On Death & Dying).
17. Kuitert,H.M. Herwaardering van de dood in
    Andersgezegd. Kampen. 1970.
18. van der Meer,C. Geneeskunduge Confrontatie met de
    Dood.Staflen,Leiden. 1970.
19. Meier,Henk J. Menswaardig sterven,euthanasie,discussie.
    Paul Brand,Hilversum,1968.
20. Mitford,J. Laatste eer naar laatste mode (transl).
    Amsterdam.1965.
21. Mochel,Henk. Een milde dood. j.h.Kok bv.Kampen. 1972.
    100pp. PB. (on active & passive euthanasia).
22. van Niftrik,G.C. Waar zijn onze doden? Den Haag,1970.
23. Rothuizen,G.Th. Afspraak met de dood:gedachten over
    ethiek en suicide. J.H.Kok b.v. Kampen. 1972. 136 pp.
24. Speijer,N. Het zelfmoordraagstuk.Een samenvattend
    overzicht van de verschillende aspecten van de
    zelf-moord. Arnhem,1969.
25. Sporken,Paul.Voorlopige Diagnose.Inleiding tot een
    medische ethiek.Ambo,Bilthoven.1969.263pp.PB.
(euthanasia,abortion,AID,&"problems around life's end")
26. Sporken,P. De laatste stervensfase: stervenshulp en
    euthanasie. Ambo,Bilthoven.1972.148pp. PB.
27. Sporken,C.P. en J.Michels. De laatste levensfase:
    Medische mogelijkheden. Ambo,Bilthoven.1972.
28. Stengel,E. Zelfmoord en poging tot zelfmoord.(transl).
    Hilversum-Antwerpen. 1967.
29. Toynbee,A. et al. Denken over de Dood (transl). Bruna,
    Utrecht. 1969.
30. Tuinier,Siegfried. Thanatologie.Ongepubliceerde
    bijdrage over een medische doodsleer.Sautpoort,1969.
31. Velema,W.H. Rondom het levenseinde.Ethische en pastorale
    overwegingen. Kok,Kampen.1971.77pp. PB.
32. Vendrik,M.H.C. & Straver C.J. Weduwen.Een verkennend
    onderzoek. Bussum. 1969. (widows & bereavement).
33. Verhoeven,C.Het leedwezen (beschouwingen over troost en
    verdriet-leven en dood).Ambo,Bilthovem.1971.
    109pp.PB.(Bereavement,consolation & grief;trust,truth
    & suicide).
34. Westerman Holstijn,A.J.Leven en Dood.Medisch-
    -Psychologische beschouwingen.Utrecht. 1939.

---oOo---

KEY JOURNAL REFERENCES

This section lists significant Journal references on topics in Thanatology where few books exist,or where no adequate book or major review is available.

1. DEATH & ADOLESCENCE,DEATH & DEVELOPMENT

Blake,R.R. Attitudes toward death as a function of developmental stages.Dissertation Abstracts,1970,30,3380.

Caprio,F.S. A study of some psychological reactions during prepubescence to the idea of death.Psychiatric Quarterly, 1950, 24, 405-505.

Collings A,W.E.Sedlacek.Grief reactions among university students.Journal of the National Association of Women Deans & Counselors,1973,36,178-183.

Hogan,RA. Adolescent views of death.Adolescence,1970,5,55-66.

Kastenbaum,R.Time & death in adolescence,in The Meaning of Death,H.Feifel,(ed).McGraw-Hill,New York,1959.

Langer,M. Object loss & mourning during adolescence. Psychoanalytic Study of the Child,1966,21,269-293.

Lowenberg,J.S. The coping behaviors of fatally ill adolescents & their parents.Nursing Forum,1970,9,269-287.

Maurer,A. Adolescent attitudes toward death.Journal of Genetic Psychology,1964,105,75-90.

Maurer,A. Maturation of concepts of death.British Journal of Medical Psychology,1966,39,35-41.

Maxwell,MB. A terminally ill adolescent & her family.American Journal of Nursing,1962,72,925-927.

Salter,CA,CD Salter.Death anxiety & attitudes toward aging & elderly among young people.Gerontology,1975,15,89.

Sarwer-Forner,G. Denial of death & the unconscious longing for indestructibility & immortality in the terminal phase of adolescence.Canadian Psychiatric Association Journal, 1972,17,51-57.

Seligman,R et al.The effect of earlier parental loss in adolescence.Archives of General Psychiatry,1974,31,475-79.

Stacey CL,Reichen ML.Attitudes toward death & future life among normal & subnormal adolescent girls.Exceptional Children,1954,20,259-262.

2. ANTHROPOLOGY (Customs & attitudes toward death & mourning in other cultures)

Ablon,J.Bereavement in a Samoan community.British Journal of Medical Psychology,1971,44,329-337.

Aginsky,BW.The socio-psychological significance of death
    among the Pomo Indians.American Imago,1940,1,1-11.
Anderson,BG.Bereavement as a subject of cross-cultural
    inquiry:an American sample.Anthropological Quarterly,
    1965,38,181-200.
Augustin,DR.Ceremonies in connection with the dead in Malolos,
    Bulacan.Philippine Sociological Review,1956,4,32-38.
Barnouw,V.Chippewa Social Atomism:Feast of the Dead.American
    Anthropologist,1961,63,1006-1013.
Bernard,HY. The Law of Death & Disposal of the Dead.
    Oceana Publications,New York.1966.
Blackman,MB.Totems to tombstones:culture change as viewed
    through the Haida Mortuary Complex,1877-1971.Ethnology,
    1973,12,47-56.
Bloch,M.Placing the Dead:Tombs,Ancestral Villages & Kinship
    Organization in Madagascar.Academic Press,London.1971.
Boas,F.The idea of future life among primitive tribes,in
    F.Boas.Race,Language & Culture.Macmillan,New York.1940.
Bohannan,P (ed) African Homicide & Suicide.Princeton
    University Press,Princeton,NJ.1960.
Brain,JL.Sex,incest & death:initiation rites reconsidered.
    Current Anthropology,1977,18,2,191-208. (96 refs).
Brown,P. Chimbu death payment.Journal of the Royal
    Anthropological Institute of Great Britain & Ireland,
    1961,91,77-96.
Caprio,FS. A psychosocial study of primitive conceptions of
    death.Journal of Criminal Psychopathology,1943,5,303-317.
Caprio,FS.Ethnological attitudes toward death:a psychoanalytic
    evaluation.Journal of Clinical & Experimental
    Psychopathology,1946,7,737-752.
Carpenter,ES.Eternal life & self-definition among the
    Aivilik Eskimos.American Journal of Psychiatry,1954,110,
    840-843.
Carstairs,GM.Attitudes to death & suicide in an Indian
    cultural setting.International Journal of Social
    Psychiatry,1955,1,33-41.
Counts,DR.Good Death in Kalidi-preparation for death in
    Western New Britain,Omega,1976,7,4,367-372.
Davis,CH.The Egyptian Book of the Dead.G.P.Putnam's Sons,
    New York,1894.
Day SB & Redshaw,TD. Tuluak & Amanlik:Dialogues on Death
    & Mourning with the Innuit Eskimo.Minneapolis,University
    of Minnesota Medical School,Bell Museum of Pathobiology,
    1973.

Devereux,G.Primitive psychiatry:Funeral Suicide and the
    Mohave social structure.Bulletin of the History of
    Medicine,1942,11,522-542.
DeVos G,Hiroshi Wagatsuma.Psycho-cultural significance of
    concern over death & illness among rural Japanese.
    International Journal of Social Psycbology,1959,5,5-19.
Dobzhansky T. Religion,death & evolutionary adaptation,in
    M.E.Spiro(ed) The Context & Meaning of Cultural
    Anthropology,The Free Press,New York,1965.
Douglass,WA.Death in Murelaga:Funeral Ritual in a Spanish
    Basque Village. University of Washington Press,Seattle.
    1969.
Fabian,J.How others die:reflections on the anthropology of
    death.Social Research,1972,39,543-567.
Frazer,JG.Belief in Immortality & the Worship of the Dead.
    Macmillan,London,1913.
Frazer,JG. The Fear of the Dead in Primitive Religion.
    Macmillan,London.1933. Arno Press,New York.1976.
Gardiner,AH.The Attitude of the Ancient Egyptians to Death
    and the Dead. Cambridge,University Press.1935.
Gluckman,M. Mortuary customs and the belief in survival
    after death among the South-Eastern Bantu.Bantu Studies,
    1937,11,117-136.
Goldschmidt,W. Freud,Durkheim & death among the Sebei,
    Omega,1972,3,227-231.
Goldschmidt,W.Guilt & pollution in Sebei mortuary rituals,
    Ethos,1973,1,73-105.
Goody,J. Death & social structure among the Lo Dagaa,
    Man,1959,59,134-138.
Goody,J. Death,Property & the Ancestors:A Study of the
    Mortuary Customs of the Lo Dagaa of West Africa. Palo
    Alto,Stanford University Press.1962.
Gough,E.K. Cults of the dead among the Nayars.Journal of
    American Folklore,1958,71,446-496.
Green,J.S. The Days of the Dead in Oaxada,Mexico:An
    Historical Inquiry. Omega,1972,3,245-261.
Henderson JL,M.Oakes.The Wisdom of the Serpent:The Myths of
    Death,Rebirth & Resurrection.Macmillan,New York.1971.
Hickerson,H. The Feast of the Dead among the 17th Century
    Algonkians of the Upper Great Lakes.American
    Anthropologist,1960,62,81-107.
Hintington,WR. Death & the social order:Bara Funeral Customs
    (Madagascar), African Studies,1973,32,650-684.
Hofer,G.Death in the primitive world (on the question of
    death suggestion in Melanesia,Confinia Psychiatrica,
    1966,9,93-114.

Huber,PB. Death & society among the Anggor of New Guinea,
    Omega,1972,3,233-243.
Jha,M. Death-rites among Maithil Brahmans, Man in India,
    1966,46,241-247.
Kane,J. The Irish Wake:a sociological appraisal.
    Sociological Symposium,1968,1,11-16.
Kelly,WH. Cocopa attitudes & practice with respect to death
    & mourning.Southwestern Journal of Anthropology,1949,
    5,151-164.
Kennard,EA. Hopi reactions to death.American Anthropologist,
    1937,29,491-494.
Kluckhohn,C.Conceptions of death among the Southwestern
    Indians,in R.Kluckhohn (ed) Culture & Behavior,
    Free Press,New York. 1962. (pp.134-139).
Lehner,E. Devils,Demons,Death & Damnation.Dover,New York.1972.
Lester,D.Fear of death in primitive societies.Behavioral
    Science Review,1975,10,229-232.
Lester,D. Voodoo death:some new thoughts on an old
    phenomenon.American Anthropologist,1972,74,786-790.
Lex,BW.Voodoo death:new thoughts & an old explanation.
    American Anthropologist,1974,76,4,818-823.
Malinowski,B. Baloma:the Spirits of the Dead,in The Trobriand
    Islands.Journal of the Royal Anthropological Institute
of Great Britain & Ireland,1916,46,353-430.
Malinowski,B. Death & the Reintegration of the Group,in
    Magic,Science & Religion.Doubleday,New York.1954.
Mastin,BA.The extended burials at the Mugharet Elhad.
    Journal of the Royal Anthropological Society of Great
    Britain & Ireland,1964,94,44-51.
Matchett,WF. Reported hallucinatory experiences as a part of
    the mourning process among Hopi Indian women,Psychiatry,
    1972,35,185-194.
Miller,S & Schoenfeld L. Grief in the Navajo:psychodynamics
    and culture.International Journal of Social Psychiatry,
    1973,19,187-191.
Mitra,DN.Mourning customs & modern life in Bengal.American
    Journal of Sociology,1947,52,309-311.
Moore,J. The Death Culture of Mexico & Mexican-Americans,
    Omega,1970,1,271-291.
Murgoci,A. Customs connected with death & burial among the
    Roumanians.Folk-Lore,1919,30,89-102.
Noon,JA.A Preliminary examination of the death concepts of
    the Ibo,American Anthropologist,1942,44,638-654.

Opler,ME.The Lipan Apache Death Complex & its extensions.
  Southwestern Journal of Anthropology,1945,1,122-141.
Opler,ME.Reactions to death among the Mescalero Indians,
  Southwestern Journal of Anthropology,1946,2,454-467.
Opler,ME,WE Bittle.The death practices & eschatology of the
  Kiowa Apache.Southwestern Journal of Anthropology,
  1961,17,383-394.
Orenstein,H.Death & kinship in Hinduism:structural and
  functional interpretations.American Anthropologist,
  1970,72,1357-1377.
Osuna P,Reynolds,DK. A funeral in Mexico:description and
  analysis.Omega,1970,1,249-269.
Paton,LB.Spiritism & the Cult of the Dead in Antiquity.
  Macmillan,New York,1921.
Paz,Octavio.The Day of the Dead,in Labyrinth of Solitude:
  Life and Thought in Mexico,Grove Press,NY.1961.pp 47-64.
Preston,JJ.Toward an anthropology of death.Intellect,
  1977,105,2383,343-344.
Racy,J. Death in an Arab culture.Annals of the N.Y.Academy
  of Sciences,1969,64,871-880.
Roll S,Brenneis,CB.Chicano & Anglo dreams of death:
  Replication.Journal of Cross-Cultural Studies,1975,
  6,3,377-383.
Reisner,GA.The Egyptian Conception of Immortality.
  Houghton Mifflin,Boston,1912.
Reynolds,F.Natural death in myth & religion:lizard,
  chameleon,& future Buddha.Hastings Center Review,
  1977,7,3,38-44.
Rivers,WHR.The Primitive Conception of Death in H.Elliott
  Smith (ed)Psychology & Ethnology,Harcourt Brace,New
  York,1926. pp. 36-50.
Savashin JS,Wimberle H. Living and dead:cross-cultural
  perspective on Jewish memorial observances.Jewish Social
  Studies,1974,36,3-4,281-300.
Swift Arrow,B. Funeral rites of the Quechan tribe.Indian
  Historian,1974,7,22-24.
Thompson,EJ. Suttee:A Historical & Philosophical Inquiry
  into the Hindu Rite of Widow Burning.G.Allen & Unwin,
  London,1928.
Tichauer,RW. Attitudes toward death & dying among the
  Aymara Indians of Bolivia,Journal of the American
  Medical Woman's Association,1964,19,463-466.
Toynbee,A. Death & Burial in the Roman World. Ithaca,NY.
  Cornell University Press,1970.

Uini,N.Tongareva death & mourning rituals.Journal of
   Polynesia,1976,85,3,367-373.
Vulliamy,CE.Immortal Man:A Study of Funeral Customs & Of
   Beliefs in Regard to the Nature & Fate of the Soul.
   Methuen,London.1926.
Yamamoto,J et al.Mourning in Japan,American Journal of
   Psychiatry,1969,125,1660-1665.

3.   DEATH & THE ARTS & LITERATURE

Abram,HS.The psychology of terminal illness as portrayed
   in Solzhenitsyn's"The Cancer Ward", Archives of Internal
   Medicine,1969,124,758-760.
Abram,HS.Death & denial in Conrad's Nigger of the Narcissus.
   Omega,1976,7,2,125-135.
Abram,HS.Death psychology,science fiction & the writings of
   SG Weinbaum.Suicide,1975,5,2,93-97.
Abramson,J. Facing the other fact of life:death in recent
   children's fiction.School Library Journal,1974,21,31-33.
Bloom,H.Death & the native strain in American poetry.
   Social Research,1972,39,449-462.
Carr,RL. Death as presented in children's books.Elementary
   Englsih,1973,50,701-705.
Crain,H.Basic concepts of death in children's literature.
   Elementary English,1972,49,111-115.
Dunne,JS. The City of the Gods:A Study in Myth & Mortality.
   Macmillan,New York,1973.
Fiedler,LA. Love and Death in the American Novel.(revised
   edition).Dell,New York.1966.
Gajdusek,RE.Death,incest & the triple bond in the later
   plays of Shakespeare.American Imago,1974,31,109-158.
Goodman,LM.Attitudes toward death in creative artists.
   Omega,1975,6,4,345-356.
Grotjahn,M.About the representation of death in the art
   of antiquity & in the unconscious of modern man,in GB
   Wilbur & W.Muensterberger(eds) Psychoanalysis and
   Culture. International Universities Press,NY.1951.p.410-424.
Heuscher,JE. Death in the fairy tale.Diseases of the
   Nervous System,1967,28,462-468.
Heuscher,JE.Existential crisis,death & changing world
   designs in myths & fairy tales.Journal of Existentialism,
   1966,6,45-62.
Hoffman,FJ.The Mortal No:Death & the Modern Imagination.
   Princeton University Press,Princeton.1964.

Jackson,M.The black experience with death:a brief analysis
   through black writings. Omega,1972,3,203-209.
Jones,B.Design for Death. Bobbs-Merrill,New York.1967.
Koeningsberg,RA. F.Scott Fitzgerald:literature & the work
   of mourning.American Imago,1967,24,248-270.
Kurtz,B. The Pursuit of Death:A Study of Shelley's Poetry.
   Octagon,New York.1971.
Lewis,O. A Death in the Sanchez Family.Random House,NY.1969.
Marshall J & V.The treatment of death in children's books.
   Omega,1971,2,36-45.
Mooney,WE. Gustav Mahler:a note on life & death in music.
   Psychoanalytic Quarterly,1968,37,80-102.
Morris,B.Young children & books on death.Elementary
   English, 1974,51,395-398.
Murphy,BW.Creation & destruction:notes on Dylan Thomas.
   British Journal of Medical Psychology,1968,41,15-67.
Nigro,DL.Death & suicide in modern lyrics.Suicide,1975,
   5,4,232-245.
Noyes,R.Montaigne on Death.Omega,1970,1,311-323.
Philiber,M. Image & language of death in Bergman's Cries
   & Whispers.Archives of Social Science & Religion,1975,
   20,175-183.
Robison,R.Time,death & the river in Dickens' Novels.
   English Studies,1972,53,436-454.
Romero,CE.The Treatment of Death in Contemporary Children's
   Literature. Long Island University,New York.1974.
Simpson,MA. Death & Poetry,in H.Feifel(ed)New Meanings of
   Death. McGraw-Hill,New York.1977.
Spencer,T. Death & Elizabethan Tragedy.Harvard University
   Press,Cambridge. 1936.
Walley,KW. Suicide in opera:a brief analysis.Omega,1971,2,
   191-194.
Walworth,JH.Conceptions of death & dying in personal poetry.
   Dissertation Abstracts International,1973,33,3327.
Weber,FP.Aspects of Death & Correlated Aspects of Life in
   Art,Epigrams & Poetry.Consortium Press,Washington,1970.
Yoeli,M.Death & compassion in medicine & literature.
   American Journal of Medical Science,1972,263,487-495.

4. ATTITUDES TO DEATH

Alexander,IE et al.Is death a matter of indifference?
   Journal of Psychology,1957,43,277-283.
Alexander,M et al.Fear of death in parachute jumpers.
   Perceptual & Motor Skills,1972,34,338.

Beard,BH.Fear of death & fear of life.Archives of General
  Psychiatry,1969,21,373-380.
Becker,HS,Bruner DK.Attitudes toward death & the dead,& some
  possible causes of ghost fear.Mental Hygiene,1931,15,828
  -837.
Bell,WD.The experimental manipulation of death attitudes:a
  preliminary investigation. Omega,1975,6,199-205.
Bengston V,et al.Attitudes toward death & dying:contrasts
  by age,sex,ethnicity,& S.E.Gerontology,1975,15,63.
Biorck,G.How do you want to die?Answers to a questionnaire
  & their implications for medicine.Archives of Internal
  Medicine,1973,132,605-606.
Bluestein,VW.Death-related experiences,attitudes & feelings
  reported by thanatology students & a national sample.
  Omega,1975,6,207-218.
Cappon,D.Attitudes of & towards the dying.Canadian Medical
  Association Journal,1972,87,693-700.
Chasin,BH.Neglected variables in the study of death
  attitudes.The Sociological Quarterly,1971,12,107-113.
Chasin,BH.Value orientations & attitudes toward death.
  Dissertation Abstracts,1968,29,1963.
Crown,B et al.Attitudes toward attitudes toward death.
  Psychological Reports,1967,20(Supplement),1181-1182.
Dickstein,L.S. Death concern:measurement & correlates.
  Psychological Reports,1975,37,262.
Dickstein,LS.Relationship between death anxiety &
  demographic variables.Psychological Reports,1975,37,262.
Dickstein,LS & Blatt SJ.Death concern,futurity &
  anticipation.Journal of Consulting Psychology,
  1966,30,11-17.
Diggory JC & DZ Rothman.Values destroyed by death.Journal
  of Abnormal & Social Psychology,1961,63,205-210.
Durlak,JA.Relationship between various measures of death
  concern & fear of death.Journal of Consulting & Clinical
  Psychology,1973,41,162.
Ermanlinski,R. Questionnaire responses regarding risk-
  taking behaviour with death at stake.Psychological
  Reports,1972,31,435-438.
Feifel,H.Attitudes toward death:a psychological perspective.
  Journal of Consulting & Clinical Psychology,1969,13,
  292-295.
Hammer,M.Relfections on one's own death as a peak experience.
  Mental Hygiene,1971,55,264-265.
Handal,PJ.The relationship between subjective life
  expectancy,death anxiety & general anxiety.Journal of

Clinical Psychology,1969,25,39-42.
Handal,PJ.Relationship between death anxiety scale &
repression.Journal of Clinical Psychology,1975,31,675-677.
Hardt,DV.Development of an investigatory instrument to
measure attitudes toward death.Journal of School Health,
1975,45,96-99.
Iammarino,NK.Relationship between death anxiety and
demographic variables.Psychological Reports,1975,37,262.
Kahana,B&E.Attitudes of young men & women toward awareness
of death.Omega,1972,3,37-44.
Kalish,RA.An approach to the study of death attitudes.
American Behavioral Scientist,1963,6,68-70.
Kalish,RA.Some variables in death attitudes.Journal of
Social Psychology,1963,59,137-145.
Kalish,RA.Of social values & the dying:a defense of
disengagement.Family Coordinator,1972,21,81-94.
Kastenbaum R & PT Costa.Psychological perspectives on
Death.Annual Review of Psychology,1977,28,225-249.(169refs)
Koocher,GP. Conversations with children about death: ethical
considerations in research.Journal of Clinical Child
Psychology,1974,3,19-21.
Kopel,K.A human relations laboratory approach to death &
dying.Omega,1975,6,219-221.
Krieger,SR,Epting FR,Leitner,LM. Personal Constructs,Throat,
& Attitudes toward death.Omega,1974,5,4,299-310.
Larsen,KS et al.Attitudes toward death:a desensitization
hypothesis.Psychological Reports,1974,35,687-690.
Lester,D. Experimental & correlational studies of the fear
of death.Psychological Bulletin,1967,67,27-36.
Lester,D.Studies on death-attitude scales.Psychological
Reports,1969,24,182.
Lester,D.Relation of fear of death in subjects to fear of
death in their parents.Psychological Record,1970,20,
541-543.
Lester,D. Attitudes toward death & suicide in a non-disturbed
population.Psychological Reports,1971,29,368.
Lester,D.Attitudes toward death today & 35 years ago.
Omega,1971,2,168-173.
Lester,D. Sex differences in attitudes toward death: a
replication.Psychological Reports,1971,28,754.
Lester,D. Studies in death attitudes-2.Psychological
Reports,1972,30,440.
Leveton,A.Time,death & the Ego-Chill.Journal of
Existentialism,1965,6,69-80.

Lonetto,R,Fleming,S.et al.The perceived sex of death and
    concerns about death.Essence,1976,1,1,66-84.
Lowry,RJ.Male-female differences in attitudes toward death.
    Dissertation Abstracts,1966,27,1607-1608.
Means,MH.Fears of one thousand college women.Journal of
    Abnormal & Social Psychology,1936,31,291-311.
Middleton,WC.Some reactions toward death among college
    students.Journal of Abnormal & Social Psychology,
    1936,31,165-173.
Moore,V.Ho for Heaven! Man's Changing Attitude Toward
    Dying. Dutton,New York. 1956.
Morison,RS.Death:process or event?Science,1971,173,694-698.
Nelson,LD & CC.A factor analytic inquiry into the multi-
    -dimensionality of death anxiety,Omega,1975,6,171-178.
Paudey,RE.Vector analytic study of attitudes toward death
    among college students.International Journal of Social
    Psychiatry,1974-5,21,7-11.
Paudey,RE,Templer DI.Use of the Death Anxiety Scale in an
    Inter-racial setting.Omega,1972,3,127-130.
Ray,JJ,Najman,J.Death anxiety & death acceptance:a
    preliminary approach.Omega,1974,5,4,311-315.
Simpson,MA.The Do-It-Yourself Death Certificate in evoking
    & estimating student attitudes toward death.Journal of
    Medical Education,1975,50,475-478.
Stacey CL,Marken K.The attitudes of college students and
    penitentiary inmates toward death & a future life.
    Psychiatric Quarterly (Supplement),1952,26,27-32.
Templer,DI.Two factor theory of death anxiety.Essence,
    1976,1,2,91-93.
Wahl,CW.The fear of death.Bulletin of the Menninger Clinic,
    1958,22,214-223.
Walker JV.Attitudes to death.Gerontologia Clinica,1968,
    10,304-308.
Walton,D.On the rationality of fear of death,Omega,
    1976,7,1,1-10.
Williams,M.Changing attitudes to death:a survey of
    contributions in Psychological Abstracts over a thirty-
    year period. Human Relations,1966,19,405-422.

5. THE DEATH OF CHILDREN

Bibring GL.The death of an infant:a psychiatric study.New
    England Journal of Medicine,1970,283,370-371.
Binger CM et al.Childhood leukemia:emotional impact on
    patient & family.New England Journal of Medicine,1969,
    280,414-418.

Bruce SJ.Reactions of nurses & mothers to stillbirths.
Nursing Outlook,1962,10,88-91.
Burgert OE.Emotional impact of childhood acute leukemia.
Mayo Clinic Proceedings,1972,273-277.
Cain AC & BS.On replacing a child.Journal of the American
Academy of Child Psychiatry,1964,3,443-456.
Chodoff P et al.Stress,defences,& coping behavior:
observations in parents of children with malignant
disease.American Journal of Psychiatry,1964,120,743-749.
Cobb BR.Psychological impact of long illness & death of a
child on the family circle.Journal of Pediatrics,
1956,49,746-751.
Crase D.Death & the young child:some practical suggestions
on support & counselling.Clinical Pediatrics,1975,
14,747-750.
Drotar D. Death in the pediatric hospital:psychological
consultation with medical & nursing staff.Journal of
Clinical Child Psychology,1975,4,33-35.
Easson WM.The family of the dying child.Pediatric Clinics
of North America,1972,19,1157-1165.
Easson WM.Management of the dying child.Journal of Clinical
Child Psychiatry,1974,3,25-27.
Emery JL.Welfare of families of children found unexpectedly
dead.British Medical Journal,1972,19,1157-1165.
Gris,DP.Mother's perceptions of care given to their dying
children.American Journal of Nursing,1965,65,105-107.
Heffion WA et al.Group discussion with parents of leukemic
children.Pediatrics,1973,52,831-840.
Karon M,Vernick J.An approach to the emotional support of
fatally ill children.Clinical Pediatrics,1968,7,274-280.
Kennell JH et al.The mourning response of parents to the
death of a newborn infant.New England Journal of Medicine,
1970,283,344-349.
Knudson AF & Natterson JM.Observations concerning fear of
death in fatally ill children & their mothers.
Psychosomatic Medicine,1960,27,456-465.
Orbach CE.The multiple meanings of the loss of a child.
American Journal of Psychotherapy,1959,13,906-915.
Orbach CE et al.The multiple meanings of the loss of a
child.American Journal of Psychotherapy,1959,13,906-915.
Singer LJ.The slowly dying child.Clinical Pediatrics,1974,
13,861-867.
Spinetta JJ.Death anxiety in leukemic children.Dissertation
Abstracts International,1972,33,1807-1808.

Spinetta JJ.The dying child's awareness of death:a review.
   Psychological Bulletin.1974,81,256-260.
Stehbens JA,Lascari AD.Psychological follow-up of families
   with childhood leukemia.Journal of Clinical Psychology,
   1974,30,394-397.
Wright L.An emotional support program for parents of dying
   children.Journal of Clinical Child Psychology,1974,
   3,37-38.

6. CHILDREN'S REACTIONS TO THE DEATH OF PARENTS

Archibald HL et al.Bereavement in childhood & adult
   psychiatric disturbances.Psychosomatic Medicine,1962,
   24,343-351.
Barnes M.Reactions to the death of a mother.Psychoanalytic
   Study of the Child,1964,19,334 ff.
Barry H & Lindemann E. Critical ages for maternal
   bereavement in psychoneuroses.Psychosomatic Medicine,
   1960,22,166-181.
Becker D,Margolin F.How surviving parents handled their
   young children's adaptation to the crisis of loss.American
   Journal of Orthopsychiatry,1967,37,753-757.
Bendiksen R,Fulton R.Death & the child:an anterospective
   test of the childhood bereavement & later behavior
   disorder hypothesis.Omega,1975,6,45-49.
Birtchnell J.The possible consequences of early parent
   death.British Journal of Medical Psychology,1969,42,1-12.
Bunch J.The influence of parental death anniversaries upon
   suicide dates.British Journal of Psychiatry,1971,
   118,621-626.
Cain AC,Fast,I.Children's disturbed reactions to parent
   suicide.American Journal of Orthopsychiatry,1966,5,873-880.
McConville BJ et al.Mourning processes in children of
   varying ages.Canadian Psychiatric Association Journal,
   1970,15,252-255.
Miller JB.Children's reactions to the death of a parent.A
   review of the psychoanalytic literature.Journal of the
   American Psychoanalytic Association,1971,19,697-719.
Wessels MA.Death of an adult & its impact upon the child.
   Clinical Pediatrics,1973,12,28-33.

7. CHILDREN'S REACTIONS TO THE DEATH OF SIBS

Cain AC et al.Children's disturbed reaction to their
   mother's miscarriage.Psychosomatic Medicine,1964,24,
   58-66.

Cain AC et al. Children's disturbed reactions to the death
  of a sibling.American Journal of Orthopsychiatry,1964,
  34,741-757.
Feinberg D.Preventive therapy with siblings of a dying
  child.Journal of the American Academy of Child
  Psychiatry,1970,9,421-425.
Holland J.Psychological response to death of an identical
  twin by the surviving twin with the same disease.
  Omega,1971,2,160-167.
Irwin R,Weston DL.The Pre-school child's response to
  death of an infant sibling.American Journal of Diseases
  of Childhood,1963,106,564-567.
Rosenblatt B.A young boy's reaction to the death of his
  sister.Journal of the American Academy of Child
  Psychiatry,1969,8,321-335.

8.   CHILDREN'S CONCEPTS OF DEATH

Alexander IE & Alderstein AM.Affective responses to the
  concept of death in a population of children & early
  adolescents.Journal of Genetic Psychology,1958,93,167-177.
Apseloff M.Death in Current Children's Fiction:Sociology
  of Literature.St Louis:Midwest Modern Language
  Association,1974.
Bolduc J. A developmental study of the relationship between
  experiences of death & age & development of the concept
  of death.Dissertation Abstracts International,1972,
  33,2758.
Bowlby J.Separation Anxiety:a critical review of the
  literature.Journal of Child Psychology & Psychiatry,
  1960,1,251-275.
Childers P et al. The concept of death in early childhood.
  Child Development,1971,42,1299-1301.
Crain H.Basic concepts of death in children's literature.
  Elementary English,1972,149,111-115.
Ferenczi S.The unwelcome child & his death-instinct.
  International Journal of Psycho-Analysis,1929,10,125-129.
Furman RA.Death & the young child:some preliminary
  considerations.Psychoanalytic Study of the Child,
  1964,19,321-333.
Gartley W & Bernasconi M.The concept of death in children.
  Journal of Genetic Psychology,1967,110,71-85.
Jackson NA.A child's preoccupation with death.American
  Nurses Association Clinical Sessions,1968,172-179.
Jackson PL.A Child's developing concept of death:implications
  for nursing care of the terminally ill child.Nursing
  Forum,1975,14,204-215.

Kastenbaum R. Childhhod:the Kingdom where creatures die.
   Journal of Clinical Child Psychology,1974,3,11-14.
Klingberg G.The distinction between living & not-living,
   among 7-10 year-old children,with some remarks concerning
   the so-called Animism controversy.Journal of Genetic
   Psychology,1957,90,227-228.
Klingensmith SW.Child animism:what the child means by
   'alive'.Child Development,1953,24,51-61.
Koocher GP.Childhood,death & cognitive development.
   Developmental Psychology,1973,9,369-375.
Koocher GP.Talking about Death with 'Normal'children:
   Research strategies & issues.Boston:Developmental
   Evaluation Clinic,The Children's Hospital Medical
   Center,1973.
Koocher GP.Talking with children about death.American
   Journal of Orthopsychiatry,1974,3,22-24.
Kubler-Ross E.The languages of dying.Journal of Clinical
   Child Psychology,1966,39,35-41.
McConville BJ,LC Boag & AP Purchit.Mourning processes in
   children of varying ages.Canadian Psychiatric Association
   Journal,1970,15,253-255.
McIntire MS,CR Angel & LJ Struempler.The concept of death in
   mid-Western children & youth.American Journal of Diseases
   od Children,1972,123,527-532.
Melear JD.Children's conception of death.Journal of Genetic
   Psychology,1973,123,359-360.
Moellenhoff F.Ideas of children about death.Bulletin of the
   Menninger Clinic,1939,3,148-156.
Nagy M.The child's theories concerning death.Journal of
   Genetic Psychology,1948,73,3-27.
Pertz A.The child's sense of death:stages in affective
   organization & notional development,in Death & Presence,
   ed.A.Godin,Brussels,Lumen Vitae,1972.
Schilder P & D Wechsler.The attitudes of children toward
   death.Journal of Genetic Psychology,1934,45,406-451.
Spinetta JJ.The dying child's awareness of death:a review.
   Psychological Bulletin,1974,81,256-260.
Spinetta JJ et al.Personal space as a measure of a dying
   child's sense of isolation.
Spinetta JJ,Rigler D,Karon M.Anxiety in the dying child.
   Pediatrics,1973,52,841-845.
Tallmer M et al.Factors influencing children's concepts
   of death.Journal of Clinical Child Psychology,1974,
   3,17-19.

von Hug-Hellmuth H.The child's concept of death.
   Psychoanalytic Quarterly,1965,34,498-514.
Waechter,EH.Children's awareness of fatal illness.
   American Journal of Nursing,1971,71,1168-1171.

9. DEATH EDUCATION

Balkin E,Epstein C,Bush D.Attitudes toward classroom
   discussions of death & dying,etc.Omega,1976,7,2,183-189.
Barton D.The need for including instruction on death & dying
   in the medical curriculum.Journal of Medical Education,
   1972,47,169-175.
Barton D et al.Death & dying:a course for medical students.
   Journal of Medical Education,1972,47,945-951.
Barton D.Teaching psychiatry in the context of dying and
   death.American Journal of Psychiatry,1973,130,1290-1291.
Barton D & Crowder MK.The use of role playing techniques
   as an instructional aid in teaching about dying,death &
   bereavement.Omega,1975,6,243-250.
Bascue LO.Counselor Responses to Death & Dying:Guidelines
   for Training.New Orleans,American Personnel & Guidance
   Association,1974.
Bell BD.Experimental manipulation of death attitudes:a
   preliminary investigation.Omega,1975,6,3,199-205.
Bennett RV.Death & the Curriculum.Chicago,American
   Educational Research Association,1974.
Berg DW & Dougherty GC.Teaching about death.Today's
   Education,1973,62,46-47.
Bloch S.A clinical course on death & dying for medical
   students.Journal of Medical Education,1975,50,630-632.
Bloch S.Teaching medical students how to care for the
   dying.Medical Journal of Australia,1975,2,24,902-903.
Bloom S.On teaching an undergraduate course on death and
   Dying.Omega,1975,6,223-226.
Bluestein VW.Death-related experiences,attitudes & feelings
   reported by Thanatology students & a national sample.Omega,
   1975,6,3,207-218.
Dickinson GE.Death education in US Medical schools.
   Journal of Medical Education,1976,51,2,134-136.
Durlak JA,Burchard JA.Preliminary evaluation of a hospital
   based continuing education workshop on death & dying.
   Journal of Medical Education,1977,52,5,423-424.
Farmer JA.Death education:adult education in the face of a
   taboo.Omega,1970,1,109-114.
Fontendt C.The subject nobody teaches.English Journal,1974,
   63,62-63.

Gaines WG et al.Attitudes of Dental & Medical students
   towards death & dying (Meeting Abstract). Journal of
   Dental Research,55 (NSIB) B281- 1976.
Griffith JA.Three medical students confront death on a
   pediatric ward:a case report.Journal of the American
   Academy of Child Psychiatry,1974,13,72-77.
Hart EJ.Death education & mental health.Journal of
   School Health,1976,46,7,407-413.
Holmes J.Teaching about death:a review of selected materials.
   Social Studies Journal,1975,4,48-50.
Knott JE,Prull RW.Death education-accountable to whom,
   for what? Omega,1976,7,2,177-181.
Kopel K.A human relations laboratory approach to death &
   dying.Omega,1975,6,219-221.
Leviton D.The need for education on death & suicide.Journal
   of School Health.1969,39,270-274.
Leviton D.A course on death education & suicide prevention.
   Journal of the American College Health Association,1971,
   19,217-220.
Leviton D.Death,bereavement & suicide education,in D.A.
   Read (ed)New Directions in Health Education.New York,
   Macmillan,1971.
Leviton D & Foreman EC.Death education for children & youth
   Journal of Clinical Child Psychology,1974,3,8-10.
Leviton D.Education for death.Omega,1975,6,183-191.
Leviton D.Death education,in W.R.Johnson (ed) Human Health
   in Action.New York,Holt,Rinehart & Winston,1976.
Leviton, D. The scope of death education.Death Education,
   1977,1,1,41-56.
Liston EH.Education on death & dying:a survey of American
   medical schools.Journal of Medical Education,1973,
   48,577-578.
Liston EH.Psychiatric aspects of life-threatening illness:
   a course for medical students.International Journal of
   Psychiatry in Medicine,1974,5,51-56.
Liston EH.Education on death & dying:a neglected area in
   the medical curriculum.Omega,1975,6,193-198.
Lonetto R,et al.The psychology of death:a course description
   & some student perceptions.Ontario Psychologist,1975,
   7,9-14.
McLure JW.Death education.Phi Delta Kappan,1974,55,483-485.
McMahon JD.Death education-an independent study unit.
   Journal of School Health,1973,43,526-527.
Mueller ML.Death education & death fear reduction.Education,
   1976,97,2,145-148.

Murray P.Death education & its effect on death anxiety levels
    of nurses.Psychological Reports,1974,35,3,1250.
Peniston DH.The importance of death education in family life.
    Family Life Coordinator,1962,11,15-18.
Pine VR.A socio-historical portrait of death education.
    Death Education,1977,1,1,57-84.
Sadwith JA.An interdisciplinary approach to death education.
    Journal of School Health,1974,44,455-458.
Shapiro,SI.Instructional resources for teaching the
    psychology of death & dying.Catalog of Selected
    Documents in Psychology,1973,3,113.
Shapiro,SI.Teaching the psychology of death:fictional and
    non-fictional resources.Catalog of Selected Documents in
    Psychology,1974,4,108-109.
Simpson MA.Teaching about Death & Dying.Nursing Times,1973,
    69,442-443.
Simpson MA. Teaching about Death & Dying:an Interdisciplinary
    Approach,in RW Raven (ed)The Dying Patient,Pitmans,
    London,1975.
Snyder M et al.Changes in nursing students attitudes toward
    death & dying:a measurement of curriculum integration
    effectiveness.International Journal of Social Psychiatry,
    1973,19,294-298.
Somerville RM.Death education as part of family life education
    The Family Coordinator,1971,20,209-224.
Somerville RM.Perspective on death:a thematic teaching unit.
    The Family Coordinator,1974,23,421.
Speer GM.Learning about death.Journal of the American
    Veterinary Medical Association,1974,165,70-73.
Staford G.Miniguide:a mini-course on death.Scholastic
    Teacher,1973,4o-44.
Swiss T.Death education in the language arts classroom.
    Language Arts,1976,53,6,690-694.
Thorson JA.Continuing education in death & dying.Adult
    Leadership,1974,23,141.
Weisskop S,JL Binder.Grieving medical students:educational
    & clinical considerations.Comprehensive Psychiatry,
    1976,17,5,623-630.
White DK An undergraduate course in death.Omega,1970,1,167-74.
Wise DJ.Learning about dying.Nursing Outlook,1974,22,42-44.
Wright L.An emotional support program for parents of dying
    children.Journal of Clinical Child Psychology,1974,3,
    37-38.

10. DEATH AND THE FAMILY

Cobb BR.Psychological impact of long illness & death of a
    child on the family circle.Journal of Pediatrics,1956,
    49,746-751.
Davis JA.The attitude of parents to the approaching death
    of their child.Developmental Medicine & Child Neurology,
    1964,6,286-288.
Emery JL.Welfare of families of children found unexpectedly
    Dead.British Medical Journal,1972,1,612-615.
Feinberg D.Preventive Therapy with siblings of a dying child.
    Journal of the American Academy of Child Psychiatry,
    1970,9,421-425.
Fond KI.Dealing with death & dying through family-centred
    care.Nursing Clinics of North America,1972,7,53-64.
Friedman SB.Care of the family of the child with cancer.
    Pediatrics,1967,40,498-507.
Goldberg SB.Family tasks & reactions in the crisis of death.
    Social Casework,1973,54,398-405.
Goldfogel L.Working with the parent of a dying child.
    American Journal of Nursing.1970,70,1675-1679.
Gordon NB,Kutner B.Longterm & fatal illness & the family.
    Journal of Health & Human Behavior,1965,6,190-196.
Hamovitch MB.The Parent & the Fatally Ill Child.Delmar
    Publishing Co.,Los Angeles.1968.
Heffron WA et al.Group discussion with parents of leukemic
    children.Pediatrics,1973,52,831-840.
Kanof A et al.The impact of Tay-Sachs disease on the family.
    Pediatrics,1962,29,37-45.
Krieger GW,Bascue LO.Terminal illness:counseling with a
    family perspective.Family Coordinator,1975,24,351-356.
Knudson AF,Natterson JM.Participation of parents in the
    hospital care of fatally ill children.Pediatrics,1960,
    26,482-490.
Langsley DG.Psychology of a doomed family.American Journal
    of Psychotherapy,1961,15,531-538.
Lewis M.The management of parents of acutely ill children
    in hospital.American Journal of Orthopsychiatry,
    1962,32,60-66.
Murstein B.The effect of long-term illness of children on
    the emotional adjustment of parents.Child Development,
    1960,31,157-171.
National Association of Social Workers.Helping the Dying
    Patient & His Family.New York,1960.

Nolfi NW.Families in grief:the question of casework
    intervention.Social Work,1967,12,40-46.
Paul NL.The role of mourning & empathy in conjoint marital
    therapy,in Family Therapy & Disturbed Families,GH Zuk
    & I Boszormenyi-Nagy (Eds).Science & Behavior Books,
    Palo Alto,1967.
Seitz PM,Warrick LH.Perinatal death:the grieving mother.
    American Journal of Nursing.1974,74,2029-2033.
Shore L.Family communication in the crisis of a child's
    fatal illness:a literature review & analysis.Omega,
    1972,3,187-201.
Sheehy DP.Rules for dying:a study of alienation & patient-
    -spouse role expectations during terminal illness.
    Dissertation Abstracts International,1973,33,3777.
Smith AG et al.The dying child:helping the family cope with
    impending death.Clinical Pediatrics,1969,8,131-134.
Tisza VB.Management of the parents of the chronically ill
    child.American Journal of Orthopsychiatry,1962,32,53-59.
Vaughan DH.Families experiencing sudden unexpected infant
    death.Journal of the Royal College of General
    Practitioners,1968,16,359-367.
Vollman RR et al.The reactions of family systems to sudden
    unexpected death.Omega,1971,2,101-106.
Welldon R.The shadow of death & its implications in four
    families,etc.Family Process,1971,10,281-302.

11. HISTORICAL ASPECTS OF DEATH

Ackerknecht E.Death in the history of medicine.Bulletin of
    the History of Medicine,1968,42,19-23.
Aries,P.Major stages & meaning of evolution of our attitudes
toward death.Archives of Social Science & Religion,1975,
    20,159-167.
Davidson GW.Basic images of death in America:an historical
    analysis.Dissertation Abstracts,1966,27,1102.
Duckett ES.Death & Life in the Tenth Century.University of
    Michigan Press,Ann Arbor,1967.
Forbes TR.Life & death in Skakespeare's London.American
    Scientist,1970,58,511-520.
Lifton RJ.On death & the continuity of life:a psycho-
    -historical perspective.Omega,1975,6,143-159.
Maurer A.Death,women & history.Omega,1975,6,131-142.
Pelikan.The Shape of Death,Life & Immortality in the Early
    Fathers. Abingdon Press,Nashville,1961.

Richmond VB.Laments for the Dead in Medieval Narrative.
    Duquesne University Press,Atlantic Highlands,NJ.1966.
Sigerist HE.The sphere of life & death in early medieval
    manuscripts.Bulletin of the History of Medicine,
    1942,11,292-303.

12. DEATH & OLD AGE

Alderson MR.Relationship between month of birth & month of
    death in the elderly.British Journal of Preventive
    Science,1975,29,151-156.
Aldrich C.Personality factors & mortality in the relocation
    of the aged.Gerontologist,1964,4,92-93.
Aldrich C et al.Relocation of the aged & disabled:a mortality
    study.Journal of the American Geriatric Society,1963,11,
    185-194.
Berezin MA.The psychiatrist & the geriatric patient:partial
    grief in family members & others who care for the elderly
    patient.Journal of Geriatric Psychiatry,1970,4,53-70.
Butler RN.The life review:an interpretation of
    reminiscence in the aged.Psychiatry,1963,26,65-76.
Christ AR.Attitudes toward death among a group of acute
    geriatric psychiatric patients.Journal of Gerontology,
    1961,16,56-59.
Corey LG.An analogue of resistance to death awareness.
    Journal of Gerontology,1961,16,59-66.
Ellison DL.Will to live:a link between social structure &
    health among the elderly.Sociological Symposium,
    1969,2,37-47.
Exton-Smith AN.Terminal illness in the aged.Lancet,1961,
    2m305-308.
Feifel H.Older persons look at death.Geriatrics,
    1956,11,127-130.
Fischer HK,Dlin BM.Man's determination of his time of
    illness or death:anniversary reactions & emotional
    deadlines.Geriatrics,1971,26,89-94.
Glaser BG.The social loss of aged dying patients.
    The Gerontologist,1966,6,77-80.
Havighurst R,Neugarten B.(eds)Attitudes toward death in
    older persons-a symposium.Journal of Gerontology,1961,
    16,44-66.
Howard E.The effect of work experience in a nursing home on
    the attitudes toward death held by Nurses Aides.
    Gerontologist,1974,14,54-56.
Jaques E.Death & the Mid-Life Crisis.International Journal
    of Psychoanalysis,1965,46,502-514.

Jeffers FC et al.Attitudes of older persons towards death:
    a preliminary study.Journal of Gerontology,1961,16,53-56.
Kalish RA.The aged & the dying process:the inevitable
    decisions.Journal of Social Issues,1965,21,87-96.
Kastenbaum,RJ.The mental life of dying geriatric patients.
    The Gerontologist,1967,7,97-100.
Killian EC.Effect of geriatric transfers on mortality rates.
    Social Work,1970,15,19-26.
Kimsey LR et al.Death,dying & denial in the aged.American
    Journal of Psychiatry,1972,129,161-166.
Lipman AG,Marden P.Preparation for death in old age.
    Journal of Gerontology,1966,21,426-431.
Marshall VW.Age & awareness of finitude in developmental
    gerontology.Omega,1975,6,113-129.
Marshall VW.Socialization for impending death in a retirement
    village.American Journal of Sociology,1975,80,1124-1144.
Pearlman J et al.Attitudes toward death among nursing home
    personnel.Journal of Genetic Psychology,1969,114,63-75.
Preston CE,Williams RH.Views of the aged on the timing of
    death.Gerontologist,1971,11,300-304.
Roberts JL et al.How the aged in nursing homes view dying
    & death.Geriatrics,1970,25,115-119.
Saul SR & S.Old people talk about death.Omega,1973,4,27-35.
Stern K et al.Grief reactions in later life American Journal
    of Psychiatry,1951,108,289-293.
Swenson WM.Attitudes toward death in an aged population.
    Journal of Gerontology,1961,16,49-52.
Templer DI.Death anxiety as related to depression & health
    of retired persons.Journal of Gerontology,1971,26,521-523.
Wolff KH.Personality type & reaction toward aging & death.
    Geriatrics,1966,21,189-192.
Wolff KH.The problem of death & dying in the geriatric
    patient.Journal of the American Geriatrics Society,
    1970,18,954-961.

13. DEATH AND PSYCHOANALYSIS

Alexander F.The need for punishment & the death instinct.
    International Journal of Psychoanalysis,1929,10,256-269.
Benson G.Death & dying:a psychoanalytic perspective.
    Hospital Progress,1972,53,52-59.
Biran S.Attempt at the psychological analysis of the fear
    of death. Confinia Psychiatrica,1968,11,154-176.
Brodsky B.The self-representation,anality & the fear of
    dying.Journal of the American Psychoanalytic Association,
    1959,7,95-108.

Bromberg W.Death & dying.Psychoanalytic Review,1933,20,
    133-185.
Burton A.Death as a Counter-transference.Omega,1971,2,
    287-298.
Carmichael B.The death wish in daily life.Psychoanalytic
    Review,1943,30,59-66.
Cochrane AL.Elie Metschnikoff & his theory of an"Instinct
    de la Mort",International Journal of Psychoanalysis,
    1934,15,265-270.
Eissler KR.Death drive,ambivalence & narcissism.
    Psychoanalytic Study of the Child,1971,26,25-78.
Federn P.The reality of the death instinct,especially in
    melancholia.Psychoanalytic Review,1932,19,129-151.
Fenichel O.A critique of the death instinct,in The
    Collected Papers of Otto Fenichel.W.W.Norton,NY.1953.
Ferenczi S.The unwelcome child & his death-instinct.
    International Journal of Psychoanalysis,1929,10,125-129.
Fleming J,Altschul S.Activation of mourning & growth by
    psychoanalysis.International Journal of Psychoanalysis,
    1963,44,419-431.
Flugel JC.Death instinct,homeostasis & allied concepts.
    International Journal of Psychoanalysis,Supplement,
    1953,34,43-74.
Fodor N.Jung's Sermons to the Dead.Psychoanalytic Review,
    1964,51,74-78.
Freud S.Dreams of the death of persons of whom the dreamer
    is fond.1900.Standard Edition,Hogarth,London.1953.Vol.4.
Freud S.Reflections on War and Death.Moffat,Yard & Co.,
    New York,1918.
Friedman DB.Death anxiety & the primal scene.Psychoanalysis,
    1961-62,48,108-118.
Furman RA.Death of a Six-year-old's mother during his
    analysis.Psychoanalytic Study of the Child,1964,19,
    377-397.
Gabel P.Freud's Death Instinct & Sartre's fundamental
    project.Psychoanalytic Review,1974,61,217-227.
Galdston I.Eros & Thanatos:a critique & elaboration of
    Freud's Death Wish.American Journal of Psychoanalysis,
    1955,15,123-134.
Garma A.Within the realm of the Death Instinct.International
    Journal of Psychoanalysis,1971,52,145-154.
Gifford S.Some psychoanalytic theories about death:a
    selective historical review.Annals of the NY Academy of
    Sciences.1969,164,638-668.

Gordon R.The Death Instinct & its relation to the Self.
    Journal of Analytic Psychology,1961,6,119-135.
Greenberg HR,Blank HR.Dreams of a dying patient.British
    Journal of Medical Psychology,1970,43,355-362.
Gyomroi EL.The analysis of a young concentration camp
    victim.The Psychoanalytic Study of the Child,1963,
    18,484-510.
Heilbrun G.The basic fear.Journal of the American
    Psychoanalytic Association,1955,3,447-466.
Jelliffe SE.The Death Instinct in somatic and psycho-
    -pathology.Psychoanalytic Review,1933,20,121-132.
Joseph F.Transference & countertransference in the case of
    a dying patient.Psychoanalysis & the Psychoanalytic
    Review,1962,49,21-34.
Leddon SC.Sleep paralysis,psychosis & death.American Journal
    of Psychiatry,1970,126,1027-1031.
Levin AJ.The fiction of the Death Instinct.Psychiatric
    Quarterly,1951,25,257-281.
Meissner WW.Affective response to psychoanalytic death
    symbols.Journal of Abnormal & Social Psychology,1958,
    56,295-299.
Ostow M.The Death Instinct-a contribution to the study of
    instincts.International Journal of Psychoanalysis,
    1958,39,5-16.
Pomedli MM.Heidegger & Freud Power of Death.Ann Arbor,
    University Microfilms,1973.
Roberts WW.The Death Instinct in morbid anxiety.Journal of
    the Royal Army Medical Corps,1943,81,61-73.
Schneck JM.Unconscious relationship between hypnosis and
    death.Psychoanalytic Review,1951,38,271-275.
Schur M. Freud:Living & Dying.International Universities
    Press,New York. 1973.
Shor RE.A survey of representative literature on Freud's
    Death-Instinct Hypothesis.Journal of Humanistic
    Psychology,1961,1,98-110.
Simmel E.Self-preservation & the Death Instinct.
    Psychoanalytic Quarterly,1944,13,16-85.
Sternbac O.Death drive & the problem of aggression and
    sadomasochism.International Journal of Psychology,
    1975,56,321-333.
Symons NJ.Does Masochism necessarily imply the existence of
    a Death Instinct? International Journal of Psychoanalysis,
    1927,8,38-46.

Wilbur GB.Some problems presented by Freud's Life-Death
    Instinct Theory.American Imago,1941,2,134-196;209-265.

14. PSYCHOSOCIAL ASPECTS OF TERMINAL CARE

Aronson M et al.The impact of the death of a leader on
    Group Process.American Journal of Psychotherapy,
    1962,16,460-468.
Fisher G.Psychotherapy for the dying:principles &
    illustrative cases with special reference to the use of
    LSD.Omega,1970,1,3-15.
Franzino M,et al.Group discussion among the terminally ill.
    International Journal of Group Psychotherapy,1976,26,
    45-48.
Fulton R & J.A psychosocial aspect of terminal care:
    Anticipatory Grief.Omega,1971,2,91-100.
Grof S et al.LSD-assisted psychotherapy in patients with
    terminal cancer.International Pharmacopsychiatry,
    1973,8,129-144.
Hackett TP.The treatment of the dying.Current Psychiatric
    Therapy,1962,2,121-126.
Hicks W,Daniels RS.The dying patient,his physician & the
    psychiatrist-consultant.Psychosomatics,1968,9,47-52.
Kast E.LSD & the dying patient.Chicago Medical School
    Quarterly,1966,26,82.
Kirtley DD,Sacks JM.Reactions of a psychotherapy group to
    ambiguous circumstances surrounding the death of a
    group member.Journal of Consulting & Clinical Psychology,
    1969,33,195-199.
Kubler-Ross E,Anderson J.Psychotherapy with the least
    expected.Rehabilitation Literature,1968,29,73-76.
Kubler-Ross E.Psychotherapy for the dying patient.Current
    Psychiatric Therapies,1970,10,110-117.
LeShan L,Gassman M.Some observations on psychotherapy with
    patients suffering from neoplastic disease.American
    Journal of Psychotherapy,1958,12,723-734.
LeShan L & E.Psychotherapy & the patient with a limited
    life span.Psychiatry,1961,24,318-323.
Norton J.Treatment of a dying patient.Psychoanalytic Study
    of the Child.1963,18,541-560.
Pahnke WN.The psychedelic mystical experience in the human
    encounter with death.Psychedelic Review,1970,11,3-20.
Preston CE.Behavior modification:a therapeutic approach to
    aging & dying.Postgraduate Medicine,1973,54,64-68.

Rosenthal HR.Psychotherapy for the dying.American Journal
    of Psychotherapy,1957,11,626-633.
Rosenthal HR.The fear of death as an indispensible factor
    in psychotherapy.American Journal of Psychotherapy,
    1963,17,619-630.
Rosenthal P.The death of the leader in group psychotherapy.
    American Journal of Orthopsychiatry,1947,17,266-277.
Shneidman ES.On the deromanticization of death.American
    Journal of Psychotherapy,1971,25,5-17.
Spalt L.Death thoughts in hysteria,antosocial personality
    and anxiety neurosis.Psychiatric Quarterly,1974,48,441-4.
Trawick JD.The psychiatrist & the cancer patient.Diseases
    of the Nervous System.1950,11,278-280.
Wagner FF.The psychiatrist & the dying hospital patient.
    Mental Hygiene,1967,51,486-488.
Wiesman AD.Misgivings & misconceptions in the psychiatric
    care of terminal patients.Psychiatry,1970,33,67-81.
Wood BG.Interpersonal aspects in the care of terminally ill
    patients.American Journal of Psychoanalysis,1975,
    35,47-53.
Wylie HW et al.A dying patient in a psychotherapy group.
    International Journal of Group Psychotherapy,
    1964,14,482-490.
Zuehlke TE,Watkins JT.Use of psychotherapy with dying
    patients:exploratory study.Journal of Clinical
    Psychology,1975,31,729-732.

15. PSYCHOSOMATIC ASPECTS OF DEATH

Achte KA & ML Vauhkonen.Cancer & the psyche.Omega,1971,
    2,45-56.
Alexander GH.An unexplained death co-existent with death
    wishes.Psychosomatic Medicine.1943.5.188-194.
Barber TX.Death by siggestion:a critical note.Psychosomatic
    Medicine.1961.23.153-155.
Barrett GU,RH Franke.Psychogenic death:a reappraisal.
    Science,1970,167,304-306.
Beigler JS.Anxiety as an aid in the prognostication of
    impending death.Archives of Neorology & Psychiatry,
    1957,Feb.,171-177.
Cannon W.Voodoo death.American Anthropologist,1942,
    44,169-181.
Dlin BM et al.Psychological adaptation to pace-maker &
    open-heart surgery.Archives of General Psychiatry,1968,
    19,599-610.

Eisendrath RM.The role of grief & fear in the death of
    kidney transplant patients.American Journal of
    Psychiatry,1969,126,387.
Goldston R,WJ Gamble.On borrowed time:observations on
    children with implanted cardiac pace-makers & their
    families.American Journal of Psychiatry,1969,126,104-8.
Hackett TP & AD Weisman.Denial as a factor in patients
    with heart disease & cancer.Annals of the NY Academy
    of Science,1969,164,802-817.
Ikemi Y et al. Psychosomatic consideration of cancer
    patients who have made a narrow escape from death.
    Dynamische Psychiatrie,1975,8,77-92.
Kastenbaum R & BK.Hope,survival & the caring environment .
    in Prediction of Life-Span (ed) F.Jeffers & E.Palmore.
    Heath,Lexington,Mass. 1971.
Lieberman MA. Psychological correlates of impending death.
    Journal of Gerontology,1965,20,181-190.
Martin HL et al.The family of the fatally burned child.
    Lancet,1968,2,628-629.
Mattson A & S.Gross.Adaptational & defensive behavior in
    young hemophiliacs & their parents.American Journal of
    Psychiatry,1966,122,1349-1356.
Noyes R,R.Ketti. Depersonalization in the face of life-
    -threatening danger:a description.Psychiatry,1976,39,
    19-27.
Pruitt RD.Death as an expression of functional disease.
    Mayo Clinic Proceedings,1974,49,627-634.
Richter CP.The phenomenon of unexplained sudden death in
    animals & man,in The Meaning of Death.(ed)H.Feifel,
    McGraw-Hill,New York.1959.
Rioch D.The psychopathology of death,in The Physiology of
    the emotions.(ed) A.Simon.C.C.Thomas,Springfield,1961.
Seligman R et al.The burned child:emotional factors &
    survival,in Proceedings of the 3rd International
    Congress for Research in Burns,ed.P.Matter.Bern,
    Switzerland: Huber.1971.
Seligman R et al. Emotional responses of burned children
    in a pediatric intensive care unit.Psychiatry in
    Medicine,1972,3,59-65.
Shontz FC,SL Fink.A psychobiological analysis of
discomfort,pain & death.Journal of General Psychology,
    1959,60,275-287.
Solnit A & F.Stark.Mourning & the birth of a defective
    child.Psychoanalytic Study of the Child,1961,16,
    523-537.

Stavraky KM et al.Psychological factors in the outcome of
    human cancer.Journal of Psychosomatic Research,1968,
    12,251-259.
Walters MJ.Psychic death:report of a possible case.Archives
    of Neurology & Psychiatry,1944,52,84-85.
Weisman AD,T.Hackett.Predilection for death:death & dying
    as a psychiatric problem.Psychosomatic Medicine,1961,
    23,232-256.
Wold DA,BD James.The adjustment of siblings to childhood
    leukemia.The Family Coordinator,1969,18,2,155-160.

16. THE DEATH OF PUBLIC FIGURES

Dorpat TL.Psychiatric observations on assassinations.
    Northwest Medicine,1968,67,976-979.
Fairbairn WRD.The effect of the King's death upon patients
    under analysis.International Journal of Psychoanalysis,
    1936,17,278-284.
Greenberg BS,Parker EB(eds).The Kennedy Assassination and
    the American Public:Social Communication in Crisis.
    Stanford University Press,Stanford CA.1965.
Heckel RV.The day the President was assassinated:patient's
    reaction in one mental hospital.Mental Hospitals,1964,
    15,48.
Kaines J.Last Words of Eminent Persons.George Routledge &
    Sons,London.1966.
Kirschner D.The death of a President:reactions of
    psychoanalytic patients.Behavioral Science,1965,10,1-6.
Krippner S.The 20-Year death cycle of the American
    Presidency.Research Journal of Philosophy & Social
    Science,1965,2,65-72.
Nemtzow J,Lesser SR.Reactions of children & parents to the
    death of President Kennedy.American Journal of
    Orthopsychiatry,1964,34,280-281.
Orlansky H.Reactions to the death of President Roosevelt.
    Journal of Social Psychology,1947,26,235-266.
Purci-Jones J et al.Temporal stability & change in
    attitudes toward the Kennedy assassination.Psychological
    Reports,1969,23,907-913.
Sheatsley OB,Feldman JJ.The assassination of President
    Kennedy:a preliminary report on public reactions and
    behavior.Public Opinion Quarterly,1964,28,189-215.
Sterba R.Report on some emotional reactions to President
    Roosevelt's death.Psychoanalytic Review,1946,33,393-398.

Wolfenstein M & G.Kliman(eds) Children & the Death of a
    President. Doubleday,New York.1965.
Wolff KH. A partial analysis of student reaction to
    President Roosevelt's death.Journal of Social
    Psychology,1947,26,35-53.

17. DEATH & RELIGION,IMMORTALITY & AFTERLIFE

Berman AL.Belief in afterlife,religion,religiosity and
    life-threatening experience.Omega,1974,5,127-135.
Ellis RS.The attitude toward death & the types of belief in
    immortality.Journal of Religious Psychology,1951,7,466.
Ettinger RCW.The Prospect of Immortality.McFadden-Bartell,
    New York.1966.
Feifel H.Religious conviction & fear of death among the
    healthy & the terminally ill.Journal for the Scientific
    Study of Religion,1973,13,353-360.
Hall,GS.Thanatophobia & immortality.American Journal of
    Psychology,1915,26,550-613.
Jelliffe SE.Review of the article"Thanatophobia & Immortality"
    Journal of Nervous & Mental Disease,1917,45,272-276.
Lester D.Religious behavior & fear of death.Omega,1970,2,
    181-188.
Lester D.Religious behaviors & attitudes toward death.in
    Death & Presence,(ed)A.Godin.Lumen Vitae,Brussels.1972.
Lifton RJ.On death & the continuity of life:a new paradigm.
    History of Childhood Quarterly:The Journal of
    Psychohistory,1974,1,681-696.
Lifton RJ.The sense of immortality;on death & the continuity
    of life.American Journal of Psychoanalysis,1973,33,3-15.
Loveland GG.The effects of bereavement on certain religious
    attitudes & behavior.Sociological Symposium,1968,1,17-27.
Martin DS,Wrightsman L.Religion & fears about death:a
    critical review of research.Religious Education,1964,
    59,174-176.
Martin DS & Wrightsman L.The relationship between religious
    behavior & concern about death.Journal of Social
    Psychology,1965,65,317-323.
Myers FW.Human Personality & Its Survival of Bodily Death.
    Longmans,Green & Co.New York.1903.
Pieper J.Death & Immortality.Herder & Herder,NY.1969.
Pollock GH.On mourning,immortality & utopia.Journal of the
    American Psychoanalytic Association.1975,23,334-362.
Pringle-Pattison SA.The Idea of Immortality.Oxford University
    Press,New York. 1922.

Street JR.A genetic study of immortality.Pedagogical
    Seminary & Journal of Genetic Psychology,1899,6,267-313.
Templer DI.Death anxiety in religiously very involved
    persons.Psychological Reports,1972,31,361-362.
Templer DI & E.Dotson.Religious correlates of death
    anxiety.Psychological Reports,1970,26,895-897.
Tuccille J.Here Comes Immortality.Stein & Day,NY.1972.
Zilboorg G.The sense of immortality.Psychoanalytic
    Quarterly,1938,7,171-199.

18.   SOCIOLOGY & DEATH

Baker GW,DW Chapman (eds) Man & Society in Disaster.
    Basic Books,New York.1962.
Blanner R.Death & social structure.Psychiatry,1966,29,328-94.
Coombs RH,PS Powers.Socialization for death:physician's
    role.Urban Life,1975,4,250-271.
Faunce WA & Fulton RL.The sociology of death:a neglected
    area of research.Social Forces,1958,36,205-209.
Habenstein RW.The social organization of death.International
    Encyclopedia of the Social Services,1968,4,26-28.
Johnston HW.Toward a phenomenology of death.Philosophy
    & Phenomenology,1925,35,396-397.
Kephart WM.Status after death.American Sociological
    Review,1950,15,635-643.
Lofland LH.Toward a sociology of death & dying.Urban Life,
    1975,11,243-249.
Marshall VW.Socialization for impending death in a
    retirement village.American Journal of Sociology,1975,
    80,1124-1144.
Orwell G.How the Poor Die,in Shooting an Elephant.
    Secker & Warburg,London.1950.
Pine VR.Social organization & death.Omega,1972,3,149-153.
Reynolds DK.Work roles in death-related occupations.
    Journal of Vocational Behavior,1974,4,223-225.
Thauberger PC,EM.A consideration of death & a sociological
    perspective on the quality of the dying patient's
    care.Social Science & Medicine,1974,8,437-441.
Vernon GM.Dying as a social-symbolic process.
    Humanitas,1974,10,21-32.
Weisman AD. The social significance of the danger list.
    Journal of the American Medical Association,1972,215,
    1963-1966.
Young FW.Graveyards & social structure.Rural Sociology,
    1960,25,446-450.

19. WIDOWS & WIDOWERS

Beck F.The Diary of a Widow:Rebuilding a Family after the
    Funeral.Beacon Press,Boston.1965.
Berardo FM.Survivorship & social isolation:the case of the
    aged widower.Family Coordinator,1970,19,11-25.
Berardo FM.Widowhood status in the United States:
    Perspectives on a neglected aspect of the family life
    cycle.Family Coordinator,1968,17,191-203.
Bornstein PE et al. The depression of widowhood after
    thirteen months.British Journal of Psychiatry,1973,
    122,561-566.
Chevan A,Korson JH.The widowed who live alone:an examination
    of social & demographic factors.Social Forces,
    1972,51,45-53.
Clayton PJ et al.Anticipatory grief & widowhood.British
    Journal of Psychiatry,1973,122,47-51.
Clayton PJ.The depression of widowhood.British Journal of
    Psychiatry,1972,120,71-77.
Cochrane AL.A little widow is a dangerous thing.International
    Journal of Psychoanalysis,1936.17,494-509.
Cooperman IG.Second careers:war wives & widows.Vocational
    Guidance Quarterly,1971,20,103-111.
Cosneck BJ.Family patterns of older widowed Jewish people.
    Family Coordinator,1970,19,368-373.
Fritz MA.A study of widowhood.Sociology & Social Research,
    1930,14,553-561.
Gerber I et al.Anticipatory grief & aged widows & widowers.
    Journal of Gerontology,1974,30,225-229.
Hiltz SR.Helping widows:group discussions as a therapeutic
    technique.Family Coordinator,1975,24,331-336.
Kraus AS,Lilienfeld AM.Some epidemiologic aspects of the
    high mortality rate in the young widowed group.Journal
    of Chronic Diseases,1959,10,207-217.
Langer M.Learning to Live as a Widow.New York,Messner,1957.
Lopata,HZ.Living arrangements of American urban widows.
    Sociological Focus,1971,5,41-61.
Lopata HZ.The social involvement of American widows.
    American Behavioral Scientist,1970,14,41-58.
Lopata HZ.Social relations of widows in urbanizing
    societies,Sociological Quarterly,1972,13,259-271.
Lopata HZ.Widows as a minority group.Gerontologist,
    1971,11,67-77.
Maddison D,Viola A.The health of widows in the year
    following bereavement.Journal of Psychosomatic Research,
    1968,12,297-306.

Mathison J.A cross-cultural view of widowhood.Omega,1970,
    1,201-218.
Pihlblad CT,Adams DL.Widowhood,social participation & life
    satisfaction.Aging & Human Development,1972,3,323-330.
Pihlblad CT et al.Socio-economic adjustment to widowhood.
    Omega,1972,3,295-305.
Schlesinger B.The widowed as a one parent family unit.
    Social Science,1971,46,26-32.
Silverman PR.Services to the widowed:first steps in a
    program of preventive intervention.Community Mental
    Health Journal,1967,3,37-44.
Silverman PR.The Widow-to-Widow Program:an experiment in
    preventive intervention.Mental Hygiene,1969,53,333-337.
Silverman PR.The widow as caregiver in a program of
    preventive intervention with other widows.Mental
    Hygiene,1970,54,540-547.
Young,M et al.The mortality of widowers.Lancet,1963,
    2,454-456.

20. NEAR-DEATH EXPERIENCES

Barrett,WF.Death-Bed Visions.Methuen,London,1926.
Canning,RR.Mormon Return-from-the-dead stories.Utah Academy
    Proceedings,1965,42,29-37.
Delacour,Jean-Baptiste. Glimpses of the Beyond. Delacorte
    Press,New York. 1973.
Dobson,M.et al. Attitudes & long-term adjustment of
    patients surviving Cardiac Arrest.British Medical
    Journal,1971,3,207-212.
Ducasse.CJ.A Critical Examination of the Belief in a Life
    After Death. Charles.C.Thomas,Springfield,Illinois.1961.
Ehrenwald,J.Out-of-the-body experiences & the denial of
    death.Journal of Nervous & Mental Disease,1974,
    159,227-233.
Hart,H.The Enigma of Survival.Charles C.Thomas,Ill.1959.
Heim,A.Notizen ueber den Tod durch Absturz.Jahrbuch des
    Schweizer Aplenklub,1892,27,327. .
Heim,A. Ditto,translated,in Noyes R & Kletti R.The
    Experience of Dying from Falls.Omega,1972,3,45-52.
Hunter,RCA.On the experience of nearly dying.American
    Journal of Psychiatry.1967,124,122-126.
Jacobson,NO.Life Without Death.Dell,New York.1973.
Jung,CG. Memories,Dreams,Reflections. Pantheon,New York,1961.
Mackenzie,A.Apparitions & Ghosts:A Modern Study.
    Barker,London.1971.

Myers,FW.Human Personality & its Survival of Bodily Death.
    (2 volumes).Longmans,Green.London.1903.
Noyes,Russell.The experience of dying.Psychiatry,1972,
    35,174-184.
Noyes,R & Kletti,R.Depersonalization in the face of life-
    -threatening danger:a description.Psychiatry,1976,
    39,19-27.
Noyes R & Kletti R.Depersonalization in response to life-
    -threatening danger.Comprehensive Psychiatry,
    1977,18,4,375-384.
Osis,K.What do the dying see? Newsletter of the American
    Society for Psychical Research,1975,Winter,24.
Osis K & Haraldsson E.Deathbed observations by physicians
    & nurses:a cross-cultural survey.Journal of the American
    Society for Psychical Research,1977,71,237-259.
Pandey,C.The need for the psychological study of clinical
    death. Omega,1971,2,1-9.
Pearce-Higgins,CJD & Whitby S. Life,Death & Psychical
    Research. Rider & Co.London.1973.
Rees WD. The hallucinations of widowhood.British Medical
    Journal,1971,4,37-41.
Roll WG.A New look at the survival problem,in J.Beloff (ed)
    New Directions in Parapsychology,Elek Science,London
    1974,pp.144-164.
Roll WG.Survival research:problems & possibilities,in E.D.
    Mitchell,& J White (eds).Psychic Exploration:A Challenge
    for Science. G.P.Putnam's Sons,New York.1974.pp.397-424.
Kalish RA.Experiences of persons reprieved from death,in
    Kutscher,A(ed).Death & Bereavement.C.C.Thomas,1969.
    pp.84-96.
Kalish,RA.Phenomenological reality & post-death contact.
    Journal for the Scientific Study of Religion,1973,
    12,209-221.
Saltmarsh HF.Evidence of Personal Survival from Cross
    Correspondences.G.Bell,London.1939.
Stevenson F.Twenty Cases Suggestive of Reincarnation.
    2nd.rev.edn.University Press of Virginia,Charlottesville
    1974.
Thurmond,C.Last thoughts before drowning.Journal of Abnormal
    & Social Psychology,1943,38,165-184.

21. DEATH AND THE PROFESSIONALS

Artiss K.Doctor-patient relations in severe illness.New
    England Journal of Medicine,1973,288,1210-1220.
Bonine,BN.Student's reactions to children's death.American
    Journal of Nursing,1967,67,1439-1440.

Bruce SJ. Reactions of nurses & mothers to stillbirths.
    Nursing Outlook,1962,10,88-91.
Caldwell D & Mishara BL.Research on attitudes of medical
    doctors toward the dying patient:a methodological
    problem.Omega,1972,3,341-346.
Degner L.The relationship between some beliefs held by
    physicians & their life-prolonging decisions. Omega,
    1974,5,223-232.
De-Nour AK,Czaczkes JW.Emotional problems & reactions of
    the medical team in a chronic haemodialysis unit.
    The Lancet,1968,2,987-991.
Fitts WT. What Philadelphia physicians tell patients with
    cancer.Journal of the American Medical Association,
    1953,153,901-904.
Fochtman D.A comparative study of pediatric nurses'
    attitudes toward death.Life-Threatening Behavior,
    1974,4,107-117.
Golub S,Reznikoff M.Attitudes toward death:a comparison
    between nursing students & graduate nurses.Nursing
    Research,1971,20,503-508.
Jones EM. Who supports the nurse? Nursing Outlook,
    1962,10,476-478.
Kazzaz DS,Vickers R.Geriatric staff attitudes toward
    death.Journal of the American Geriatric Society,
    1968,16,1364-1371.
Klagsbrun S.Cancer,emotions & nurses.American Journal of
    Psychiatry,1970,126,1237-1244.
Lester D,et al.Attitudes of nursing students & nursing
    faculty toward death.Nursing Research,1974,Jan-Feb.,
    50-53.
Livingston PB,Zimet CN.Death anxiety,authoritarianism &
    choice of specialty in medical students.Journal of
    Nervous & Mental Disease,1965,140,222-230.
Lutticken CA et al.Attitudes of Physical Therapists
    toward death & terminal illness.Physical Therapy,
    1974,54,226-232.
Magni K.Reactions to death stimuli among theology students.
    Journal for the Scientific Study of Religion,
    1970,9,247-248.
Marshall J et al. The doctor,the dying patient & the
    bereaved.Annals of Internal Medicine,1969,70,615-621.
Margin LB & Collier PA.Attitudes toward death:a survey of
    nursing students.Journal of Nursing Education,1975,
    14,28-35.
Matse J.Reactions to death in residential homes for the
    aged.Omega,1975,6,21-32.

Miller LB,Erwin E.A study of attitudes & anxiety in medical
    students.Journal of Medical Education,1959,34,1089-1092.
Morris CM.The nurse & the dying patient.American Journal
    of Nursing,1955,55,1214-1217.
Murray P.Death education & its effect on the death anxiety
level of nurses.Psychological Reports,1974,35,1250.
Oken D.What to tell cancer patients:a study of medical
    attitudes.Journal of the American Medical Association,
    1966,195,36-37.
Quint JD,Glaser B.Improving nursing care of the dying.
    Nursing Forum,1967,6,368-378.
Reynolds DK.Work-roles in death-related occupations.
    Journal of Vocational Behavior,1974,4,223-225.
Rich T,Kalmanson GM.Attitudes of medical residents toward
    the dying patients in a general hospital.Postgraduate
    Medicine,1966,40,127-130.
Rothenberg MB.Reactions of those who treat children with
    cancer.Pediatrics,1967,40,507-512.
Schusterman LR,Sechrist L.Attitudes of registered nurses
    toward death in a general hospital.Psychiatry in
    Medicine,1973,4,411-426.
Simmons S,Given B.Nursing care of the terminal patient.
    Omega,1972,3,217-225.
Strauss AL.Family & staff during last weeks & days of a
    terminal illness.Annals of the NY Academy of Sciences,
    1969,164,687-695.
Travis TA et al.The attitudes of physicians toward
    prolonging life.Psychiatry in Medicine,1974,5,17-26.
Wagner B.Teaching students to work with the dying.American
    Journal of Nursing,1964,64,128-131.
Wodinsky A.Psychiatric consultations with nurses on a
    leukemia service.Mental Hygiene,1964,48,282-287.
Yeaworth RC et al. Attitudes of nursing students toward
    the dying patient.Nursing Research,1974,23,20-24.

—————oOo—————

FILMS AND AUDIO-VISUAL MEDIA AVAILABLE IN GREAT BRITAIN

A. FILMS

1. THE RIGHT TO LIVE:WHO DECIDES? B&W,reviewed above.
   £1.50.Available from Scottish Central Film Library.
2. DEATH:HOW CAN YOU LIVE WITH IT? 19 min. Extract from
   the feature film Napoleon & Samantha,with Will Geer;
   about what a boy learns from his dying grandfather.
   Guild Sound & Vision.
3. LIVING WITH DEATH. 30 min. 1969.From BBC-TV Man Alive.
   General discusion of terminal illness,somewhat dated.
   BBC Enterprizes.
4. DEAD MAN. 5 min. B&W. Reviewed above.£2.00.Concord.
5. SUICIDE:BUT JACK WAS A GOOD DRIVER.15 min.Color.
   Reviewed above. McGraw-Hill,UK.
6. DO I REALLY WANT TO DIE?30 min.Color.Dutch film,1976.
   English sub-titles.Discussion by people who have
   attempted suicide,of the problems they encountered.
   Concord,& Contemporary. £ 10.00
7. A CASE OF SUICIDE. 30 min. B&W.1969.From BBC-TV Man
   Alive.Katie killed herself at 17:explores how she might
   have been helped by those near her. Concord,CFC,BBC-sales.
8. TO DIE WITH DIGNITY. 25 min.Color. About a Miami doctor's
   proposals to withdraw life-support systems from incurable
   patients,allowing the patient more freedom in his last
   choices. Rental:£6.00 Film Forum,London.
9. WHY DID STUART DIE? 50 min. B&W.1976. Stuart Fisher,
   aged 2 months,died without warning on New Years Day,1975.
   He was a victim of "cot-death",the Sudden Infant Death
   Syndrome.Explores the commonness and nature of this
   condition,and how it might be dealt with.From BBC-TV
   Horizon. Rental:£7.00. Concord.
10. DEATH BY REQUEST. 30 min. Color.1977. From Granada TV,
    World in Action.An elderly woman with an incurable
    illness is campaigning for a change in the law to allow
    her to choose suicide,and to be helped to commit suicide
    when she wishes.Her family & opponents comment.
    £ 6.60. Concord, & Granada.
11. THE MERCY KILLERS. 30 min.B&W.1967.From BBC-TV Man
    Alive.Euthanasia discussed by doctors,lawyers & clergy;
    a man with severe paralysis,& the problem of a malformed
    baby.Not altogether up to date. Sale:£50,Rent:£3.00
    BBC or Concord.

12. THE EQUATION OF MURDER.40 min.Color.From BBC-TV Horizon.
    Murder:discussed by psychiatrists who have treated
    murderers,by criminologists,sociologists,geneticists,
    general public---and murderers. BBC-Enterprizes.Film or
    VCR.
13. A WALK UP THE HILL. 30 min.Color. Discussion of
    Euthanasia based on the case of Dr Allen Wakefield at
    77 who suffers a severe stroke after retiring.The
    family struggle with the decision about whether to keep
    him alive by extraordinary measures. Concordia.
14. THE LIFE THAT'S LEFT.29 min.Color.1977.Reviewed above.
    Religious Films,Ltd.
15. 40 YEARS OF MURDER. 52 min.Color.From BBC-TV Horizon.
    Film or VCR. Profile of Prof.Keith Simpson,Britain's
    leading forensic scientist,who has investigated over
    100,000 deaths.He doesn't find his job macabre,but an
    exciting series of puzzles to solve.BBC Enterprizes
    Sale only.
16. SOON THERE WILL BE NO MORE ME.10 min.Color.Reviewed
    above.Emotional film,with mainly still pictures,of a
    woman reviewing how she feels about her fatal cancer,
    for her baby daughter. Sale:£89,Rent:£3.60.Concord.
17. THE PARTING.16 min.Color.Yogoslavian community meets
    death,& everyone is involved in the customary rituals.
    CFC,Concord.
18. REMEMBER ALL THE GOOD THINGS. 30 min.B&W.1974. Tony
    Whiteley was 34 when he was told he had incurable lung
    cancer & 3 months to live.His son was 3,& his wife
    expecting their 2nd child.About their plans and ways of
    coping.Also available is "Vivian Whiteley on Her Own",
    the sequel. Sale:£90.Rental:£4.6o. Concord.
19. AVRIL.20 min.Color.1976. A woman of 50 is interviewed
    about her attitudes towards how she & her family cope
    with her terminal illness.Dept.of Teaching Media,Univ.
    of Southampton,& B.M.A.Library.
20. SADIE.28 min. Color.1974. Dialogue between patient,her
    daughter,& doctor;the interrelationship & ways of
    talking about the unspoken.Sympathetic & complex. Poor
    sound quality. Cicely Saunders,St Christopher's Hospice,
    & Behr Cinematography.
21. GRIEF.50 min. B&W.From Thams-TV Report.1973. Several
    people discuss their experiences of grief,& how others'
    ineptness made it more difficult.Concord. Sale:£100,
    Rental:£ 4.40.

22. PAULA.34 min.Color.1972. A cancer patient talks about
    her reactions to her illness & her approaching death.
    The constant panning & zooming of the camera is
    distracting & the sound is sometimes difficult.
    St Christopher's Hospice.
23. SUDDEN INFANT DEATH SYNDROME:AFTER OUR BABY DIED.
    21 min.USA 1975. Reviewed elsewhere. BMA Library.
24. OUT OF TRUE.41 min.B&W.1951.Fictional account of a
    young woman who attempts suicide & receives psychiatric
    treatment.Very out of date. Concord Films.
25. THE ADMITTANCE. 44 min. B&W.Divorced woman in her 30's
    & drinking,attempts suicide,& receives treatment.Dull.
    National Film Board of Canada.
26. A CRY FOR HELP. 14 min.B&W.1973.Made for a drug company,
    interview by psychiatrist of patient who has survived
    an overdose,stressing dangers of barbiturates.Rather
    too long for its purpose. Guild Sound & Vision.
27. OVERDOSE.20 min. Color. Dramatic reconstruction of
    interview between social worker & suicide survivor.
    Film Australia.Sale £100,Rental:£6.00
    Concord,& Film Forum.

B. FILM DISTRIBUTOR'S ADDRESSES

BBC Enterprizes:Hire. Woodstone House,Oundle Road,
    Peterborough,PE2 9PZ.Tel:0733 52257/8.
BBC Enterprizes.Sale. Villiers House,The Broadway,London
    W5 2PA.Tel:01 743 8000 Telex:934-678-265781.
British Medical Association/BLAT Film Library, Film
    Librarian,BMA House,Tavistock Square,London WC1.
    Tel: 01 387 4499.
Concord Films Council,Nacton,Ipswich,Suffolk.IP10 0JZ.
    Tel:0473 76012 Bookings & accounts,0473 77747 despatch.
Concordia Publishing House Ltd.,Viking Way,Bar Hill Village,
    Cambridge,CB3 8EL. Tel: 0954 81011.
Contemporary Films Ltd.,55 Greek Street,London W1.
    Tel: 01 734 4901.
Film Forum (DBW)Ltd.,56 Brewer St.,London W1.Tel:01 437 6487
Granada Television Film Library,Manchester M60 9EA.
    Tel: 061 832 7211,ext.207 or 332.
Guild Sound & Vision Ltd.,Woodston House,Oundle Rd,
    Peterborough PE2 9PZ. Tel:0733 63122,Telex 32659.
McGraw Hill Publishing Co.Ltd,McGraw-Hill House,
    Shoppenhangars Road,Maidenhead,Berks.
National Film Board of Canada,1 Grosvenor Square,London W1X
    0AB. Tel: 01-629-9492.

Religious Films Ltd.,Foundation House,Walton Road,Bushey,
    Watford WD2 2JF, Herts. Tel. 92 35444
Saint Christopher's Hospice,51-53 Lawrie Park Road,
    Sydenham,London SE26 6DZ Tel: o1-778-9252
Scottish Central Film Library,16/17 Woodside Terrace,
    Charing Cross,Glasgow G3 7XA. Tel:041 332 9988.

C. AUDIOTAPES,VIDEOTAPES,FILMSTRIPS & TEACHING MATERIALS
   IN BRITAIN

1. WHO CARES? The Case of Helen Johnstone. Rather complex
   to set up,but a good kit for use with students.A role
   play around Helen who,it is discovered near the end of
   the exercise,has committed suicide.Explores many
   problems of adolescence,including sexual identity,
   feelings of inadequacy,variations of the norm,loneliness,
   friendship,VD & Pregnancy.Not to be used lightly.
   Cockpit Press.

2. SUICIDE. Filmstrip-50 frames,Color.+ Audiotape. Suicide
   in adolescents & college students,causes,warning signs
   & sources of help.FS-£2,Tape-£2,Audiocassette-£2.50
   Concordia.

3. THE PATIENT WHO IS NOT GOING TO GET BETTER. 19 min.
   tape + 20 slides.1971.Long-term illness,stationary,
   progressive or terminal.Aimed at the family,on how to
   plan & cope:nursing care,bed-baths,skin-care,attitudes,
   help from doctors & district nurse.Graves (71-78)

4. PATIENTS' ATTITUDES TO DEATH.Tape,reel or cassette.31 min
   Talk by a patient with terminal cancer.1976.Graves.
   (76-17)

5. MAINLY MURDER. Dr A.Usher.60min.75 slides & tape.1970.
   Forensic medicine talk on aspects of death.Trent RHA.

6. DEATH CERTIFICATION. Dr John Havard.20 min.audiotape.
   1977.Discusses functions of Death Certificate,and the
   Broderick Committee Report,problems in investigation
   of unexplained deaths. Graves (77-40)

7. CARE OF THE BEREAVED.30 min. Audiotape.1971. Rev.M.
   Wilson.Bereavement,mourning,preparation & helping.
   Graves. (71-71)

8. TALKING TO RELATIVES. Miss EA Williamson,Nursing Tutor.
   21 min.Audiotape.1970. On a children's ward,talking to
   parents,especially about emergencies & death.Graves.
   (70-54).

9. SHOULD A DOCTOR TELL? Dr FR Gusterson.26 min.Audiotape
   1976.Personal opinions of what is best,in terminal
   malignant disease,to tell to patient & relatives.
   Graves (76-24)

10. AM I DYING,DOCTOR? Dr R.Tredgold.14 min.Audiotape.
1975. Psychiatrist discusses reactions to fears of
dying & their management. Like most of the Graves
tapes in this area,unexceptional,and none of them by
recognized experts in the subject area.Graves.(75-52)
11. TEAM WORK IN CARE OF THE DYING.33 min.Audiotape.1973.
Panel discussion:doctor,chaplain,nurse,physiotherapist
& social worker.Graves, (73-46).
12. CHILDREN & DEATH. Dr.S.Yudkin,pediatrician.40 min.
Audiotape.1967.Preparing children for death in
themselves,friends & family.Graves (67-32).
13. THE BASIC PRINCIPLES OF TERMINAL CARE.Dr FR Gusterson
28 min.Audiotape.1976. Some basic points,not terribly
well dealt with. Graves (76-73)
14. PSYCHIATRIC ASPECTS OF BEREAVEMENT. 48 min,tape+8 slides
1968. Dr Colin Murray Parkes. Trent RHA.
15. LIVING WITH DYING.155 slides in 2 carousel cartridges,
2 tape cassettes,Teacher's Guide.Sunburst Communications,
reviewed elsewhere.1974. Edward Patterson,UK.
16. TALKING ABOUT DYING.Videotape.25 min. 1972. 38 min.
Barbara McNulty of St Christopher's,in conversation
with 2 patients.Introduced by Michael Simpson.
London University AV Centre.
17. BEREAVEMENT.5 slides,25 min tape.1967. Dr Colin
Murray Parkes discusses the results of his studies of
bereavement.Graves (67-34),Centre for Med.Ed,Dundee.
18. THE THERAPEUTICS OF TERMINAL PAIN.R Twycross.1976.
Univ.of London AV Centre. Videotape.
19. A TIME TO DIE.34 min.videotape.Color. Recorded at
terminal care unit,aimed at helping social work
students understand their potential contribution.
Universities of Sheffield & Aberdeen.Aberdeen
Univ.TV Service.
20. THE NATURE & MANAGEMENT OF PAIN IN TERMINAL MALIGNANT
DISEASE. 3rd edn.1975. Dr Cicely Saunders,St Christophers.
42 min.Tape/slides. (reel or cassette).+handout.Sale or
Loan.Detailed discussion of methods.Graves (75-72)
21. THE THERAPEUTICS OF TERMINAL PAIN. Videocassette.
NHS Training Aids Unit.
22. LIVING WITH DEATH.Dr Macadam.Videotape.Ampex 1".
University of Leeds AV Service.
23. LABELLING SUICIDE.Tape D291-02/07.Interview with
coroner about inquests,suicide,unexplained deaths.
Open University.

24. THE CONCEPT OF SUICIDE. 60 min.Audiotape.Prof.E.
    Stengel. 1972. Trent RHA.
25. SUICIDE--THE GREAT ESCAPE. 27 min. audiotape +6 slides.
    1969. Reasons for suicide,& how we respond to it.
    Graves (69-20). Somewhat out of date.
26. SUICIDE--A SAMARITAN DOCTOR TALKS.40 min.Audiotape.
    1970.Dr George Day.Who does it?Why?Where can they
    turn?. Graves (70-52).
27. ATTEMPTED SUICIDE (Parasuicide):EPIDEMIOLOGICAL &
    SOCIAL FACTORS. 41 min.B&W videotape.various formats
    available.1972.Definitions,differences in rates,
    ecological & family linkage studies.Trends in
    parasuicide,speculation about causes.Prevalence in
    community. Univ.of London AV Centre.
28. SUICIDE: EPIDEMIOLOGICAL & SOCIAL ASPECTS.31 min.
    B&W. Videotape. various formats.1972. Similar review
    of completed suicide,changes since 1900,& causes.
    Univ.of London AV Centre.
29. WINTHROP SERIES. The Winthrop Laboratories, a
    pharmaceutical company,produces an audiotape magazine
    for General Practitioners.These have included several
    relevant talks,including:---
    --Suicide.Dr Michael Simpson.
    --Cot deaths.Dr Douglas Chambers.Vol.4.No.3. 8 min.
    --Cot deaths.Dr Bernard Knight. Vol.4. No.5. 4 min.
    --Terminal Care-Dr M.Garrett.Vol.1.No.6. 9 min.
    --Care of the Dying.Dr R.Lamerton.Vol.6.no.6.9min.
    Care of the Dying.Dr.L.Goldie.Vol.2.No.5.
    What do we mean by Death? Dr John Zorab.Vol.3.No.2.1976.
    The Fact,the time,& the cause of death.Prof.Donald Teare.
       1977,Vol.4.No.1.
    --Homicide & Sudden Death.Dr CA St Hill,Vol.6.No.4.9min.
    --Death Certificates.Dr JM Torry.Vol.5.No.6. 6 min.

D. AV SUPPLIERS ADDRESSES
Aberdeen University TV Service,King's College,Old
    Aberdeen,Aberdeen AB9 2UB.Tel.0224 40241 ext 6500/1
    Tel. 0224 491979 (direct line)
Cockpit Press,Gateforth Street,Marylebone,London NW8
Concord Films Council,Nacton,Ipswich,Suffolk. IP10 0JZ
Edward Patterson Associates Ltd.,68 Copers Cope Road,
    Beckenham,Kent. Tel: 01 658 1515
Graves Medical Audiovisual Library,PO Box 99, Chelmsford,
    CM1 5HL. Tel: 0245 83351.

London University Audiovisual Centre, 1 Bedford Square,
    London WC1B 3RA. Tel:01 636 3104
Open University Education Enterprizes (purchase),
    12 Cofferidge Close,Stony Stratford,Milton Keynes,
    MK11 1BY.Tel. 0908 566744
Open University Hire--c/o Guild Sound & Vision.
St Christopher's Hospice,151 Lawrie Park Road,
    Syndenham,London SE 26
Trent Regional Health Authority,The Librarian,Falwood
    House,Old Falwood Road,Sheffield,S10 3TH.
    Tel: 0742 306511.
University of Leeds Television Service (DJG Holroyde,
    Director). Television Centre, Leeds, LS2 9JT
    Tel: 0532 31751
Winthrop Medikasset,Winthrop House,Surbiton-Upon-Thames,
    Surrey. Tel. 01 399 5252.

———o0o———

STOP PRESS ADDITIONS

1. AND A TIME TO LIVE:TOWARD EMOTIONAL WELL-BEING DURING THE CRISIS OF CANCER. Robert Chernin Cantor.Harper & Row,New York. 1976.276 pp. $ 9.95.
2. COPING WITH TRAGEDY:SUCCESSFULLY FACING THE PROBLEM OF A SERIOUSLY ILL CHILD. J.L.Schulman.Follett,Chicago, 1976.335 pp. $ 9.55.
3. DISCOVERING SUICIDE:STUDIES IN THE SOCIAL ORGANIZATION OF SUDDEN DEATH. J.Maxwell Atkinson.Macmillan Press, $ 8.95.
4. THE DYING CHILD. Jo-Eileen Gyulay.McGraw-Hill,New York. 1978. 192 pp. $ 8.95.
5. ETHICAL ISSUES IN DEATH & DYING. ed.R.F.Weir. Columbia University Press,New York.1977.405pp.$20,$8 PB.
6. ETHICS AT THE EDGES OF LIFE:MEDICAL & LEGAL INTERSECTIONS. The Bampton Lectures in America.Yale University Press, New Haven.1978. 353 pp. $ 15.00.
7. FUNERAL CUSTOMS IN TOLKIEN'S TRILOGY. Karen Rockow. 973. 30pp. PB. $ 1.50.Obtainable via Highly Specialized Promotions,Brooklyn NY.
8. GIFT OF LIFE:THE SOCIAL & PSYCHOLOGICAL IMPACT OF ORGAN TRANSPLANTATION. RG Simmons,SD Klein,RL Simmons. John Wiley & Sons.1977. 526 pp. £ 16.
9. HEALING: IMPLICATIONS FOR PSYCHOTHERAPY.ed.J.L.Fosshage & P.T.Olsen.Human Sciences Press,NY.1978. 359 pp.$15.95. A very variable collection of pieces on psychic healing, meditation,TM,LSD,etc.Includes Chogyam Trungpa on Acknowledging Death.
10. IF YOU WILL LIFT THE LOAD,I WILL LIFT IT TOO. A guide to the Creation of a Widowed-to-Widowed Service in Your Community. Phyllis R.Silverman(with A.Musicant & S.Richter.(Supplement to Helping Each Other in Widowhood,for Funeral Directors).The Jewish Funeral Directors of America,Inc.1977.125 pp. $ 8.95.
11. LEGISLATIVE MANUAL ,1976 Edition.Society for the Right to Die,Inc.New York. 1976.96pp.PB. Excellent review of current Right-To-Die legislation, reprinting & summarizing all current US Bills & Statutes,comparing their characteristics.An important job well done.

12. <u>LOSS AND GRIEF IN MEDICINE</u>. P.Speck. Bailliere Tindall,
    London.1978.106 pp. PB.
    Grief,normal,abnormal,anticipatory;in medical contexts:
    obstetrics & gynaecology,general surgery & medicine;
    cultural factors & grief;with some references. By a
    hospital chaplain not previously known for his work
    in this area. **
13. <u>THE MANY FACES OF GRIEF</u>. Edgar N.Jackson.Abingdon
    <u>Press,1977.174 pp. $ 7.95.</u>
Yet another book on grief by the inexhaustable Jackson.
14. <u>MEDICAL HUBRIS :A Reply to Ivan Illich.David Horrobin,</u>
    reviewed above,is now also published by Churchill
    Livingstone,Edinburgh & London,1978. £ 3.00.
15. <u>NÉMÉSIS MEDICAL:L'EXPROPRIATION DE LA SANTE.Ivan</u>
    <u>Illich.</u> Editions du Seuil,Paris.1975.
16. <u>THE PSYCHODYNAMICS OF PATIENT CARE.LH & JL Schwartz.</u>
    Prentice-Hall,NY.1972.£3.25.Includes a chapter on
    relevant problems in the ICU,as well as death & grief.
17. <u>PSYCHOSOCIAL CARE OF THE DYING PATIENT.Ed.Charles A.</u>
    Garfield. McGraw-Hill,NY.1978.480pp. $ 13.95.
18. <u>PSYCHOSOMATIC MEDICINE— ITS CLINICAL APPLICATIONS.</u>
    Ed.E.Wittkower & H.Warner.Harper & Row,NY. 1977.
    356 pp. $ 14.95. Chapter 2,Grief in General Practice,
    by Bernard Schoenberg.Brief & not very special review.
19. <u>THE PRIVATE WORLDS OF DYING CHILDREN.Myra Bluebond-</u>
    -Langner. Princeton University Press.1978.
    Simply outstanding:sound observation,good theoretical
    grasp of the complex situations,exceedingly well
    written. *****
20.<u>READINGS IN ADULT PSYCHOLOGY:CONTEMPORARY PERSPECTIVES.</u>
    1977-78 Edition.Ed.DT Jaffe & LR Allman.1977. 320pp.
    illus.PB £ 5.20. Harper & Row.
    A collection of articles reprinted from magazines,
    journals & books.Stresses the developmental approach
& aging.Its section on death includes Lifton & Olson on
immortality,Kubler-Ross on Dying(the JAMA article),& Norman
Paul on Grief (rather weak).Also includes Jacques' Death &
the Mid-Life Crisis.
21. <u>READINGS IN AGING & DEATH.Ed.SH Zarit.Harper & Row,1977.</u>
    Similar.

22. RELIGIOUS ENCOUNTERS WITH DEATH:INSIGHTS FROM THE
    HISTORY & ANTHROPOLOGY OF RELIGIONS. Ed.FE Reynolds &
    EA Waugh.Pennsylvania State University Press,
    University Park,PA.1977. 244pp. $ 14.50.
Ethnographic & historical essays based on 1973 conference
of the American Academy of Religion (very late).15 essays.
Weak definition of terms,but wide range of models.
23. RESPECTFUL TREATMENT:THE HUMAN SIDE OF MEDICAL CARE.
    Martin R.Lipp. Harper & Row,NY.1977,232pp.PB.
24. THE SANCTITY OF SOCIAL LIFE:PHYSICIANS' TREATMENT
    OF CRITICALLY ILL PATIENTS. Diana Crane.
    reviewed above.Also published:Transaction Books,
    New Brunswick,NJ.1977.285pp. $ 4.95.
25. SEELSORGE IM KRANKENHAUS. Josef Mayer-Scheu.
    Grünewald,Mainz. 1977. 110pp. PB.
Imaginative text of pastoral care by a leading German
expert,includes discussions of"Das Tabu des Todes, und
Wahrheit am Krankenbett".
26. SEPARATE PATHS:WHY PEOPLE END THEIR LIVES.Linnea
    Pearson,with Ruth B.Pertilo. Harper & Row,NY.
    1977.171pp. $ 7.95.
Chatty exchange of letters between Christian academics,
on matters relating to suicide. I'm not sure why.
27. THE SHADOW BOX.(A Play) Michael Cristofer.Drama Book
    Publishers,NY.1977.$ 7.95.
    Play set in a 'colony'for terminal patients & families.
Discusses truth-telling & denial,etc.,but very unlikely
cast & plot.
28. SHAME,EXPOSURE & PRIVACY. Carol D.Schneider.Beacon
    Press,Boston.1977.180pp. $ 9.95.
Odd book,extolling the social utility of shame as an agent
of social control,with much inappropriate filler material
& a muddled thesis: but,some discussion of death as an
embarrassment,& other relevant factors,including exposure
of the body,privacy,& similar issues crucial for the
patient & often ignored.
29. SOCIAL SERVICES FOR THE AGED DYING & BEREAVED.Celia
    Berdes.International Federation on Aging,1900 K St.,
    NW,Washington DC 20049.1978.82pp.$3.00. PB.
An unnexessary & superfluous publication,devoid of
perspective & wisdom,inadequate & amateurish.A brief & trite
review of attitudes to death & aging;home health care in

29 ctd). terminal illness of the aged;the Hospice movement
(ill-informed & out of proportion);Counselling for the Aged
Dying & Bereaved (simplistic models of grief);suicides &
suicide prevention;dignified death & euthanasia;education
& training for dealing with aged death & bereavement
(peculiar grammar abounds); & some recommendations of
unknown origin & no great originality or authority or
usefulness.Even if well-meaning,an author simply cant put
together a good report just by collating bits & pieces
from other people.Uncritical & naive. *

30. SUICIDE & THE SOUL. James Hillman.Spring Publications,
    Switzerland. 1976. 191 pp. PB.
    Odd booklet,from Jungian point of view.

31. SUICIDE:IN & OUT- Reynolds & Farberow (reviewed above)
    now in Paperback,at $ 3.95.

32. TOMBSTONE LETTERING IN THE BRITISH ISLES. Alan Bartram.
    Lund Humphries,U.K. 1978. £ 3.95.
A design study of the lettering on tombstones (one of a
series also studying Street Names & Fascia/Shop Front
Lettring). Of somewhat specialist interest,perhaps?

33. WHY ME? What Every Woman Should Know About Breast
    Cancer to Save Her Life. Rose Kushner.Harcourt,Brace
    Jovanovich.1977. Paperback edition ($2.50)of the
    earlier:Cancer:A Personal History & An Investigative
    Report,hard cover 1975,413 pp.$10.00.
Hectically exhorting & exhausting,not always very modest.

34. THE WIDOWER.Jane Burgess & Willard K.Kohn.Beacon
    Press,Boston.1978. 192 pp. $ 8.95. The forgotten man.

35. VULNERABLE INFANTS:A PSYCHOSOCIAL DILEMMA.JL & LH
    Schwartz. McGraw-Hill,NY.1977.378pp. PB.

36. YOU CAN FIGHT FOR YOUR LIFE:EMOTIONAL FACTORS IN THE
    CAUSATION OF CANCER. Lawrence LeShan. M.Evans & Co,NY
    (Lippincott). 1977. 192 pp.$ 7.95.Hopeful & simplistic.

37. LISTEN TO THE CHILDREN.Cancer Care Inc,1 Park Avenue,
    New York,NY 10016. $ 2.50. Report of a study on the
need for professional help for children with a seriously
ill or dying parent,conducted by Cancer Care Inc & the
National Cancer Foundation,reviewing 40 families with 88
children.They found a significant incidence of behavior
problems;what the child is told is less important than how.

38. THE MORBID STREAK:DESTRUCTIVE ASPECTS OF THE
    PERSONALITY. Ann Dally. Wildwood House,London.1978
    140pp. £ 4.95.
Considers various aspects of self-destructive behavior,
though at times it seems more a moralistic sermon than
a scientific or intellectual study.

39. THE THANATOLOGY BOOK CLUB is run by Roberta Halporn
    at Highly Specialized Promotions,P.O.Box 989,
    Brooklyn,NY 11202, from whom further details can be
    obtained. She also publishes the news pamphlet,The
    Thanatology Librarian.

40. ETHICAL ISSUES IN DEATH & DYING. ed.TL Beauchamp and
    S.Perlin.Prentice-Hall,Englewood Cliffs,NJ. 1978
    368 pp. $ 8.95. PB.

41. SHOULD THE CHILDREN KNOW?ENCOUNTERS WITH DEATH IN THE
    LIVES OF CHILDREN. Marguerita Rudolph,Schocken Books,
    New York. 1978. 110 pp. $ 8.95.

42. HELP FOR THE BEREAVED. Kathleen Smith. Duckworth,
    London. 1978. 96 pp. £ 1.50.

43. WRITE YOUR OWN WILL. Keith Best. Elliot Right Way
    Books,Tadworth,Surrey,England.1978. 50 pence.

44. THE GRIEF PROCESS. Yorick Spiegel. SCM Press Ltd.,
    London. 1978. 384 pp. £ 6.50.
Also published by the Abingdon Press,Nashville,1977,and
originally published as Der Prozess des Trauerns:Analyse
und Beratung.Christian Kaiser Verlag,Munich,& Matthias
Grünewald Verlag,Mainz,1973. A heavy tome,with dense writing.
Relates grief processes,understood in terms of dynamic
psychology,to Christian ritual and theology regarding
death,& finds marked inadequacies.Considers developing new
and appropriate approaches.Considers the Gospel of St John,
& Christ's preparation of His Apostles for his own departure
& their grief. Demanding but rewarding.

45. TO LIVE UNTIL WE SAY GOOD-BYE.Elizabeth Kübler-Ross.
Photographs by Mal Warshaw.Prentice-Hall,NY.1978.160pp.
    100 B&W photographs.Hardback only.
An account,illustrated in detail,of Kubler-Ross' counseling
work with terminally ill patients,depicting her method of
therapy.An important record of one personal style of work.
****

46. WILLS AND PROBATE. Consumers' Association,London,U.K.
    1978. £ 1.75 (£1.50 to members).
The principle British guide to wills and probate,with clear
guidance and good examples.

47. WHAT TO DO WHEN SOMEONE DIES. Consumers' Association,
    London,U.K. 1978. £ 1.50 (£1.25 to members).
Very practical guidance on such points as:getting a death
certificate,registering the death,arranging the funeral
and burial or cremation,claiming National Insurance
Allowances,pensions and grants.Consumers'Association,
Caxton Hill,Hertford,SG13 7LZ,U.K.

48. THE GRIEF PROCESS:ANALYSIS & COUNSELLING. Yorick
    Spiegel.Also published by Abingdon Press,Nashville,
    1977. 384 pp. $ 13.95.

49. THE PURITAN WAY OF DEATH:A Study in Religion,Culture
    & Social Change. David E.Stannard.Oxford University
    Press,New York. 1977. 236 pp. $ 11.95.

50. SUICIDE RESEARCH:Proceedings of the Seminars on Suicide
    Research by the Yrjö Jahnsson Foundation,1974-1977.
    (Ed)Kalle Achté & Jouko Lönnqvist.Preface Norman L.
    Farberow.1976.179 pp. $ 8.50. PB.
22 articles.Available from:Yrjö Jahnsson Foundation,
Ludwiginkatu 3-5,SF-00130,Helsinki,Finland.

51. SUICIDE IN HELSINKI:An Epidemiological & Social
    Psychiatric Study of Suicides in Helsinki in 1960-61
    and 1970-71.Jouko Lönnqvist.Monographs of Psychiatria
    Fennica. Fmk 35. $ 9.00

52. THE CAUSES OF SUICIDE.Maurice Halbwachs.Translated by
    H.Goldblatt.Routledge & Kegan Paul,London.1978.£7.75.

53. THE PENALTY OF DEATH:THE CANADIAN EXPERIMENT.C.H.S.
    Jayewardene.Lexington Books,Lexington,Mass.1977.
    125 pp. $ 13.00

54. DYING:FACING THE FACTS,Ed.Hannelore Wass.will now be
    published by McGraw-Hill,New York with Hemisphere,
    Washington DC,available 1979.Price estimate $10.00
    PB & $ 15.00 Hardback.

55. LYING:MORAL CHOICE IN PUBLIC & PRIVATE LIFE. Sissela
    Bok. Pantheon,New York. 1978. 326 pp. $ 10.95.